Para Eduardo,

Un fuerte abrazo

# Dendritic Spines

# Dendritic Spines

**Rafael Yuste**

The MIT Press
Cambridge, Massachusetts
London, England

MIT Press books may be purchased at special quantity discounts for business or sales promotional use. For information, please email special_sales@mitpress.mit.edu or write to Special Sales Department, The MIT Press, 55 Hayward Street, Cambridge, MA 02142.

This book was set in Times New Roman on 3B2 by Asco Typesetters, Hong Kong. Printed and bound in the United States of America.

Library of Congress Cataloging-in-Publication Data

Yuste, Rafael.
Dendritic spines / Rafael Yuste.
    p. ;   cm.
Includes bibliographical references and index.
ISBN 978-0-262-01350-5 (hardcover : alk. paper) 1. Dendrites.  I. Title.
[DNLM: 1. Dendritic Spines. WL 102.5 Y95d 2009]
QP376.Y87   2009
616.07′9—dc22                                        2009012440

10   9   8   7   6   5   4   3   2   1

A mis padres

# Contents

We learn a lot from books, but we will learn more from contemplating nature, cause and reason for all books. The direct observation of phenomena has a somewhat perturbing effect in our mental inertia, certain exciting and enlivening virtue, which is absent or very weak even in the most faithful copies or description of reality.
—Santiago Ramón y Cajal (1897)

The future will prove the great physiological role played by the spines.
—Santiago Ramón y Cajal (1904).

Preface

This book describes a personal journey through the biology of spines, small dendritic protrusions that cover most neurons in the brain. I think it is fair to say that, more than a hundred years since their discovery, the reason for their prevalence in the nervous system is not yet clear. Dozens of different functions have been proposed for spines, and any reader of this literature will likely be confused by all these hypotheses, many of which appear to contradict one another. At the same time, spines probably must play a key role in neural circuits, given that they are so ubiquitously used in them. Because of this, I suspect that unless we understand what spines actually do, we will not understand how the brain works.

I am a neurobiologist who has been fascinated by these structures since I first encountered them in my experiments. Over the years, together with my students and collaborators, I have studied their development, structure, biochemical and biophysical properties, and function. This book is an attempt to solve the "spine problem," to search for this fundamental function of spines by analyzing spines systematically from different angles. The book originated from a series of reviews, written mostly with close collaborators, discussing spine structure, biochemistry, development, motility, plasticity, calcium compartmentalization, electrophysiology, computation, and also the early history of spine research. Although partly based on these reviews, this book is not a comprehensive summary of this extensive literature, but more of a personal search for the function of the spines by highlighting some aspects of their biology that I find particularly interesting. In this spirit, following the old medical dictum of seeking a single disease to explain many disparate symptoms, I have attempted to synthesize all the information I have gathered about spines into a coherent picture, linking their function with that of circuits in which they operate. My argument is that, once viewed from the circuit perspective, all the various pieces of the spine puzzle will fit together nicely into a unified, overarching function. As I will argue in this book, it is not a coincidence that the brain uses spines, since it is precisely because of the spines that these circuits could have significant computational strengths. Spines would, at the same time, make circuits quite versatile and mediate the robust functioning of many regions of the brain. But before diving into the argument, which I will do in the first chapter, I want to state from the outset that the book is a personal synthesis which draws from our own research on the spines from pyramidal neurons in mammalian cortex, with illustrations taken from our own work or that of our close collaborators. I do not mean to ignore the contributions of other colleagues, but to use the book format as a forum to reflect on and discuss the data that I myself have examined closely. Also, because key experiments have not yet been performed for many parts of the argument, this discussion is very speculative compared with articles in the primary literature. I don't apologize for speculating, but warn the reader to understand this book more as an essay on spines rather than a comprehensive review of all the work done on the topic.

A stimulus to write this book was the need for a text for an advanced undergraduate seminar I teach at Columbia University, a course that has often focused on the "spine problem." The comprehensive frame of mind inculcated into Columbia undergraduates through their Core Curriculum has probably stimulated me to synthesize a coherent picture for them. Besides being broad "thinkers in training," Columbia students are fun, and full of fresh ideas, and they have made me revise my opinions and raise my own standards. I am thankful for their questions, their insights and irreverence, and also their serious work and interest in these apparently obscure topics. I had them in mind when I imagined the primary readers of this book.

In addition to my undergraduate students, too many to name after 14 years of teaching at Columbia College, I want to thank graduate and postdoctoral students who have worked in my laboratory on spine structure, development, and function. In particular, I would like to mention Ania Majewska, Ayumu Tashiro, Anna Dunaevsky, Sila Konur, Vivian Ferstermaker, Boaz Nemet, Vovan Nikolenko, Mustuo Nuriya, Jiang Jiang, Roberto Araya, Wei Gan, Emiliano Rial-Verde, Tim Vogels, Darcy Peterka, and Hiroto Takahashi. Indeed, this book is based on an understanding of spines that results from their experiments, their data, and our lab discussions, and, because of this, the book is essentially illustrated with their data, as my tribute to their work. When I write "we" I really mean "them."

I should mention that their work, and therefore this book, would not have been possible without the support of the National Eye Institute and, more recently, the Howard Hughes Medical Institute, institutions that have financed spine research in my laboratory over the years. In addition, Mor Dar and Sarah Mack are responsible for many of the drawings in the book. Also, Susan Buckley, Julie Lavoie, Katherine Almeida, and other colleagues from MIT Press were instrumental in supporting the long process of assembling, revising, editing, and eventually publishing the book.

Besides wonderful students, Columbia has also provided me over the years with the freedom to pursue my dreams. It is difficult to imagine a more supportive and exciting neuroscience community in the world, a tribute to Columbia's past and present academic leaders and administrators. My gratitude to them and to my colleagues and collaborators, including Eric Kandel, Steve Siegelbaum, Tom Jessell, Richard Axel, Gerry Fischbach, Carol Mason, Peter Scheiffelle, Micky Goldberg, Larry Abbott, Wes Gruber, Brian McCabe, Dan Salzman, Randy Bruno, and Charles Zuker in Columbia's Medical School; and the "downtown" crowd of Darcy Kelley, Marty Chalfie, Stuart Firestein, Jian Yang, Mike Sheetz, Julio Fernández, Brent Stockwell, Rae Silver, Aurel Lazar, Louise Brus, Ken Shepard, Elizabeth Hillman, Liam Paninsky, Paul Sadja, Dimitris Anastassiou, and Ken Eisenthal; and to many others members of the larger neuroscience community on both campuses with whom I am constantly interacting. I cannot go to work without encountering intellectual challenges, support, advice, camaraderie, and humor. Larry Abbott, in particular, provided key advice during the final editing of the manuscript, and I am especially indebted to him for his clear thinking and common sense.

Outside Columbia, my special thanks go to three colleagues in particular: Rodolfo Llinás for his pointed criticisms, historical perspective, and encouragement to rise to the highest scientific challenges, regardless of the opinion of others; Kevan Martin, for his altruistic support of my work over the years and his careful comments on previous versions of the text; and finally, my dear friend and colleague Javier De Felipe and members of his laboratory for their hospitality at the Cajal Institute in Madrid, where I found a second scientific home in the last summers. The time spent at the Cajal helped connect me with the rich Spanish tradition of spines studies, starting from the seminal contributions from Cajal himself, but also including key work from Marín-Padilla, Valverde, Ruiz-Marcos, Sotelo, Nieto-Sampedro, and De Felipe, among many others. Indeed, a mural in the seminar room at the Cajal Institute features Valverde's beautiful drawings of dendrites from pyramidal neurons, illustrating the effects of sensory deprivation of spine densities and morphologies, a striking statement that challenges the audience to understand the role of these structures in brain function and plasticity.

As mentioned, many chapters are based on reviews that were originally written with coauthors. I am not only grateful to these coauthors, but eager to recognize their important contribution to this text. In particular, I want to credit Tobias Bonhoeffer, who has been a wonderful colleague and friend since we first met in 1988, and who wrote with me three of the original reviews. Knut Holthoff, Ania Majewska, Carlos Portera-Calliau, Ayumu Tashiro, David Tsay and Rochelle Urban, wrote other reviews with me and thus have had a major influence in this text.

As Ortega y Gasset said, I am "me and my circumstances." The way I think and how I work and write is a direct reflection of the environment in which I grew up as a scientist. So credit (though not blame) for my efforts should reflect back on my mentors, starting with Alberto Sols, Alberto Ferrús, Claudio Cuello, Leslie Barnett, Sydney Brenner, Larry Katz, Torsten Wiesel, David Tank, and Winfried Denk. I work and write in a constant mental discussion with my memories of my interactions with each of them and with many of the people they attracted to the stimulating environment they helped created at the Universidad Autónoma, Cajal Institute, McGill, LMB, Rockefeller, Duke and Bell Labs. Often, our old lunch conversations and debates resurfaced and weaved themselves into the argument of the book.

Finally, my deepest gratitude goes to my parents, whose constant support and help over the years made this book possible, and also to all my family. To Keka and Clara for illuminating my days and especially to Steph, for all her love and support, to whom I owe so much, including many dinners at Arzak.

**Dendritic Spines**

# 1 Introduction

Dendritic spines (hereafter referred to as spines) are small protrusions that arise from dendrites of many neurons, covering them like leaves on a tree (figure 1.1). Although they are quite heterogeneous in size and shape, on average they consist of a small head (~1 μm in diameter), connected by a thin neck (~0.2 μm in diameter, and from 0.5 up to several micrometers in length) to the parent dendritic trunk. Spines are found in many species, from annelids to primates, and are particularly abundant in the central nervous system of vertebrates. Their prevalence indicates that they must be essential for brain function. Indeed, in most brain areas, spines are dominant structural elements, covering the dendrites of the majority of principal neurons. For example, spines can exist in great numbers, even more than 200,000 spines per neuron on cerebellar Purkinje cells, and are also extraordinarily abundant on pyramidal neurons' dendrites in the cortex and on the "spiny" neurons in the striatum, for example. At the same time, spines are absent, or present at much lower densities, on some classes of neurons such as inhibitory interneurons in the forebrain. Why do some cells have so many spines, yet others have none? More generally, what is the function of the spines?

## The Spine Problem

It has been more than a hundred years since Santiago Ramón y Cajal first described the existence of spines, yet it is still unclear exactly what they do. Cajal proposed that spines serve to connect axons with dendrites, and that synaptic connections are made on spines, rather than directly on dendritic shafts. The reason for this would be because spines would increase the amount of dendritic membrane available for synaptic contacts, similar to how intestinal villae increase the absorbing surface area in the digestive system (Berkley, 1896; Ramón y Cajal, 1899c). Indeed, it is now clear that spines receive most excitatory inputs (Gray, 1959b) and, moreover, that practially all spines have an excitatory synapse on their head (Arellano et al., 2007b;

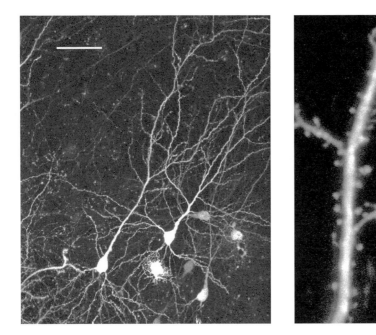

**Figure 1.1**
Imaging living spines. (Left) Two-photon image from living GFP-transfected neurons in a hippocampal slice culture. Scale bar: 50 μm. (Right) Individual dendritic spines are clearly resolved at high magnification. Note the small size and variability in shape of the dendritic spine morphologies. Scale bar: 5 μm. Reprinted with permission from Dunaevsky et al., 1999.

Colonnier, 1968). This makes it fair to assume that, in the mature nervous system, each spine essentially corresponds to one excitatory synapse. Not only do excitatory axons terminate on spines, but, interestingly, in many spiny neurons, there are practically no excitatory axons connecting directly with the dendritic shaft, as if it were to be avoided (Colonnier, 1968). Moreover, although spines significantly increase the surface area of dendrites (Wilson, 1986), there appears to be plenty of free surface area on the dendritic shaft to receive additional inputs (Colonnier, 1968). This is something that one can even appreciate in Cajal's own drawings (see chapter 2), so it is surprising that Cajal held the view that spines were necessary to increase the surface area of the dendrite available to receive synaptic inputs. Spines therefore must have a different function than merely increasing dendritic area.

What could this function be? A variation of Cajal's idea is that spines could still serve to enhance circuit connectivity, albeit in a different way than by increasing the area of the dendrite. By producing spines, dendrites could connect with more axon terminals than without them, because the additional length provided by the spine neck could allow dendrites to reach axons passing by at some distance from the dendrite (Peters and Kaiserman-Abramof, 1970; Swindale, 1981). This "virtual dendrite" (Ziv and Smith, 1996), created by spines, could help sample the neighboring volume and also provide a wider selection of axons available to a dendrite, helping to make synaptogenesis more selective (see chapters 5 and 6; Stepanyants et al., 2002). This design might minimize the wiring for neural circuits, given that axons could course through the nervous system in straight trajectories, without local detours, and still encounter adequate numbers of synaptic partners. Indeed, inspection of any Golgi stain clearly shows how most excitatory axons have relatively straight courses over short distances. The lack of tortuosity in axons of excitatory cells, which are the majority of the neurons in the CNS, supports the "principle of economy" in the design of the nervous system (Ramón y Cajal, 1899c), because straight axons would minimize the distance that the electrical signals need to travel. A nervous system with shorter wiring will not only be more economical to build and maintain, but also lead to increased speed in the processing of neural signals. Nevertheless, although it appears quite logical, the hypothesis that spines help connect dendrites with axons does not explain why most inhibitory inputs are made onto dendritic shafts, rather than spines (Fairen et al., 1984; Somogyi et al., 1998). If spines were so advantantageous for connectivity, why don't all neurons have spines? Why are only some neurons spiny? Thus, the function spines serve could be more sophisticated, one perhaps specific to particular classes of cells and particular types of inputs—excitatory ones.

To solve this conundrum, in addition to the idea that the spines increase connectivity, dozens of other proposals have been put forward over the decades, ranging from the idea that spines having no particular function, being perhaps an epiphenomenon of the development or the cell biology of the neuron, to the hypotheses that spines serve as biochemical compartments, electrical compartments, neuroprotective devices, diffusional buffers, or even digital logic elements (Shepherd, 1996). From this multitude of proposals, the most widely considered ones relate to the role that spines could play in functional compartmentalization, that is, making a spine the functional unit of the dendrite, one that encompasses a single synaptic input. In particular, the peculiar morphology of a typical spine, with a small head that receives the synaptic input and which is connected to the dendritic shaft by a thin neck, has led to the idea that spines are biochemical compartments. For example, spines could restrict calcium accumulations to individual synapses and, therefore, localize calcium-dependent synaptic plasticity to individual inputs (Holmes, 1990; Koch and Zador, 1993; Lisman, 1989; Rall, 1974b; Wickens, 1988). Indeed, imaging experiments have demonstrated that spines are calcium compartments, and therefore, ideally poised to isolate long-term synaptic plasticity (calcium mediated) to individual inputs (see chapters 7 and 8; Yuste and Denk, 1995). At the same time, a calcium compartmentalization that is equally restricted to individual synaptic inputs can be found in neurons without spines, where excitatory inputs occur directly on the dendritic shaft (Goldberg et al., 2003b). Therefore, in addition to calcium compartmentalization, spines must provide additional functional advantages to neurons that have them or to inputs that use them.

Besides calcium, spines could compartmentalize other biochemical signals (chapter 7; see also Yasuda et al., 2006). At the same time, as an alternative to biochemistry, spines could isolate inputs electrically (chapter 9; Tsay and Yuste, 2004). Indeed, a rich tradition of theoretical studies has explored the potential that spines could have to implement an electrical function (Chang 1952; Coss and Perkel, 1985; Jack et al., 1975). Spines could act as passive electrical filters (Rall, 1974b), or boost and amplify synaptic inputs (Rall and Segev, 1988), or even function as gates for Boolean logic (Koch, 1999; Shepherd, 1996). These theoretical ideas were generally discarded in the late 1990s, because of the low estimates of spine neck resistances based on morphological reconstructions (Koch and Zador, 1993) and of the strong diffusional coupling between spines and dendrites (Svoboda et al., 1996). The argument against electrical compartmentalization is that a high spine neck conductance (or a low neck resistance) would make the spine isopotential with the dendrite anyhow. Thus, the spine would always faithfully follow the dendrite voltage and transmit synaptic or dendritic potentials without any significant alteration. Nevertheless, recent work has challenged these arguments, reviving again the electrical compartmentalization thesis. Estimates of a strong electrical coupling between spines and dendrites are based on passive membrane models, and it is becoming clear that every part of the neuron, including spines, is covered with active membrane conductances. Therefore, it is possible that the existence of channels on spines or on spine necks, or, given the small dimensions of spines, even a few of them, could make these theoretical calculations erroneous. Moreover, the electrical behavior of spines has recently been directly probed with voltage imaging and glutamate uncaging experiments, and results from these experiments are indicating that spines are indeed electrical compartments, endowed with active conductances (Tsay and Yuste, 2004; see also Araya et al., 2006b; Araya et al., 2007). Moreover, this electrical compartmentalization appears to underlie the linear integration of excitatory postsynaptic potentials (EPSPs) by dendrites (Araya et al., 2006a) and changes in this electrical compartmentalization could perhaps modify synaptic plasticity (Tsay and Yuste, 2004; see also chapter 9).

It does seem, therefore, that when we consider the structure of the nervous system we are facing a significant mystery with respect to the spines. The majority of neurons are covered with morphological specializations which are mediating essentially all excitatory connections in many regions of the brain, yet we are still ignorant as to why this is happening. This is what I would call the "spine problem," and the goal of this book is to attempt to solve it, by gathering different types of information about spines and bringing it together into a unified explanation.

## Overview of the Book

My key assumption is that spines are key circuit elements and that their function must be linked to the logic of the circuits that use them. A corollary is that we may never understand how the brain works without understanding the specific function of spines. My aim in this book is to integrate all current knowledge on spines with information on key features of the circuits in which they operate, and search in this light for the elusive function of the spine.

Toward that goal, the book progresses through a discussion of different aspects of the biology of spines. I first review Cajal's original work of spines, in chapter 2, illustrating his seminal ideas and their impact on future research on spines. I continue in chapter 3 by discussing the morphological structure of spines. This chapter highlights not only the heterogeneity of spine shapes (a hint to a potential heterogeneity and versatility of spine functions), but also the correlation between the size of the spine head and the size of the synapse (an indication of the link between form and function explored in more detailed in later chapters). In light of these structural data I put forward the idea that spines are essentially as small as possible, as if neurons were maximizing their numbers and, therefore, increasing their connectivity. Chapter 4 then reviews the large number of studies on the molecular and biochemical cascades present in spines. This specialized biochemistry highlights what must be a fundamental role of the spine in chemically isolating excitatory synapses and thus providing them with a molecular identity that can be regulated independently by the neuron. This chapter should be particularly interesting to researchers who want to make use of the increasingly sophisticated molecular toolbox for manipulating spines, given that altering some of these molecules can lead to changes in spine structure or function.

Chapters 5 and 6 discuss two closely related topics: spine development and spine motility. Chapter 5 focuses on the initial developmental emergence of spines and dendritic filopodia, the highly motile protrusions that could be spine precursors. I will argue that, in some classes of neurons, spine development appears to be cell autonomous, whereas in other neurons, spine densities are regulated by the synaptic development and by the past history of neural activity at the spine. In addition, this chapter reviews imaging studies that demonstrate that spines are remarkably stable in the adult brain and could persist over the life of an animal. Finally, I discuss the massive developmental pruning of spines (and of corresponding synaptic connections) that occurs postnatally, representing perhaps the most significant event in the development of brain circuits. Chapter 6 reviews the relatively recent discovery of spine and filopodial motility. By actively moving around, spines and filopodia could sample larger territories and thus acting as "virtual dendrites," perhaps enabling the dendrite to connect to nearby axons. This motility agrees well with the previously mentioned hypothesis that spines increase the connectivity of the nervous system and simplify its wiring by preventing detours in axonal trajectories.

Next, chapter 7 examines what is perhaps the most widely assumed function of spines: the compartmentalization of calcium, which is the basis of input-specific synaptic plasticity. I review calcium dynamics of spines and discuss how calcium compartmentalization in spines arises from a combination of functional and morphological features. In spines, local calcium influx and extrusion mechanisms are aided by the diffusional barrier of the thin spine neck to generate isolated calcium accumulations, highly localized to the activated spine. Therefore, spines create an isolated microcompartment for calcium biochemistry. Given the small size of the spine, this microcompartment should be well-mixed and operate close to diffusional equilibrium. This chapter also discusses the enhanced accumulations of calcium that occur when spines simultaneously receive synaptic inputs and backpropagating action potentials (APs) from the dendrite. This calcium "supralinearity," mediated by the $N$-methyl-D-aspartic acid (NMDA) receptor, can result in long-term potentiation (LTP). Thus, it could represent the biochemical detection of the temporal coincidence of input and output of the neuron and therefore have a significant computational meaning for the cell.

At this point in the book I consider the role of spines in long-term synaptic plasticity, a follow-up of their role in the calcium compartmentalization, incorporating many of the results discussed in previous chapters. Starting with Cajal, it has been argued that physical changes in spines may underlie learning. Chapter 8 examines the potential relation between LTP and morphological changes in spines, a focus of many recent experiments which have often produced contradictory results and interpretations. Because it deals with morphological plasticity, this chapter is closely related to chapters 5 and 6. I concur with those that hypothesize that LTP leads to increases in spine size and shortening or widening of the spine neck, whereas I suggest that the spinogenesis occasionally observed after synaptic stimulation likely has a different function. Indeed, the increases in spine size during LTP nicely explain the relation between spine size and synaptic strength. At the same time, experiments carefully examining the role of the spine neck on synaptic plasticity are only starting to be carried out.

Chapter 9 focuses on the electrical function of the spines. This is a topic in which key experiments, such as measurement of voltage in the spine head or neck during synaptic activation, have only recently begun. This chapter is therefore based mostly on theoretical studies and computer simulations of spines. Several potential effects of spines on the transmission of excitatory potentials are discussed, from filtering of synaptic inputs to their amplification or even the generation of dendritic action potentials. In addition, I discuss the correlation between the size of the spine head and the strength of the synapse, by which larger spines appear to inject larger currents into the dendrite than smaller spines. An additional, inverse correlation appears between the length of the spine neck and synaptic strength. Both correlations, beautifuly demonstrating the marriage of form and function, are so clear that spine morphology might be used to calculate synaptic strength.

## Spines and Neural Networks

The final chapter is a speculation on the computational function of spines, searching for the logic of their existence in brain circuits. This chapter brings together the two threads of the book—the roles of spines in implementing a distributed circuit and in enabling the independent regulation of the strength of each synapse—into a personal proposal for the solution of the spine problem. As previously mentioned, I reason that the best light in which to understand the function of spines is in their role in the circuit. Starting from that premise, and assuming that many of the roles discussed in the previous chapter are indeed valid, I then attempt to link them into a common, unified function. Considering the biophysical design of spines, I argue that spines slow down the synaptic inputs and enable the neuron to better integrate them. This slow integration appears designed to enable the temporal summation of inputs, and the electrical isolation provided by the spine neck allows this summation to occur without significant interference, leading to a linear addition arithmetic for inputs. Indeed, spines are found primarily in neurons that receive high convergence of inputs (e.g., Purkinje cells, cartwheel and pyramidal cells in the cochlear nucleus, spiny cells in striatum, pyramidal neurons of all cortical regions). This is likely not coincidental, and I argue that each spiny neuron type is essentially acting as a linear integrator of a large distributed input matrix. Moreover, spine motility during synaptogenesis, by increasing the diversity of the connectivity, could help implement this large distributed matrix of inputs and make it even more distributed. Therefore, distributed matrices of connections, together with linear integration of inputs, would both be facilitated by spines, whose ultimate purpose is to help build biological neural networks, ones in which the sampling of all possible inputs could be maximized. As I will discuss in this chapter, neural networks, first proposed as purely theoretical entities in the 1940s, are distributed circuits where the computation becomes an emergent property of the connectivity matrix and the temporal dynamics it can sustain. By using spines, biological circuits could make this strategy possible.

Moreover, for a distributed neural network, input-specific synaptic plasticity with implementation of a local learning rule appears necessary, since this would help set up and fine-tune these networks and thereby give them the capacity to learn. Thus, the fundamental function of spines could be to first distribute synaptic inputs, then to help integrate them faithfully and, finally, make them plastic. My hypothesis is that all previously discussed functions, including synaptic plasticity, are part of this larger common design plan and that spine-laden circuits are biological neural networks.

Like in many neural network models, where input integration is linear, spiny dendrites could implement the mathematical function of an integral. Spines could therefore represent the anatomical signature of a type of distributed circuit in which all inputs are summed up linearly. Being distributed, these circuits would be particularly robust to perturbation. In a way, they could operate like a democracy, in which every citizen is polled and the contributions of all members are added arithmetically to reach a decision. Like in a democracy, the distribution of the "power" to all elements makes the system robust, since in principle, not any one element is absolutely key. Moreover, to ensure the full benefit of the distribution of information to every member of the network, counting of the "votes" has to be as complete and accurate as possible, so it may not be surprising that neurons in distributed circuits should aim to perform an equally complete and accurate integration of their inputs. But in contrast with political democracies, votes in this "neuronal democracy" would not have identical values, since synaptic weight varies from synapse to synapse. Although every single vote would be faithfully counted, all votes would not be equal. In neural networks endowed with plasticity learning rules, the weight of the vote from each member would change over time, based on the past history of events. These circuits would therefore be analogous to a "plastic democracy." This plasticity is crucial, since it would endow this type of circuit with the ability to learn from its past activity, thus creating a veritable "learning machine." The effect of such a distributed operation on the neural circuits could be profound, and the spine's function, after all their apparent complexities, could actually be quite simple: as building blocks of the brain circuits, they would implement a robust, plastic, and emergent form of computing, that is, a neural network.

# 2 Discovery

Our story starts in the spring of 1888, in Barcelona. At that time, this progressive city was undergoing a febrile creative period in literature, arts, architecture, and industrial development, taking the leadership in the creation of modern Spain. A similar revolution was occurring in the relative obscurity of the Department of Histology of Barcelona's Medical School, in the laboratory of Santiago Ramón y Cajal, a newly arrived professor of Histology and Pathology, who was starting his scientific career after a relatively tumultuous youth.

One of Cajal's personality traits was apparently his strength of character and perseverance. Indeed, Cajal was from the region of Aragón and, in the popular culture of Spain, Aragonese are considered to be particularly single-minded and persistent. This is captured in a story of an Aragonese farmer (a "*baturro*") riding his donkey on the train tracks and, when faced with an oncoming train at full speed and blowing its whistle to warn him, tells the train that "blow as much as you want, but you are the one who needs to step out of the tracks." Cajal combined such single-mindedness and persistence with superb observational capabilities and intuition. Indeed, Cajal himself credited his scientific successes not to his intelligence, education, or training, but instead to his "will-power," aided by good experimental techniques, laboriousness, and plain common sense (Ramón y Cajal, 1923). In fact, exercising the will was the recipe for success he recommended to young investigators, in his book, appropriately named, "Tonics of the Will" (Ramón y Cajal, 1923).

On May 1, precisely on the day of his thirty-six birthday, Cajal published a monograph entitled *Estructura de los centros nerviosos de las aves* (Structure of the Nervous Centers in Birds) in the first issue of a journal that he himself produced, edited, financed and published (Ramón y Cajal, 1888). As he later wrote, the publication of this journal used up all his savings and prevented him and his wife from affording household help to care for their many children (Ramón y Cajal, 1923). In his monograph, a brief communication with two figures, Cajal described the application of the Golgi stain to the cerebellum of bird species. He had just been taught the Golgi staining method by his friend Luis Simarro in Madrid, who himself had recently learnt it from Ranvier in Paris, one of the premier neuroscientists of the time. The Golgi impregnation enabled, for the first time, the relatively complete staining of the dendritic trees of neurons and is, even today, a very useful tool for the morphological analysis of dendrites. To a greater extent than any of his peers, Cajal had been struck by the potential of the Golgi technique, particularly when applied to the embryonic nervous system, to reveal neuronal morphologies. In his brief article, Cajal noted that the surfaces of Purkinje cells were covered with small protrusions, which he called *espinas* (i.e., "spines," as in the spines of a rose, or "thorns"). In his own words:

Also, the surface of the Purkinje cells' dendrites appear ruffled with thorns or short spines, which on the terminal dendrites look like light protrusions. Early on we thought that these eminences were the result of a tumultuous precipitation of the silver; but the constancy of their existence and its presence even in preparations where the staining appears with great delicacy in the remaining elements, incline us to consider them as a normal disposition. (Cajal, 1888; trans. by author; see figures 1.2, 2.1, and 2.2).

In this relatively brief communication, written in Spanish, a language not commonly used by international scientists, spines were described and named for the first time. The choice of the word "spine" was apparently based on the similarities with the spines of a rose bush (figure 2.3, plate 1), although in dendritic spines sharp terminations are not common; indeed, even in Cajal's drawings, spine heads are normally represented as a ball (figure 2.2). As we will see below, at the end of his life, when writing to his disciple Rafael Lorente de Nó, he may have had misgivings about this terminology which implies that dendritic spines have sharp endings. At the same time, interestingly, recent imaging data indicate that living dendritic spines do actually have sharp edges (see chapter 5 for the discussion on the morphology of living dendritic spines), so the name "spine" may be appropriate, after all.

Cajal's brief 1888 paper had other surprises. In this same publication, he could not detect the presence of anastomoses between axons and dendrites, hypothesized to exist by Golgi and other investigators, and proposed, also for the first time, that neurons are independent units in the nervous system. This assertion laid the basis of his "neuron doctrine," an opposing hypothesis to Golgi's established reticular theory, which postulated that neurons would form a continuous network of physically joined cells (see Shepherd, 1991). Thus, in the same publication, he revolutionized neuroscience, with two fundamental and apparently unrelated observations: Neurons are independent from each other, and they are covered with spines. As we will see, in his later career he proceeded to link both facts into a single conception of the brain.

Cajal was not the first to use the Golgi method and also not the first to observe spines. Other investigators such as Kölliker, Dogiel, Meyer, and even Golgi himself, were more established than Cajal and working in well-recognized centers of

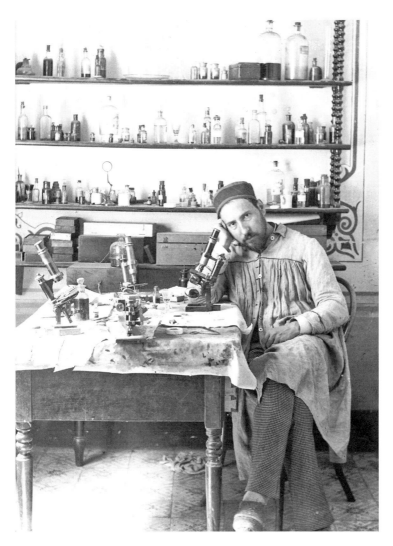

**Figure 2.1**
Cajal in his laboratory. Reproduced with permission from "Herederos de Santiago Ramón y Cajal."

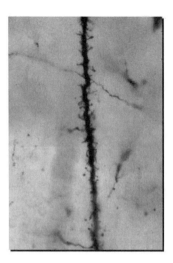 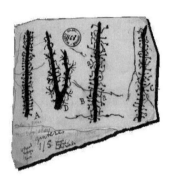

**Figure 2.2**
(Left) Photomicrograph of an original Golgi preparation from Cajal. The image shows a pyramidal neuron with abundant spines (courtesy of Cajal Institute, Madrid). (Right) Drawings of different types of spines by Cajal: "Types of collateral spines of cerebral pyramids. A, rabbit; B, child of two months; C, spines of a one-month-old cat (visual region); D, portion of a dendrite of a spinal motor neuron of a cat in a phase before end feet are formed." Reproduced with permission from "Herederos de Santiago Ramon y Cajal."

anatomical research at the time, and had observed spines before him. However, these researchers regarded spines as artifacts of fixation or silver precipitates which were outside the neuronal membranes. Indeed, in their scientific publications they represented neurons with smooth dendritic trees, devoid of spines. Since spines are still clearly visible in Golgi's original preparations (D. Purpura, personal communication), obviously Golgi chose to ignore them by drawing neurons with smooth surfaces. This was not such an unreasonable choice, considering that the Golgi method is notoriously capricious and variable in results (figure 2.4). In fact, even today it is still unclear how Golgi impregnations work. To make things more confusing, Cajal thought that other observable structures on the surface of neurons, such as dendritic varicosities, were artifactual (Ramón y Cajal, 1904). So it is understandable how Cajal's proposal that spines were real structures was met with skepticism.

In spite of these doubts, maybe because of Cajal's character, he pressed on. Rather than buckle under the pressure of his contemporaries, and perhaps shielded from them by his relative isolation, far from the centers of scientific inquiry of his time, he continued with his studies on the structure of spines, in a flurry of publications that followed. Shortly afterwards, Cajal revealed that spines are not particular to birds but are also present in the dendrites of many neurons of the cerebral cortex of mammals (Ramón y Cajal, 1891b). Importantly, he speculated that spines must

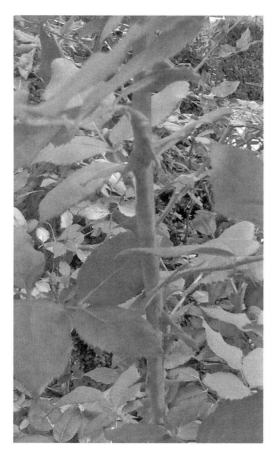

**Figure 2.3 (plate 1)**
Spines in a rose bush.

receive axonal inputs from other neurons, and thus serve as the main point of contact between axons and dendrites (Ramón y Cajal, 1894). This is the point where his neuronal doctrine came full circle: Neurons are independent from each other, but they connect to one another through their axons and spines.

As mentioned in chapter 1, Cajal wondered what the advantage was of using spines as recipient sites for axonal connections, given that axons could, in principle, connect directly to the dendritic trunk. He proposed the idea that spines would greatly extend the surface of the dendrites, and therefore dramatically increase their capability to receive axons. This hypothesis was based on the comparison to intestinal villi, since their highly branched structure increases the surface area devoted for absorption of nutrients. In addition, Cajal also proposed that physical changes in

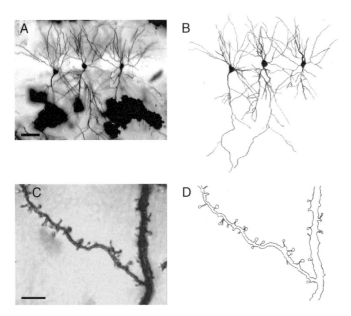

**Figure 2.4**
The Golgi method stains dendritic spines. (A) Photomicrograph of a section of mouse hippocampus, stained with the rapid Golgi method. Note how neurons impregnated by the Golgi stain often have additional dark artifacts (silver deposits). Scale bar: 50 μm. (B) Camera lucida drawing of the same field, where the neuronal morphologies of three CA1 pyramidal neurons are clearly visible. Reprinted with permission from Konur et al., 2003. (C) Higher magnification photomicrograph of one of these neurons. Spines can be detected as small protrusions emanating from the dendrites. (D) Camera lucida drawing of the same dendrite. Scale bar: 5 μm. From Konur and Yuste, unpublished material.

spines could be associated with neuronal function and learning (Ramón y Cajal, 1891a, 1893). Imagining that his histological preparations were alive, he argued that, in the living animal, spines would move and change, growing with activity and retracting during inactivity or sleep. So physical movements of the spines could be capable of connecting or disconnecting neurons. As he wrote: "Since it seems rather likely that the named spines represent points of charge or of current gathering, their retraction (which in this fashion would isolate them from the terminal nerve fibers, with which they are in contact) would give rise to the individualization or separation of neurons" (Ramón y Cajal, 1899c). Indeed, as I discuss in chapters 5, 6, and 8, one of the most exciting recent findings has been the discovery that spines are indeed constantly moving and experience morphological plasticity in vivo and in vitro (see Dunaevsky et al., 1999; Fischer et al., 1998). So the ideas from Cajal are, one hundred years later, still central to the study of the function of spines.

In 1896, partly to defend himself from attacks that his so-called spines were artifacts of the Golgi method and did not appear with other staining procedures, Cajal extended his studies on spines using a different method, the Ehrlich methylene-blue stain (Ramón y Cajal, 1896a, b). In these articles, he refined this technique and showed that, when properly used, it could also reveal spine morphologies.

In subsequent years, Cajal described with great detail spines in motor, visual, auditory, and olfactory human cortices (Ramón y Cajal, 1899a, b, 1900a, b). In 1899, he summarized many of his observations in his book *Histology of the Nervous System of Man and Vertebrates*, where he restated his view that spines increase the surface area of dendrites and thus serve as site of contact between dendrites and axons. In an additional effort to convince his colleagues, he collected together all his arguments that spines could not be artifactual, because:

1. Spines are shown by different methods, such as Golgi, Cox, or methylene blue stains.

2. They always arise in the same position of the neuron, from the same regions of the brain.

3. Spines are never or rarely found in certain parts of the neuron (e.g., the axon, soma, or initial dendrites).

4. Spines do not resemble crystal deposits when viewed with higher-power objectives.

5. Spine pedicles (necks) can occasionally be detected.

Moreover, noting that cells from more highly evolved animals have more spines, he argued that spines were linked to intelligence (Ramón y Cajal, 1899c, 1904).

Finally, in one of his last contributions to the problem, Cajal discussed which axons specifically contact spines (Ramón y Cajal, 1933), arguing that spines, in fact, could be contacted by different types of axons. According to his data, in cortical pyramidal neurons, spines can be contacted by (i) axonal collaterals from other pyramidal cells, (ii) axons from some interneurons (Golgi type II cells), and (iii) axons from other associative neurons.

It is not an exaggeration to argue that Cajal was obsessed with spines, and that he undertook a personal crusade, pretty much alone and until his death, to convince his peers that spines were not only real, but also crucially important. As a testament to his indomitable character, on his deathbed, Cajal was still arguing about spines. On October 15, 1934, two days before he died, he wrote a letter, in shaky handwriting, to his disciple Lorente de Nó (figure 2.5). After reporting that he was so sick he could no longer leave his bed or work, he advised Lorente to pay close attention to spines and their morphologies. He wrote, "Note that spines are not irregular protrusions but instead genuine spines ending in a ball. The neck is sometimes too lightly stained" (copy of autograph letter to Lorente, courtesy of Dr. Francisco Álvarez, Creighton University, trans. by the author). In this letter, he even had the stamina to draw some examples of spines with clear ball endings (figure 2.5).

América du Nord.

Docteur R. Lorente de Nó
Institute for the Deaf of
The Rockefeller Foundation
878 South Kings Higle Way
St Louis Missouri
U.S.A.

Madrid 5 de Octubre 1934.

Estimado compañero y amigo:

Yo me encuentro muy grave con una colitis que dura ya cerca de dos meses y que no me permite abandonar el lecho, ni comer ni escribir.

Sirve esta para decirle que recibí su trabajo sobre el asta de Ammon del ratón, agradeciéndole el regalo.

Dos observaciones no más: 1ª Espinas.

cerebro

Cox
conejo
adulto
cerebro.

note 1 que no se trata de excrecencias puntiagudas o mazuda verasino de genuinas espinas terminadas por una bola. El pedúnculo a veces es demasiado pálido.

2. asta de Ammon. El ratón es poco favorable para un estudio estructural. Es difícil descubrir las células de axon corto, y ofrece una tendencia excesiva a dar macizos de fibras sin detalles de origen ni terminación.

¿Por qué no ha trabajado V. en el conejo de 20 a 40 días? El Cox me proporcionó magníficas arborizaciones sueltas de células de axon corto y multitud de detalles, que no siempre se ven bien con el método de Golgi.

Le saluda cariñosamente su viejo amigo

Cajal

In spite of this string of arguments and the combined weight of his evidence, Cajal's conclusions took a long time to be accepted. Eventually, many of his contemporaries, such as Retzius, Schaffer, Edinger, Azolay, Berkley, Monti, and Stefanowska, came to agree with him and confirmed the appearance of spines in their preparations.

At the same time, spines were not considered to be particularly important or interesting, and for decades not much work was carried out on them. Indeed, Cajal's proposal of the role of spines in connecting axons and dendrites would have to wait half a century for confirmation. This occurred due to the introduction of a new technique, electron microscopy (EM), which enabled the visualization of the fine structure of cells with unprecedented spatial resolution (see chapter 3). Using EM, De Robertis and Palay performed the first ultrastructural description of synapses (DeRobertis and Bennett, 1955; Palay, 1956), and shortly afterwards, synapses were demonstrated on spines (Gray, 1959a, b). Cajal was proven correct, and spines became a bona fide topic of interest for neurobiological studies.

As we discuss in the following chapters, each decade since the 1950s brought an increased number of studies of spines, which has accelerated since 1990 due to the introduction of novel imaging techniques that have allowed experimentation with living dendritic spines. Nevertheless, the specific function of the spine, more than a century after its discovery, is still subject to great debate. Many different hypotheses have been proposed, often in contradiction with one another (Alvarez and Sabatini, 2007; Bourne and Harris, 2008; Harris, 1999; Harris and Kater, 1994; Peters and Kaiserman-Abramof, 1970; Shepherd, 1996; Swindale, 1981; Yuste and Majewska, 2001; Yuste et al., 2000). In the subsequent chapters I examine advances in our knowledge of spine morphology, ultrastructure, biochemistry, development, dynamics, calcium compartmentalization, biophysical properties, and electrophysiology from the point of view of reconciling this increasingly large phenomenology and attempting to close in on the specific function of the spine.

◀ **Figure 2.5**
Letter from Cajal to Lorente. (Top) Envelope addressed to R. Lorente de Nó. (Bottom) Manuscript letter. Note the drawing of dendritic spines. Paragraph is translated in the text. Reproduced with permission from "Herederos de Santiago Ramón y Cajal."

# 3 Structure

*As Cajal predicted, spines are primary recipients of synaptic inputs. Indeed, practically every spine has an excitatory synapse. The small proportion of spines that do not have a synapse lack a clear head, resembling dendritic filopodia. Some spines have both an excitatory and an inhibitory synapse. Also, spines are occasionally branched, holding two synaptic terminals. Spines often have smooth endoplasmic reticulum and ribosomes, but appear to exclude rough endoplasmic reticulum and microtubules.*

*Spine morphology is very diverse, with no clear quantitative evidence for different subtypes of spines. The spine head volume reflects the size of the synapse, being correlated with the area of the postsynaptic density and the number of presynaptic docked vesicles. The morphologies of the spine head and neck are generally not correlated with each other, and the spine neck length is also not correlated with its diameter.*

*Differences in spine size and density exist across cells types, brain areas, and animal species. In fact, even within a given cell, the size of the spine heads and the dimensions of their necks vary greatly. The spine head size is regulated by the interspine distance and, in some cases, also by distance from the soma.*

*Spines are particularly small, as if the neuron were maximizing their number. Moreover, spines can be located along the dendrite forming helixes, as if they were maximizing the sampling of the adjacent neuropil. Spiny neurons receive inputs from many different axons, and neighboring spines are generally not contacted by the same axon. Moreover, some spiny neurons receive only a single synaptic contact from each presynaptic cell, maximizing the number of presynaptic inputs it integrates. Because of this, as a first approximation, each spine can be thought of as an independent input line, and spiny dendrites appear designed to help integrate inputs from as many different sources as possible. This integration could approach, in some cases, the maximum theoretical limit of sampling every presynaptic neuron in a local circuit.*

As mentioned in the previous chapter, the introduction of electron microscopy in the 1950s provided a definite confirmation of Cajal's proposal that spines received synaptic inputs. Since then, many ultrastructural studies have examined spines from

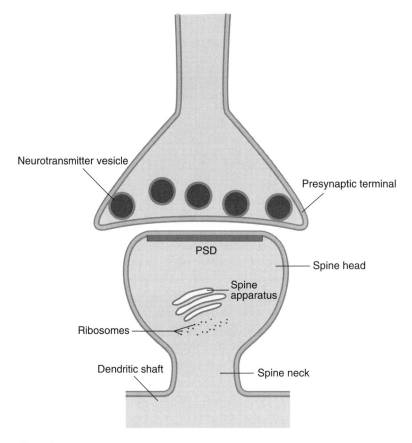

**Figure 3.1**
Schematic diagram of a dendritic spine with basic nomenclature.

different cell types. In this chapter I attempt to summarize common morphological features of spines. I will draw heavily from the literature on pyramidal and Purkinje cells, and especially from our own studies. As will be apparent, spines are morphologically very heterogeneous, although at the same time, they are conspicuously small. These facts, and their particular spatial arrangement in some cases, suggest a functional interpretation of their structure, as if they were designed to maximize input integration.

**Ultrastructure of Spines**

Let us define some basic nomenclature: Spines emerge from dendritic *shafts*, and can be divided into a spine *neck* and a spine *head* (figure 3.1). The head contains the syn-

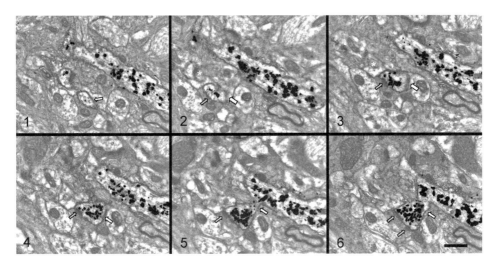

**Figure 3.2**
Ultrastructural analysis of a dendritic spine. Images are photographs of sequential 50-nm thick sections through a preparation of mouse visual cortex. Arrows mark the appearance of a dendritic spine, which is connected to the dendrite in section 6. The neuron has been stained with a gold-toned Golgi method. Unpublished material from Arellano et al., 2007a. Scale bar: 350 nm.

apse, composed of the presynaptic terminal, and the postsynaptic density (PSD). Spines are typically small (typically less than 3 μm in length, from the dendritic attachment to the tip of the head), with a roughly spherical head (0.5–1.5 μm diameter) connected by a narrow neck (<0.5 μm diameter) to the dendritic shaft. These are miniaturized structures (~1 femtoliter [fl] or less in volume), not much bigger than a synapse. In fact, one can think of the spine as the minimal cytoplasm associated with a synapse, since most spines receive a single asymmetric excitatory synapse on their heads (figures 1.3 and 3.2).

**Subtypes of Spines**

Spines display a large diversity of morphologies (figure 3.3). There have been many proposals to classify spines according to their morphological characteristics, although it has been also argued that this diversity is part of a continuum without clearly distinct classes (see below; Arellano et al., 2007a). Nevertheless, perhaps the most accepted classification is the one proposed by Peters and Kaiserman-Abramof in 1970. According to them, spines could be morphologically categorized into three essential types: thin, mushroom, and stubby spines (Peters and Kaiserman-Abramof, 1970; figures 3.4 and 3.5). *Thin* spines are most common and have a thin, long neck and a small bulbous head. *Mushroom* spines are those with a large head and are

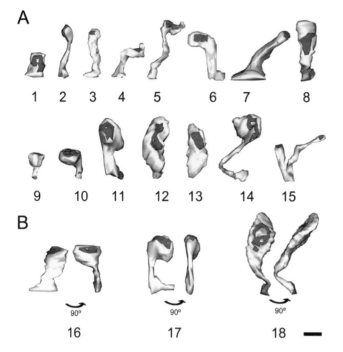

**Figure 3.3**
Three-dimensional reconstruction of spines showing the variability in their morphology. (A) Different spine types: stubby (1), thin (2), mushroom (9–11), and ramified (15). Most reconstructed spines were atypical or intermediate types (3–8, 12–14). (B) Spines appear different depending on the angle of observation. 16–18 illustrate three spines from two points of view after 90° rotation. Dark areas = PSDs. Scale bar: 0.5 μm. Reprinted from Arellano et al., 2007a.

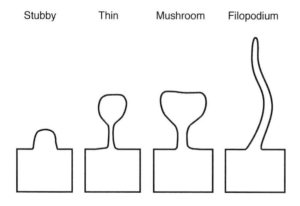

Stubby    Thin    Mushroom    Filopodium

**Figure 3.4**
Morphological subtypes of spines. Schematic drawing of spine morphologies in four traditional categories (Peters and Kaiserman-Abramof, 1970).

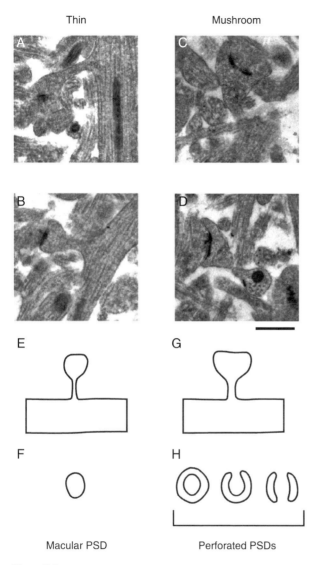

Thin                          Mushroom

Macular PSD              Perforated PSDs

**Figure 3.5**
Morphological subtypes of spines and PSDs. Electron micrographs of different types of dendritic spines in hippocampal slice cultures. (A, B) Thin spine with macular PSDs. (C, D) Mushroom spine with perforated PSDs. Scale bar: 500 nm. (E–H) Schematic drawings of thin and mushroom spines and macular and perforated PSDs. Reprinted from Tashiro and Yuste, 2004.

typically found in adult samples. *Stubby* spines are devoid of a neck (Jones and Powell, 1969; Peters and Kaiserman-Abramof, 1970), and are particularly prominent during early postnatal development (Harris et al., 1992), although they are still found in the adult (Benavides-Piccione et al., 2002). In addition, dendritic *filopodia* are longer and normally have no clear head (figure 3.4, right). Smaller "thin" spines generally have macular postsynaptic densities (PSDs), whereas larger, mushroom-like spines have more complex, perforated ones (Harris et al., 1992). Not surprisingly, larger spines have more structural components: more glutamate receptors (Matsuzaki et al., 2001; Nusser et al., 1998), smooth endoplasmic reticulum (SER) and polyribosomes (Bourne et al., 2007b; Ostroff et al., 2002; Spacek and Harris, 1997), endosomes (Cooney et al., 2002; Park et al., 2006), and astroglial contacts (Witcher et al., 2007).

Excitatory synapses, also known as Gray type 1, are characterized by an electron-dense thickening, the PSD, located on the cytoplasmic surface of the synaptic membrane (figures 3.1 and 3.2), a relatively wide intermembrane distance between pre- and postsynaptic membranes, and a thin presynaptic density (active zone) with neurotransmitter vesicles (Gray, 1959a, b). The PSD is an electro-dense protein band located immediately beneath the postsynaptic membrane (Kennedy, 2000). PSDs can be either continuous (disklike or "macular"; figure 3.5, left), or large and irregular (figure 3.5, right). In single thin sections, PSDs are often visualized as if they were multiple separate structures, but following three-dimensional (3-D) reconstructions, they are in many cases actually found to be connected together and "perforated" by the presynaptic grid (Cohen and Siekevitz, 1978; Peters and Kaiserman-Abramof, 1969; figure 3.2 and 3.5, right).

In contrast to excitatory synapses, which occur typically (but not exclusively) on the spine heads, symmetric synapses (Gray 2) with pre- and postsynaptic densities of similar thickness (Gray, 1959a, b) occur mostly on dendritic shafts. Occasionally some spines also receive inhibitory "symmetric" synapses on their neck or sometimes even their head, in addition to an excitatory synapse (figure 3.6, plate 2). As we will discuss, the function of these inhibitory synapses on spines is still unclear.

**Do All Spines Have a Synapse?**

Since the studies of Gray, most researchers have assumed that every spine has a synapse. At the same time, while using single-section electromicroscopy it is easy to demonstrate when a spine has a synapse, it is difficult to show conclusively that a spine *lacks* a synaptic contact, since to do so one needs a complete serial thin-section reconstruction (figure 3.7). A recent reconstruction study examining this issue directly in adult mouse neocortex (Arellano et al., 2007b) has found that only a very small proportion (~4%) of all spines lacked a synaptic contact. Interestingly, spines

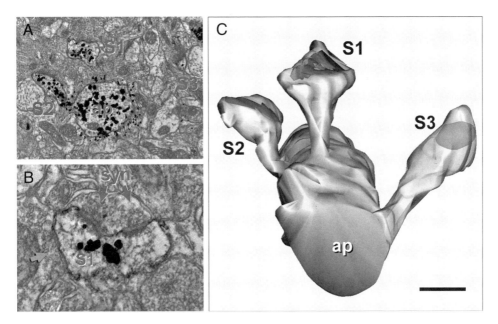

**Figure 3.6 (plate 2)**
Inhibitory synapse on spine. (A) Ultrastructural section through the head of two spines from an apical dendrite of a mouse neocortical pyramidal neuron. (B) Detail of the asymmetrical synapse on one of them;
note the perforated PSD, the synaptic cleft and the presynaptic terminal with rounded vesicles (syn). This
spine also established a symmetrical synapse (left membrane). (C) Three-dimensional reconstruction
of the same segment, displaying three spines (S1–3); the rendering has been slightly shifted down to show
the synaptic junctions and S3 is partially transparent to show the location of the PSD. S1 has an inhibitory
synaptic contact (green), in addition to an excitatory one (red). Scale bar 0.6 µm. Reprinted from Arellano
et al., 2007a.

that lacked a synapse had a particular morphology, being slender, small, and without
a clear head (figures 3.8 and 3.9, top row). It therefore seems that the globular shape
of the spine head is created by the synaptic contact. These "nonsynaptic" spines were
not located in a particular region of the dendrite, and could represent a newly formed
spine that is acquiring a synapse (see chapter 5). In any case, they are a small minor-
ity, so in practice, one can assume that essentially all spines have a synapse. This
strict correlation suggests the idea that spinogenesis and synaptogenesis must be
closely linked and regulated phenomena.

   In contrast to typical spines, thin, long protrusions without a clear head are called
filopodia (figures 3.4 and 3.10). These are mostly developmentally transient structures that disappear after the peak period of synaptogenesis (Fiala et al., 1998; Miller
and Peters, 1981). I will discuss them in depth in chapters 5 and 6, but at this point
we would argue that their lack of a clear head might reflect a lack of synaptic contact. Indeed, some investigators have described that filopodia lack synapses (Linke

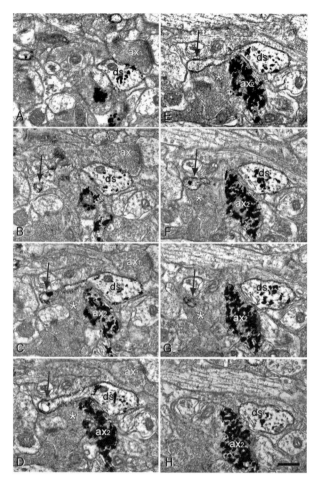

**Figure 3.7**
Nonsynaptic spine. Electron micrographs showing serial sections (70 nm thick) through a gold-toned Golgi-impregnated spine (arrow) lacking a PSD arising from a dendrite. Note the absence of a PSD in the labeled spine, observed just after it first appears and before it disappears. Scale bar: 350 nm. Reprinted from Arellano et al., 2007b.

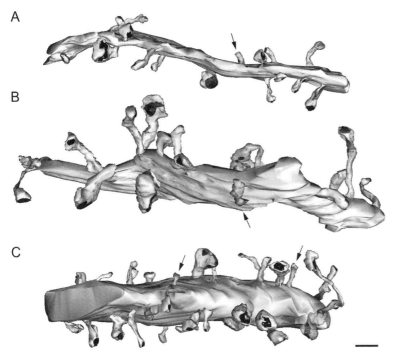

**Figure 3.8**
Most spines have synaptic contacts. Reconstructions of electron micrographs from serial sections of dendritic segments to illustrate the distribution of some nonsynaptic spines (arrows). The remaining spines establish synaptic contacts (shaded, PSD). (A, B) Basal dendrites; (C) apical dendrite. Scale bar: 2 μm. Reprinted from Arellano et al., 2007b.

et al., 1994). On the other hand, others find synaptic features in filopodia during early development (Fiala et al., 1998; Vaughn et al., 1974), although these synapses were described as immature, without the typical PSDs found in mature spines.

A majority of spines have single heads. However, a small but significant proportion of all spines are branched (figure 3.9, fourth spine in lower row). This is found in dentate granule cells (Trommald and Hulleberg, 1997), CA1 pyramidal neurons (Harris et al., 1992; see also Fiala and Harris, 1999), and mouse neocortical pyramidal neurons (Arellano et al., 2007a). The morphologies of the two spine heads, stemming from the same neck, are not correlated and show variations similar to those found among individual spines. No cases have been reported where two heads of branched spines make synapses with the same axon (Harris et al., 1992; Sorra and Harris, 1998; Trommald and Hulleberg, 1997). Why would some spines have two heads? Given that branched spines are correlated with spine density, and that they are independently connected by different axons, one possibility is that they represent

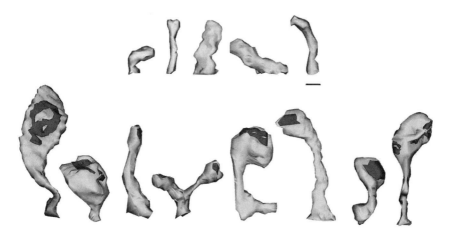

**Figure 3.9**
Morphology of nonsynaptic spines. Reconstructed nonsynaptic spines (top) and examples of synaptic spines (bottom; PSDs are shaded). Note how nonsynaptic spines are smaller and lack a clear head. From Arellano et al., 2007b. Scale bar: 250 nm.

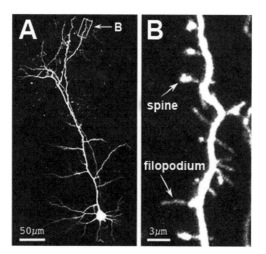

**Figure 3.10**
Dendritic filopodia in a pyramidal cell. (A) Two-photon microscopy image of a mouse layer 5 neocortical pyramidal neuron. (B) Higher magnification from the dendritic segment. Note that dendritic spines have clear spine heads, and filopodia lack them. Reprinted from Portera-Cailliau, and Yuste, R. (2004).

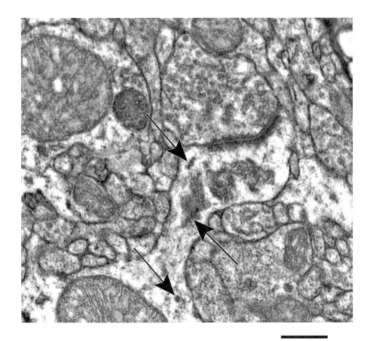

**Figure 3.11**
Spines have ribosomes and smooth ERs. Ultrastructural section of a dendritic spine with ribosomes (arrows) and SER (intracellular membranes in the head of the spine). Scale bar: 250 nm. From Arellano et al., unpublished data.

axonal "mistakes," whereby an axon makes a synapse with an already existing spine, as if it were a dendritic shaft, and a second spine eventually emerges from the first one. This would also suggest that axons play an instructive role in the emergence of spines (see chapter 5).

**Inside the Head of a Spine**

Spines are often associated with polyribosomes, so they must be capable of protein synthesis (figure 3.11). Polyribosomes are found most commonly at the bases of spines, but occasionally also in spine heads or necks (Spacek, 1985a; Steward and Levy, 1982; figure 3.11). Protein synthesis occurs locally in dendrites (see chapter 4; Steward and Schuman, 2001), although it is unclear how much can occur inside spines. Since some synaptic proteins, such as CaMKIIα, FMRP, and Arc, are synthesized depending on synaptic activity, the close association of ribosomes with spines could, in principle, enable protein synthesis to be locally regulated in individual

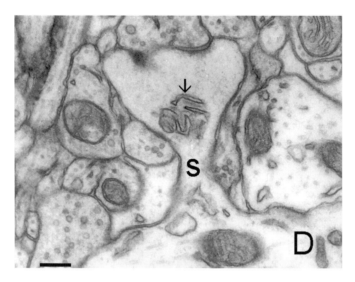

**Figure 3.12**
Spine apparatus. Ultrastructural section of a dendritic spine, showing the stack of membranes that represents the spine apparatus (arrow). S, spine; D, dendrite. Reprinted from Portera-Cailliau, and Yuste, R.
(2004).

spines (Steward and Schuman, 2001). At the same time, the thin spine neck could
constitute a significant barrier for linear polymers such as a typical mRNA molecule
(1–3 μm, longer than many spines in fact), so the small morphological features of
spines may not be particularly well suited for the translation of mRNA.

Many spines also contain SER, which is continuous with the SER in dendritic
shafts and can extend through the spine neck to the head, sometimes also continuously (A. Merchan and J. De Felipe, unpublished data). The spine SER is presumably involved with intracellular trafficking and also with the regulation of
intracellular calcium stores. In the hippocampus, about half of all spines contain
some SER, and in the cerebellum most spines have SER. SER can take the form of
vesicles, tubules, or a "spine apparatus"—a stack of SER cisternae and dense plates
between them (figure 3.12; Gray, 1959a). Larger spines, which also have perforated
synapses, often contain a spine apparatus, and the number of cisternae in it is correlated with the PSD area (Spacek and Harris, 1997). Spine apparati are common in
cortex and hippocampus, but rarely found in cerebellum (Spacek and Hartmann,
1983). The function of the spine apparatus is unknown, although its absence in
synaptopodin-deficient mice is correlated with alterations in long-term synaptic plasticity (Deller et al., 2003).

It is interesting to discuss what spines *do not* have. Apparently, there is no rough
endoplasmic reticulum (RER) in spines. Given the importance of RER in the assem-

bly of membrane-targeted proteins, this implies that all membrane proteins in the postsynaptic density, or in the spine, might be synthesized elsewhere, and then either diffuse along the membrane or are shipped to the spine as membrane bound units (see chapter 4). Also interesting to note is that mitochondria are normally excluded from spines, although dendrites have many. Although one could argue that spines are too small to accommodate mitochondria, presynaptic terminals, which are similarly sized as spines, do have them. Finally, spines have no microtubules, as if to avoid rigidity in their structure. In fact, as explained in the next chapter, spines are full of actin, and this makes them extremely plastic.

Finally, some spines are associated with astroglial processes, but others are not (Spacek, 1985b). Because large spines have more astroglial contacts than smaller ones, it is possible that glia can participate in the modulation of synaptic transmissions only in these spines.

### What Is the Real Ultrastructure of Spines?

To finish this survey of the morphologies of spines, it should be mentioned that ultra-structural studies of fixed tissue are subject to potential artifactual alterations in morphology created by fixatives. In the case of spines, it has been argued that the traditional view of the spherical shape of a typical spine head may partly result from the use of aldehyde fixatives. In fact, living spines, or those fixed under more gentle conditions, resemble more an open hand, with fingers protruding upwards, surrounding the presynaptic terminal (Roelandse et al., 2003). As mentioned in chapter 2, whether the heads of the spines are ball-shaped or sharp fingerlike protrusions (as implied by their name) was discussed by Cajal and Lorente de Nó (figure 2.5). Nevertheless, high-resolution imaging experiments of living spines in vitro and in vivo document small fingerlike filopodial protrusions ("spinules") emanating from most spines and arranged in a concave cup-shape (Dunaevsky et al., 1999; Fischer et al., 1998; Lendvai et al., 2000). These "hand with fingers"—shaped morphologies represent the real morphology of the spine. The function of these spinules is mysterious, and perhaps could provide a retrograde signaling mechanism, perhaps mediating transendocytosis, between the PSD and the presynaptic terminal.

### Correlations between Spine Shape and Synaptic Function

Spine morphology is highly variable from spine to spine, even within the same dendrite, and this diversity has baffled researchers since Cajal. For example, spine head volumes, as shown in a recent database of reconstructed spines from mouse neocortical neurons (figure 3.13A), can range from 0.01 to 0.4 $\mu m^3$, with most of it (>80%) composed of spine head volume. The spine neck can vary in length from 0.1

A

B

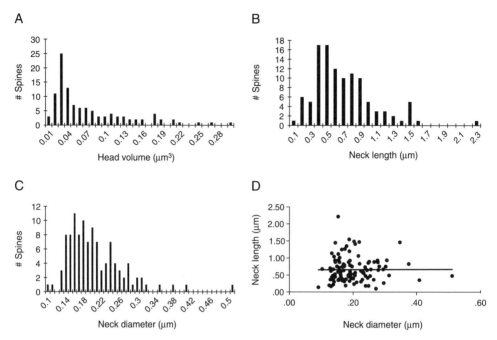

C

D

**Figure 3.13**
Distribution of morphological variables of spines. Data from serial ultrastructural reconstructions of spines from mouse neocortical pyramidal neurons. Reprinted from Arellano et al., 2007a.

to more than 2 μm, and its diameter from 0.09 to 0.5 μm (figure 3.13B, C). Interestingly, the spine neck length and its neck diameter are uncorrelated with each other, as if they were regulated by independent processes (figure 3.13D).

Inspection of these distributions of spine variables reveals unimodal distributions with long tails, without any clear evidence for morphologically distinct classes of spines such as "stubby," "thin," and "mushroom" types (see also figures 3.3 and 3.8). Therefore, because quantitative measurements of reconstructions display rather a continuum of morphologies (Arellano et al., 2007a), these traditional spine classifications should be perhaps used only as a shorthand for discussing spine morphologies.

Quantitative ultrastructural studies have demonstrated strong correlations between some morphological variables of the spine and the synaptic structure. The area of the PSD, as the spine head volume, displays a great variability compared across spines, also with a unimodal distribution with a long tail (figure 3.14A). But interestingly, the spine head volume (and also the total spine volume) is positively correlated with the PSD area, with a remarkably small variance (figure 3.14B). This result is very robust, found in cerebellar Purkinje cells (Harris and Stevens, 1988), CA1 pyra-

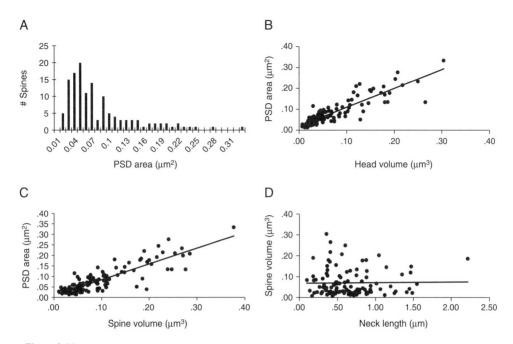

**Figure 3.14**
Correlations between spine morphological variables. Reprinted from Arellano et al., 2007a.

midal neurons (Harris and Stevens, 1989), and neocortical pyramidal cells (Arellano et al., 2007a). Moreover, the PSD area is also positively correlated with the number of presynaptic vesicles (Harris and Stevens, 1988), with the number of docked vesicles, and also the size of the presynaptic active zone (Schikorski and Stevens, 1999). The number of docked vesicles corresponds closely to the readily releasable pool of vesicles, which, in turn, correlates with the release probability (Rosenmund and Stevens, 1996; Schikorski and Stevens, 2001). Also, the PSD area is correlated with the number of postsynaptic receptors, which is itself correlated with the current injected at the synapse (Nusser et al., 1997; Nusser et al., 1998). Finally, glutamate uncaging experiments have demonstrated that the larger spines inject more current into the dendrite (Matsuzaki et al., 2004).

Given these correlations, it is interesting to inquire whether there are similar correlations between the spine neck morphology and synaptic strength. In mouse pyramidal neurons, the spine neck length and diameter seem to be uncorrelated to each other (figure 3.13D). The morphology of the spine neck is also uncorrelated with the spine head size or the size of the PSD (Arellano et al., 2007a; Benavides-Piccione et al., 2006). Nevertheless, for spines in the apical dendritic tree, the spine neck diameter, but not the neck length, is positively correlated with the area of the PSD and the spine head volume (Arellano et al., 2007a). Thus, it is safe to assume that, while for most spines, the spine neck and head appear to be independently regulated, for a subset of spines, those with larger heads tend to have broader necks. The significance of this special case is unclear, and will be addressed in later chapters.

As will be discussed later as well (chapters 7, 8, and 9), the spine neck length also has a direct functional relevance, since it can regulate the degree of biochemical isolation of the spine from its parent dendrite and play a major role in the electrical filtering (or amplification) of synaptic currents injected at the head of the spine.

A corollary of these correlations is the possibility of quantitative prediction of functional properties of synapses based on morphological measurements of spines. A larger spine volume implies more docked vesicles, a higher probability of release, and more postsynaptic receptors, whereas a longer spine neck could mean a slower diffusional equilibration time with the dendrite and a stronger degree of electrical isolation. The structure of the spine could, therefore, reveal its functional role. Images such as those drawn by Cajal could directly reflect synaptic function, since different spine head sizes or neck lengths could generate different functional regimes of operations of the spine (figure 3.15). Therefore, it becomes interesting to quantify spine morphological parameters across different cell types and even across different portions of a neuron. This search could lead to systematic correlations that would be helpful in understanding the biophysical properties of pyramidal neurons and the function of cortical circuits.

**Regulation of Spine Size and Densities**

Is there a relationship between the morphology of the spine and its position within the dendritic tree? An early qualitative study reported that in neocortical pyramidal cells, spines located farther away from the soma had longer spine necks (Jones and Powell, 1969). Similar claims were made for dentate granule cells in hippocampus (Laatsch and Cowan, 1966). A recent ultrastructural study has quantitatively re-examined this possibility in pyramidal neurons from mouse neocortex (figure 3.16; Arellano et al., 2007a). For spines located close to the soma, encompassing most of the spines in basal dendrites, there does not appear to be any clear correlation between spine head and neck dimensions and distance from the soma (figure 3.16).

While ultrastructural reconstructions can be used to accurately measure spine head and neck dimensions, they suffer from the problem that it is painstakingly difficult to accumulate data from many spines. Light microscopic measurements of spines, on the other hand, are easy to perform in large numbers, although they suffer from the limitation that spine dimenstions approach the spatial resolution of light microscopes. A light-microscopic study using Golgi impregnations also explored quantitatively spine head diameter and spine density versus spine position along the dendrite,

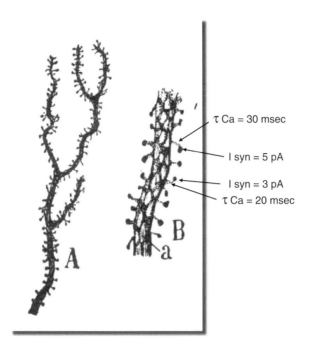

τ Ca = 30 msec

I syn = 5 pA

I syn = 3 pA

τ Ca = 20 msec

**Figure 3.15**
Potential relation between morphological and functional parameters in spines. Original illustration from Cajal, displaying dendritic spines from a cerebellar Purkinje cell, as drawn from Golgi material. From Ramón y Cajal, 1899c. Reproduced with permission from "Herederos de Santiago Ramón y Cajal." The hypothetical synaptic currents (I syn) and calcium decay time constant (tau Ca) for two spines are illustrated, highlighting the relation between spine morphology and synaptic strength and calcium decay kinetics.

dendritic morphology, and laminar position of the neuron (Konur et al., 2003). The study was performed reconstructing and measuring approximately 23,000 spines from several types of neurons (figure 3.17). This work revealed systematic differences in spine head diameters and densities between cell types, but these differences were on top of a large variability in spine head diameters and densities, even among cells from the same region and even across different parts of a neuron.

**Subtypes of Spines, Revisited**
At the light level, the distribution of spine sizes within a single neuron approximates a single-peak distribution with no clear evidence of different size subpopulations of spines (figure 3.18A, plate 3). Thus, in agreement with the ultrastructural reconstructions discussed earlier, it seems that the variability of spine size (reflecting synaptic strength) is part of a continuum. In this study (Konur et al., 2003), apical and basal dendrites displayed similar average head diameters. In fact, a significant correlation

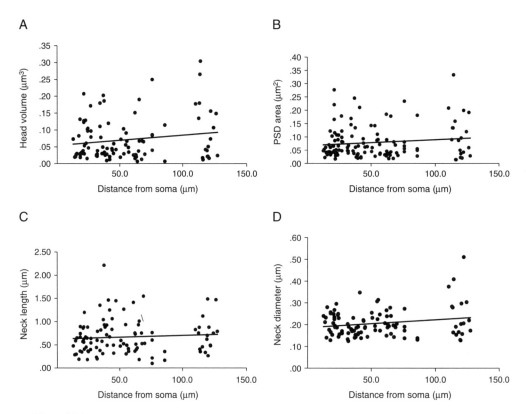

**Figure 3.16**
Apparent lack of correlation between spine morphological variables and distance from the soma.
Reprinted from Arellano et al., 2007a.

between head diameters of apical and basal dendrites was found for individual spines, as if neurons were regulating the average spine size throughout the cell.

Is the placement of spines along dendritic trees random or regulated? Like spine head diameters, in this Golgi survey (Konur et al., 2003), interspine distances displayed a unimodal distribution, which was similar for apical and basal dendrites (figure 3.18B). Strikingly, in practically all cells, significant correlations were found between spine head diameter and interspine distance, indicating that larger spines are spaced further away from each other, on average, than smaller spines (figure 3.18C). This correlation was also observed when analyzing the average spine head diameter and interspine distance for all neurons (figure 3.18D). Therefore, since the spine head diameter (and therefore its volume and PSD area) is correlated with the interspine distance, it appears that dendrites may be able to control the total synaptic strength they receive and maintain a constant amount of it.

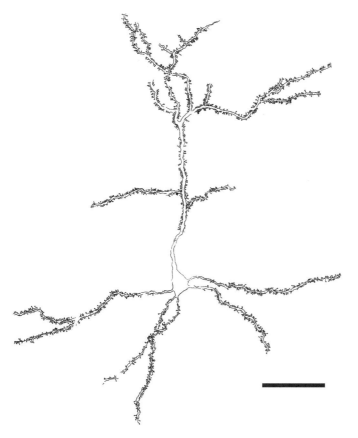

**Figure 3.17**
Reconstruction of spines present in a pyramidal neuron. Camera lucida drawing from Golgi-impregnated mouse CA1 pyramidal neuron. Reprinted from Konur et al., 2003.

## Spine Size and Distance to the Soma

An interesting finding that emerged from this Golgi survey of spines was that the spine head diameter increased with increasing distance from the soma (figure 3.19, plate 4). This increase was particularly significant for apical dendrites of CA1 pyramidal neurons (see also Megias et al., 2001). One could argue that spines located in the distal dendrite are electrically further away from the soma and could therefore compensate for their distance by becoming larger and injecting more current into the dendrite. Indeed, in CA1 pyramidal neurons, inputs located further away from the soma are functionally stronger (Andersen et al., 1980; Magee and Cook, 2000). Nevertheless, it is unclear whether the stronger synaptic weights in those studies are explained solely by the morphologies of the spines, since the modulation of the spine

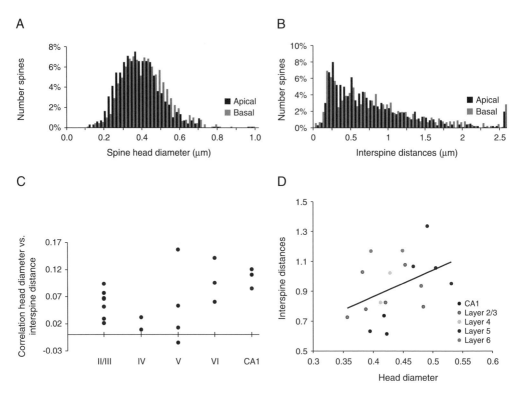

**Figure 3.18 (plate 3)**
Distribution of spine sizes and densities in pyramidal neurons and correlations between spine size and densities. (A) Apical (black) and basal (red) dendritic spine head diameter histogram of a layer 2/3 pyramidal neuron. Histogram is normalized such that apical and basal head diameter values add up to 100%. (B) Apical (black) and basal (red) interspine distance histogram. (C) The correlation coefficients between interspine distances and spine head diameters plotted with respect to the layer that the cell belongs to. In 18 out of 19 cells a positive correlation is observed. (F) Average spine head diameter plotted against its average interspine distance. Reprinted from Konur et al., 2003.

head diameter was only strong in a subpopulation of pyramidal neurons (Konur et al., 2003). Finally, based on the link between spine head diameter and interspine distance, one could also expect corresponding increases in interspine distances in distal dendrites.

Altogether, these results indicate that spine head size and densities, and therefore synaptic properties, are modulated in the neocortex and hippocampus in relation to cortical regions, laminar position, and, in some cases, even the distance from the soma along the dendritic tree. One interpretation of this regulation is the possibility that there are intracellular mechanisms that jointly control the number of spines and their size; these mechanisms could match the average synaptic size between apical and basal dendrites and regulate the distribution of excitatory synapses and their

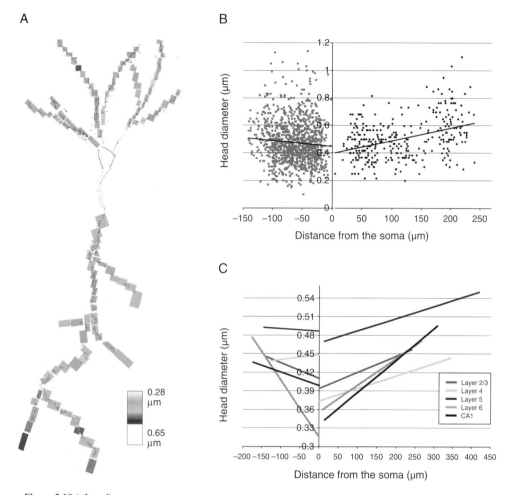

A

B

C

Head diameter (μm)

Distance from the soma (μm)

Head diameter (μm)

Distance from the soma (μm)

0.28
μm

0.65
μm

Layer 2/3
Layer 4
Layer 5
Layer 6
CA1

**Figure 3.19 (plate 4)**
Spine size increases in distal dendrites. (A) Topographical distribution of spine head diameters along a
CA1 pyramidal neuron. Each dendritic segment is color coded according to the average head diameter of
the spines within that segment. Bluer hues correspond to larger heads whereas yellowish hues signify
smaller heads. Note how blue regions predominate in the distal dendritic tree, in the stratum lacunosum-
moleculare region. (B) Measurement of spine head diameter as a function of distance from the soma from
this CA1 neuron. Note how spines become larger in the distal dendritic tree. (C) Average relations for CA1
cells and neocortical pyramidal neurons from different layers. Reprinted with permission from Konur et al.,
2003.

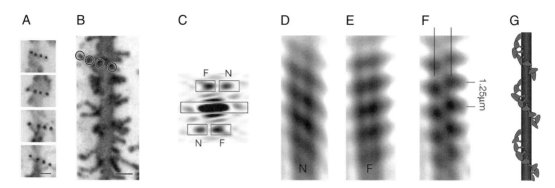

**Figure 3.20**
Spine helixes. Spines can be located in helical arrangements in Purkinje cells. (A) Spine necks forming regular linear arrays over the shaft surface, revealed in confocal sections. (B) Periodic arrangement of spines (circles). (C) Diffraction pattern of (B), showing two pairs of peaks arranged with approximate mirror symmetry about a vertical axis. (D and E) Filtered images revealing paths traced by lines of spines on the near (N) and far (F) sides of the shaft, made by including only spatial Fourier terms associated with the separate pairs of peaks in the diffraction pattern. (F) Filtered image made by including terms within all of the masked areas in (C); pair of vertical lines indicate the radius at which the modulations have the greatest contrast. Scale bars: 1.0 μm. Reprinted from O'Brien and Unwin, 2006. (G) Schematic rendering of a helical pattern of spines along a dendrite.

total strength on pyramidal cells. This possibility, emerging from light microscopy studies, could be tested and investigated at the ultrastructural level. In fact, such large-scale ultrastructural studies are starting to become feasible due to the introduction of focused ion beam milling electron microscopy, which enables automatic ultrastructural reconstructions while preserving synaptic features (Merchan-Perez et al., 2009).

**Nonrandom Distribution of Spines along Dendrites**

From the previous data one could argue that spines tend to be spaced at a minimal distance from each other (see the refractory distance in figure 3.18B). Also, as explained, in many pyramidal neurons the interspine distance is inversely correlated with the spine size, so their position may be precisely regulated (figure 3.18C). This appears to be true at least for some cases: In Purkinje cells, spines are distributed according to a helical topology along the dendritic shaft (figure 3.20; O'Brien and Unwin, 2006). The helixes have no particular rotational preference, are often missing "steps," and are broken into small segments. Interestingly, sometimes spines are arranged in double helixes, like DNA. Helical spine patterns are also found in human and mouse neocortical pyramidal neurons, so this result could reflect a general property of spines (Yuste et al., in prep.). It is as yet unknown why spines would be arranged in helixes, but, as in the case of DNA and other polymers, a helical topology appears to be a very efficient design principle to systematically fill a volume.

By being positioned in helixes around the dendrite, spines could maximize their efficiency at capturing axons from the neighboring neuropil (see below). This striking result confirms that the exact position of many spines could be determined intrinsically by the neuron, even though one would expect that this basic helical scaffold could be altered by many factors, both during development and during the rest of the life of the animal.

Further evidence for an additional nonrandom positioning of spines comes from studies of spine distribution in neocortical neurons (Marín-Padilla, 1967; Elston and De Felipe, 2002). It appears that, for all species, spine density along the basal dendrites from layer 3 pyramidal neurons starts at a very low value near the soma, reaches a peak approximately 70 to 100 μm from the soma, and then gradually decreases toward the tips of the dendrite (figure 3.21A and B). Along apical dendrites from layer 5 pyramidal neurons, spine density also starts at zero near the soma, then increases to a peak and gradually decreases (Ruiz-Marcos and Valverde, 1969). This distribution can be fitted by a double exponential function and is altered by sensory deprivation or disease (Ruiz-Marcos and Valverde, 1969). It is possible that different spine densities could reflect different laminar densities of axonal terminals, or differences in extracellular signals regulating spine develoment and maintenance (Marín-Padilla, 1967). In any case, differences in spine densities along the dendrites, as they course through different layers, indicate the potential for external regulation of spinogenesis in pyramidal neurons.

Spine sizes and densities also appear to be differently regulated across cortical areas (figure 3.21C). Neurons in visual cortex, for example, have smaller spines than those in frontal cortex (Benavides-Piccione et al., 2006; Elston et al., 2005; Elston and De Felipe, 2002). Finally, spines also have systematically different densities and sizes across different species. Human spines are larger and exist at higher densities than those of mice, for example (figure 3.22; Benavides-Piccione et al., 2002). Although one might expect larger spines in humans than mice because a larger body and neuron size, an increased spine density indicates that excitatory inputs are actually more abundant in humans, as if we had a more dense connectivity matrix in our brain circuit. In fact, Cajal already noted that humans are a particularly "spiny" species, and he speculated that our intellectual capabilities could be related to the spiny-ness of our circuits (Ramón y Cajal, 1899c). One could argue that, whatever function spines are carrying out, it is one more developed in the human brain.

**Functional Interpretation of Spine Structure: Spines Maximize Connectivity**

I would like to conclude the chapter by discussing the functional meaning of spine morphologies. These ideas are necessarily speculative and seek to analyze all the information presented in this chapter from a unified viewpoint.

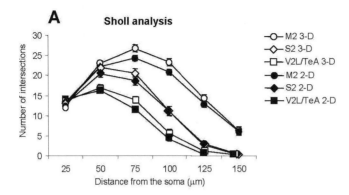

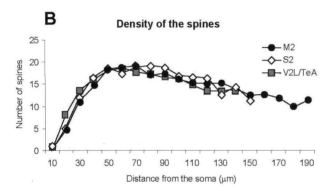

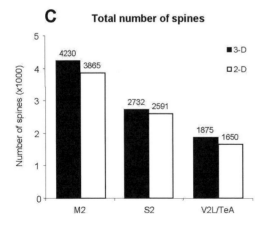

**Figure 3.21**
Distribution of spines in different cortical regions. (A) Number of 2D and 3D Sholl intersections of basal dendritic trees from mouse neocortical pyramidal neurons, according to cortical area. (B) Calculated spine density per 10 μm segment of the dendrite from the soma to the tip of the dendrite. (C) Total number of spines estimated from 3D and 2D reconstructions. Reprinted from Ballesteros-Yánez et al., 2006.

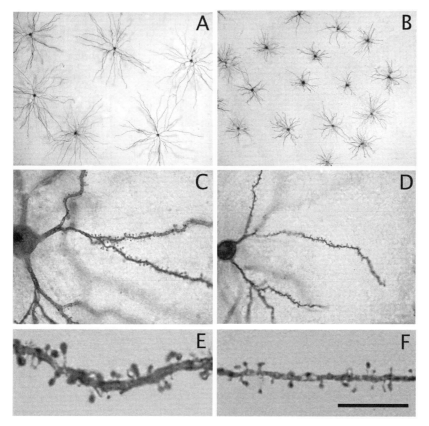

**Figure 3.22**
Spines in humans are larger and more abundant than in mice. (A, B). Low-power photomicrographs of
layer 3 pyramidal cells from human (A) and mouse (B) temporal cortex, injected in fixed sections with
Lucifer Yellow. Note the smaller size of mouse neurons. Sections are parallel to the cortical surface. (C,
D) Photomicrograph of horizontally projecting dendrites of a human (C) and mouse (D) pyramidal cells.
(E, F) High-power photomicrographs of the basal dendrite segments of human (E) and mouse (F) pyramidal cells, illustrating individual dendritic spines. Note the smaller size of the mouse spines. Scale bars:
425 μm in A and B; 45 μm in C and D; 10 μm in E and F. Reprinted from Benavides-Piccione et al., 2002.

My first reflection relates to the ultimate structural design logic for spines. Why are
spines built the way they are? Why do they have these particular shapes and dimensions? Obviously, spines are built to accommodate synapses, and essentially each
spine has an excitatory synapse. But it seems that spines are miniaturized devices,
and are as small as possible to hold a synapse. Inspection of their morphological
reconstructions (figure 3.3) reveals that the PSD occupies a significant proportion of
the surface of the head of the spine. One could argue that there is hardly any space
left on a typical spine to fit another synapse, particularly if synapses require additional components to the PSD.

It is possible, too, that synapses themselves are as small as possible, given the signal-to-noise limitations associated with the very small number of receptors they possess, and also the small numbers of presynaptic vesicles released (often individual ones). One could therefore argue that evolution is maximizing the number of synapses and of spines. Moreover, it is very telling that, at least in some instances, spines are arranged in helixes, maximizing the sampling of the neuropil. I would argue that this is a seminal observation, one that gives away the logic of the spine function. Their structural goal would be not only to connect with axons, but to sample as many axons as possible, maximizing their interactions. In this respect, it is quite interesting to note that synapses tend to be located at the tips of the spines, as if they were just as long as needed to "catch" a passing axon (figure 3.3).

But if this is the case, why aren't spine necks longer, since this could enable spines to sample the neighboring neuropil even better? The fact that spine necks have a length limit can be interpreted as an indication that further elongating the spine neck must have a negative effect on the synapse, as if there were a particular length of the neck beyond which the electrical signals would not reach the dendrite. As I discuss in chapter 9, recent evidence indicates that spines that have very long necks have a negligible electrical effect on the dendrite.

Also, why aren't there more spines, given that dendritic shafts appears to be devoid of synapses? Perhaps the amount of current that a given piece of dendrite can integrate is limited. Given that dendrites have a particular electrical structure, this is not such an unreasonable assumption. Indeed, the joint regulation of inter-spine size and spine head diameters points to this possibility. It is also possible that the spine distribution along a dendrite is an optimal geometrical solution to the phys-ical constrains of sampling the neuropil, in which case, the ultimate reason for their distribution could lie in the topology of the axonal fields.

Thus, one could argue that spines appear designed to maximize connectivity and integrate information from many sources. This idea, perhaps implicit in Cajal's orig-inal suggestion that spines increase connectivity, has seen many reincarnations in the last decades (Anderson and Martin, 2001; Chklovskii et al., 2002; Peters and Kaiserman-Abramof, 1970; Stepanyants et al., 2002; Swindale, 1981). However, if this were the case, one would expect that the structure of the presynaptic components would also reflect this same design logic. Is there any evidence for this? Indeed, it seems that the presynaptic axons follow precisely the same logic to maximize connec-tivity, since the excitatory axons that contact spines originate on neurons that project in a distributed manner. Moreover, axons that contact spines rarely make more than a few synaptic contacts with the same postsynaptic neuron. For example, granule cell fibers contact Purkinje cell spines, making apparently only a single contact with the recipient neuron. In this case, the flat and orthogonal geometry of the Purkinje cell ensures that a given parallel fiber has one, and only one, chance to contact any given Purkinje cell. This has as clear a structural logic: the cerebellum appears to have optimized the distributed connectivity principle to the maximum theoretical limit. That is, each granule cell makes, at most, a single contact with each Purkinje cell, and, in turn, each Purkinje cell receives axons from as many granule cells as possible (hundred of thousands). This beautiful arrangement is also probably present in other spine-laden circuits. For example, the projections from CA3 to CA1 pyramidal neurons, which terminate on spines from the stratrum radiatum of the hippocampus, are most likely mediated by single spine contacts (P. Somogyi, personal communication). In neocortex the number of contacts received by a spiny neuron from a single axon can be higher than one, but is generally very small (Markram, 1997). Moreover, the connections made by a single excitatory axon in the necortex do not normally occur on the same dendritic branch (although occasionally exceptions are found, J. De Felipe, unpublished data).

Thus, I would argue that spine-laden circuits are designed to maximize the distribution of connections, and that this design is apparent in both the structural design of the postsynaptic dendrites with their spines and the geometry and connectivity patterns demonstrated by presynaptic axons. Spiny circuits are distributed matrices of connectivity, and in some cases they could approach the maximum theoretical limit, as one could expect from the helical patterns, which are a most efficient manner to sample space.

A second reflection relates to the morphological heterogeneity of the spine shape and its relation with synaptic strength. The morphology of spines is highly variable, suggesting that it may be of functional importance. Indeed, in the last decade, it has become clear that not only does the spine structure reflect the functional features of the spine synapses, but the correlation between spine morphology and its function is remarkably strong. This underscores the close relation between spines and synapses, to the point that one can imagine the spine as the membrane recipient that holds the synapse. These correlations become obvious: the larger the synapse, the larger its holder. But why would the pre- and postsynaptic morphologies need to be so tightly correlated? Perhaps this should be expected, given how interactive synaptogenesis appers to be. In any case, these strong correlations between structure and function of the spine and synapse are a very useful tool for neurobiologists, allowing one to functionally interpret the morphology of a dendrite.

In this light, the diversity in spine size tells us also something more: synapses have very different strengths, presumably as a consequence of their plasticity. Thus, in this distributed matrix of connectivity, each axon and each synapse could have a different weight on a postsynaptic neuron. While maximizing the sampling of axons, a neuron also keeps their functional influence different from one another. As I argue in the last chapter, combining maximum connectivity with the functional individuality and plasticity for each connection could provide spiny circuits with increased flexibility and computational power.

# 4 Molecules

*Hundreds of molecules have been described in spines, involving many biochemical pathways. This molecular richness must endow synapses with a flexible biochemical machinery, one that likely makes synapses biochemically independent from other synapses and the rest of the neuron. In particular, the prominent actin and Rho pathways appear to play a central role and are ideally positioned to finely control spine morphological and functional plasticity.*

*One function of the spine thus might to be to biochemically organize and isolate the synapse. Given their small size and the complexity of their biochemical machinery, spines are paramount examples of biological nanotechnology, supporting a role that spines could have in implementing distributed connectivity with local learning rules in biological circuits.*

After discussing the morphological structure of the spine, it is pertinent to delve deeper into its molecular structure, focusing in particular on the types of proteins present in spines. The sheer amount of information being gathered about spines from molecular studies makes this a very fast-moving field, so by the time this book is published, it is likely that numerous additional molecules will have been characterized in spines.

I recognize that this promises to be a difficult chapter to read, and some readers may not find it particularly illuminating and will be tempted to skip it. At the same time, it is essential to discuss the molecular components of the spine for several reasons. First, molecules are, after all, the fundamental structural components of spines. Second, molecular biology is the common language of biology, and protein engineering through molecular genetic methods is an essential tool to experimentally manipulate and probe spine function. And third, from a bird's eye view, by considering not just which individual molecules or families of molecules spines have, or do not have, one may gain important insights into what spines can, or cannot, do functionally.

Significant overlap exists between molecular studies of spines and molecular studies of synapses. This makes the literature on the topic particularly large and often confusing. The reader is encouraged to consult recent reviews (Calabrese et al., 2006; Ethell and Pasquale, 2005; Kennedy et al., 2005; Tada and Sheng, 2006, Fend and Zhang, 2009). Also, recent proteomics studies are providing an increasingly complete molecular description of the spine and the synapse (Cheng et al., 2006; Grant et al., 2004; Husi et al., 2000; Li et al., 2004; Walikonis et al., 2000; Yoshimura et al., 2004).

I will briefly discuss, in order, proteins associated with glutamate receptors, NMDA-PSD95 complexes, AMPA-GRIP complexes, calcium homeostasis, actin regulation, adhesion molecules, kinases, phosphatases, neurotrophins, Rho GTPases, proteases, and channels (for a overview, see figure 4.1). To conclude, I will propose a potential functional interpretation of these findings.

**Glutamate Receptors**

As major sites of glutamatergic inputs, spines have all four types of glutamate receptors: NMDA, $\alpha$-amino-3-hydroxy-5-methyl-4-isoxazole-propionate (AMPA), kainate, and metabotropic glutamate (mGlu) receptors (figure 4.2).

The NMDA receptor (NMDAR) is a heterotetramer composed of NR1, NR2A-D, or NR3 and is invariably found in the PSD (Takumi et al., 1999). In addition to glutamate binding, NMDAR activation requires postsynaptic depolarization to remove blockade by $Mg^{2+}$, and when this happens, it generates a significant calcium influx into the neuron. This property is important for the detection of temporally coincident pre- and postsynaptic activity by spines (see chapters 7 and 8; Yuste and Denk, 1995; Yuste et al., 1999), which is necessary for many forms of synaptic plasticity (Malenka and Nicoll, 1999; Markram et al., 1997b). AMPA receptors (AMPAR), also heterotetramers, are made from the GluR1–4 subunits. Most AMPARs are $Ca^{2+}$-impermeable, and this property is controlled by the incorporation of the GluR2 subunit. Whereas AMPARs composed of GluR1, 3, and 4 show some $Ca^{2+}$-permeability, GluR2-containing AMPARs are generally not $Ca^{2+}$-permeable (Hollmann et al., 1991). This is due to RNA editing, which converts a glutamine residue in the channel pore forming domain to a positively charged arginine, rendering the receptor $Ca^{2+}$-impermeable (Hume et al., 1991; Sommer et al., 1991).

Interestingly, the presence or absence of GluR2 in a neuron correlates quite well with the presence or absence of spines. In many areas of the nervous system, neurons that express GlurR2 (and whose AMPARs are therefore calcium-*impermeable*) are highly spiny, whereas neurons that do not express GluR2 are sparsely spiny or aspiny (Goldberg et al., 2003a). This correlation holds true for neurons in hippocampus, neocortex, amygdala, retina, spinal cord, and auditory brainstem. Also, calcium-impermeable AMPARs endow aspiny interneurons with the ability to generate fast synaptic transients, whereas NMDARs generate particularly slow synaptic poten-

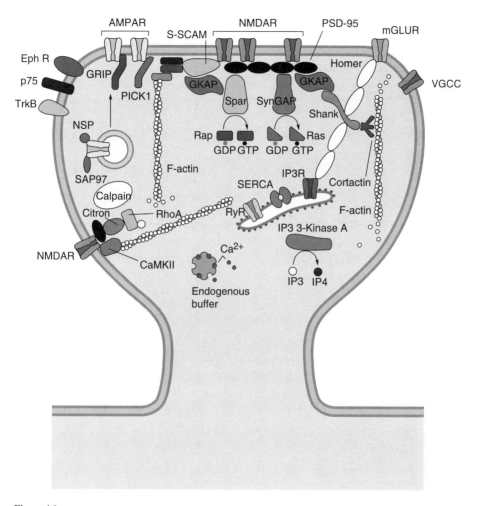

**Figure 4.1**
Major molecular components of a spine. Subsequent figures focus on particular pathways.

tials. Therefore, fast synapses generally use calcium-permeable AMPARs located on dendritic shafts, whereas slower synapses use calcium-impermeable AMPAR and NMDARs, located on spines (Goldberg et al., 2003a). Moreover, the artificial expression of GluR2 can turn aspiny interneurons into spiny ones (Passafaro et al., 2003), as if GluR2 were itself part of the switch used to control spinogenesis.

A number of electrophysiological experiments indicate a large variability in the number of functional AMPARs from synapse to synapse, although every spine appears to contain NMDARs (Malenka and Nicoll, 1999). Indeed, immunoelectron microscopy shows that the number of AMPARs in single synapses is variable from

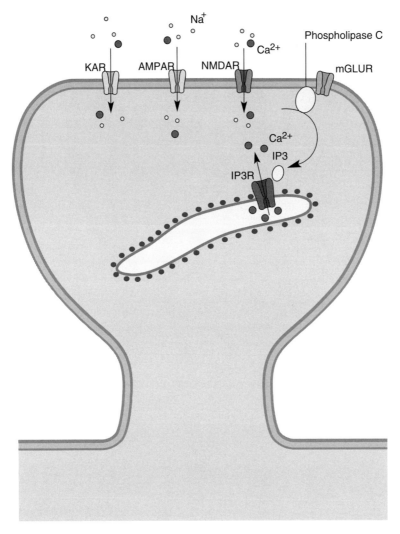

**Figure 4.2**
Glutamate receptors in dendritic spines. Na$^+$ ions are represented by small white circles, and Ca$^{2+}$ ions by larger darker ones.

spine to spine and correlates with the PSD area (Nusser et al., 1998). Approximately 15% of asymmetric synapses in CA1 spines have no AMPARs, perhaps representing silent synapses, formed exclusively of NMDARs (Liao et al., 1995; Malenka and Nicoll, 1999). These electrophysiological and morphological findings are consistent with two-photon imaging of calcium accumulations in spines, mediated by NMDARs and AMPARs (see chapter 7; Kovalchuk et al., 2000; Yuste et al., 1999). Mapping of functional AMPARs by two-photon uncaging of caged glutamate has also been used to estimate the number of glutamate receptors present in each spine (Matsuzaki et al., 2001). This work has also revealed a large variability in the number of AMPARs present in different spines, with a significant proportion of them having no detectable AMPARs. In addition, in agreement with the correlation between structural and functional parameters of the spine (see figure 3.14), there appears to be a correlation between the volume of the spine and the number of AMPARs present at the synapse.

Kainate receptors (KARs), a separate type of glutamate receptors, are composed of GluR5–7 (also known as KA1–2) subunits (Chittajallu et al., 1999) and are also found in the PSDs (Huntley et al., 1993; Roche and Huganir, 1995). Like the GluR2 subunit of AMPARs, GluR5 and 6 subunits undergo RNA editing, which regulates $Ca^{2+}$-permeability (Chittajallu et al., 1999).

Finally, metabotropic glutamate receptors (mGluR) are G-protein coupled receptors. Spines contain mGluR1 and 5 (Baude et al., 1993; Lujan et al., 1996), which are coupled to phospholipase C and phosphoinositide hydrolysis, producing inositol triphosphate (IP3) (Finch and Augustine, 1998; Takechi et al., 1998). Interestingly, mGluRs are found in the periphery, but not in the center, of the PSD (Baude et al., 1993; Lujan et al., 1996), hinting at the potential existence of functional subcompartments within the spine.

**NMDAR-PSD-95 Complex**

In addition to glutamate receptors, various proteins are found in the PSD of glutamatergic synapses (figure 4.3; table 4.1).

The proteins PSD-95/SAP90, PSD-93/Chapsyn-110, SAP97, and SAP102 are part of the membrane-associated guanylate kinases family (MAGUKs), characterized by multiple protein-binding domains, including three PDZ domains, a src homology 3 domain, and a guanylate kinase–like (GK) domain (Sheng and Sala, 2001). Through these protein-binding regions, PSD-95 and other members of the PSD-95 family interact with a variety of proteins and are thought to work as a molecular scaffold (Sheng and Sala, 2001). Specifically, the PDZ domains of PSD-95, PSD-93, and SAP102 bind to the C-terminal of NR2 subunit (Kim et al., 1996; Kornau et al., 1995; Mèuller et al., 1996). Moreover, the C-terminal sequence of NR2 appears to

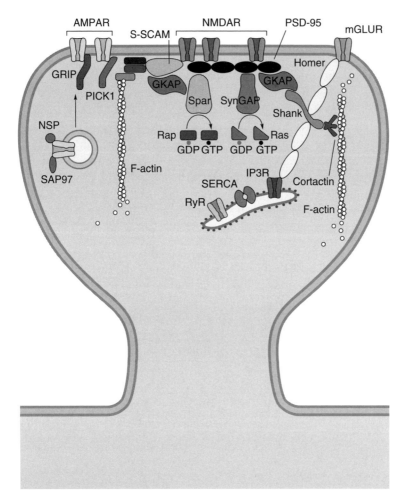

**Figure 4.3**
PSD-associated proteins in spines.

be required for the localization of NMDARs to the PSD (Mori et al., 1998; Steiger-wald et al., 2000). However, the interaction between NMDARs and PSD-95 does not seem important for the synaptic localization of NMDARs, since it is intact in PSD-95 knockout mice (Migaud et al., 1998). Also, when the synaptic targetting of PSD-95, PSD-93 and presumably other PSD-95 family proteins, is prevented using a mutant of CRIPT, a microtubule-binding protein found in spines (Niethammer et al., 1996), the synaptic clustering of NMDARs is still normal (Passafaro et al., 1999). Thus, PSD-95 may not just cluster NMDARs, but also link them to intracellular sig-naling machinery (Migaud et al., 1998).

**Table 4.1**
Proteins in NMDAR/PSD-95 complex

**PSD-95/SAP90, PSD93/Chapsin-110, SAP97, SAP102**
Members of PSD-95 family of MAGUK proteins. They contain three PDZ domains, one GK domain, and one SH3 domain, and interact with a variety of membrane and cytoplasmic proteins. Binding partners of PSD-95 include $K^+$ channels, kainate receptor subunits (GluR6 and KA1), neuroligin, neuronal NO synthase, PMCA4b, and citron (Sheng and Sala, 2001).

**GKAP/SAPAP**
GKAP consists of four members, GKAP 1–4 (Sheng and Kim, 2000). The PDZ domain of GKAP binds to the GK domain of PSD-95 (Kim et al., 1997; Naisbitt et al., 1997; Satoh et al., 1997; Takeuchi et al., 1997) and of S-SCAM (Hirao et al., 1998). The C terminal of GKAP binds to the PDZ domain of shank (Naisbitt et al., 1999).

**Shank**
Characterized by a variety of protein-binding domains such as multiple ankyrin repeats, an SH domain, a PDZ domain, a proline-rich region, and a SAM domain. Shank comprises three known members, Shank 1, Shank 2, and Shank 3 (Sheng and Kim, 2000). Shank binds to Homer (Tu et al., 1999) and actin-binding protein, cortactin (Naisbitt et al., 1999).

**Homer**
Products of three genes: Homer 1, Homer 2, and Homer 3. Homer contains an EVH1 domain and a C-terminal coiled coil (CC) domain (Xiao et al., 2000). One of splice variants, Homer 1a, is a product of immediate early gene regulated by synaptic activity (Brakeman et al., 1997), whereas Homer 1b and 1c are constitutively expressed (Kato et al., 1998; Xiao et al., 1998). Homer 1b and 1c contain a CC domain and show self-multimerization, but Homer 1a lacks a CC domain (Kato et al., 1998; Xiao et al., 1998). Homer binds to mGluR, IP3R, and Shank (Tu et al., 1998; Tu et al., 1999).

**SynGAP**
A Ras GTPase-activating protein (GAP). SynGAP binds to the PDZ domains of PSD-95, and its GAP activity is inhibited by CaMKII (Chen et al., 1998; Kim et al., 1998).

**SPAR**
A Rap GTPase-activating protein. SPAR binds to the GK domain of PSD-95 and may regulate spine morphology (Pak et al., 2001).

**S-SCAM**
S-SCAM contains five or six PDZ domains, a GK domain and two WW domains (Hirao et al., 1998). Three isoforms—S-SCAMα, β, and γ—are found (Hirao et al., 2000). S-SCAM binds to GKAP through the GK domain (Hirao et al., 1998), and PSD-95 (Hirao et al., 2000), neuroligin, NMDAR (Hirao et al., 1998), and β- and δ-catenin (Ide et al., 1999; Nishimura et al., 2002) through the PDZ domains.

Through PSD-95, NMDAR links with a variety of proteins including GKAP, Shank, Homer, SynGAP, SPAR, and S-SCAM (figure 4.3). Also, through the PSD-95/GKAP/Shank/Homer complex, NMDARs are connected to mGluRs and IP3R (Tu et al., 1999; Tu et al., 1998). This linkage may enable functional interactions between these receptors, and their close association may allow $Ca^{2+}$ influx through NMDARs and IP3, generated in an mGluR-dependent manner, to access IP3Rs and regulate its function (Tu et al., 1999). This coupling can be regulated by neuronal activity through the activity-dependent expression of Homer 1a, which is thought to work as an endogenous dominant negative regulator for constitutive forms of

Homer (Xiao et al., 1998). Also, the proximity of NMDARs to SynGAP (Kim et al., 1998) and SPAR (Pak et al., 2001) may enable synaptic activity to regulate the Ras and Rap signaling pathways (see below).

## AMPAR-Binding Proteins

The synaptic expression of AMPARs is dynamically regulated by neuronal activity (Malinow and Malenka, 2002). Several proteins interact with specific subunits of AMPAR and may mediate this dynamic regulation of trafficking and stabilization of AMPARs (see figure 4.3, left). AMPAR subunits have PDZ-binding motifs in their C-terminal and, through these motifs, bind to PDZ proteins (Sheng and Sala, 2001). Whereas GluR1 binds to SAP97 (Leonard et al., 1998), GluR2 and GluR3 bind to PDZ-containing proteins, GRIP/ABP (Dong et al., 1997; Srivastava et al., 1998) and PICK1 (Xia et al., 1999). The disruption of these interactions prevents the synaptic localization of AMPARs (Hayashi et al., 2000; Osten et al., 2000). In addition to PDZ proteins, GluR2 also binds to NSF, an ATPase with an important role in membrane fusion (Nishimune et al., 1998; Osten et al., 2000; Song et al., 1998). GluR1 binds also to an actin-binding protein, protein 4.1N (Shen et al., 2000). The disruption of these bindings reduces the surface expression of AMPAR (Noel et al., 1999; Shen et al., 2000). Finally, stargazin, a protein that interacts with the AMPAR, influences AMPA receptor trafficking and synaptic responses by slowing channel deactivation and desensitization (Tomita et al., 2005).

## $Ca^{2+}$ Homeostasis

In addition to $Ca^{2+}$ influx through ionotropic glutamate receptors, $Ca^{2+}$ influx into spines occurs through voltage-gated $Ca^{2+}$ channels (VGCCs) (Yuste et al., 2000; figure 4.4; see also chapter 7). VGCCs have been detected in spines using labeled ω-conotoxin, a selective antagonist for VGCCs (Mills et al., 1994). The number of VGCCs in individual spines has been estimated to vary between one to twenty individual proteins, with fluctuation analysis of $Ca^{2+}$ transients induced by action potentials (Sabatini and Svoboda, 2000). Interestingly, spine VGCCs appear to be regulated differently from those located even a few micrometers away, in the dendritic shaft.

The spine intracellular free calcium concentration ($[Ca^{2+}]_i$) can also be increased through release from internal stores, which can be activated by metabotropic receptors, such as mGluRs. Inositol triphosphate receptors (IP3Rs) and ryanodine receptors (figure 4.4), involved in the release of $Ca^{2+}$ from internal stores, are found in the SER of spines (Martone et al., 1997; Sharp et al., 1993; Walton et al., 1991).

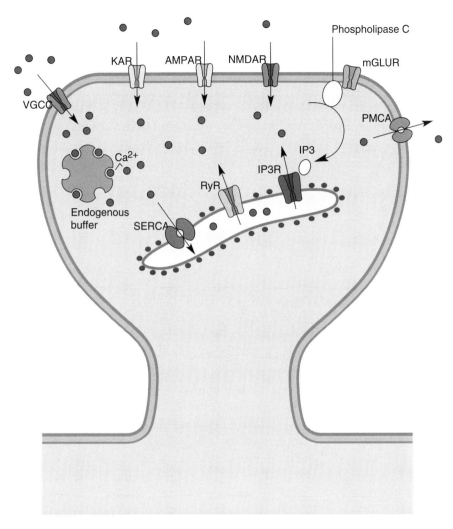

**Figure 4.4**
Molecules related to $Ca^{2+}$ homeostasis in dendritic spines. $Ca^{2+}$ ions are represented by dark circles.

However, this differs according to brain region. For example, in rat hippocampus, ryanodine receptors, but not IP3 receptors, are found in spines (Sharp et al., 1993). On the other hand, both receptors are found in neostriatal spines (Martone et al., 1997). Finally, IP3 receptors, but not ryanodine receptors, are present in cerebellar spines (Walton et al., 1991).

Molecules involved in the extrusion of cytoplasmic $Ca^{2+}$ can be also found in spines (see figure 4.4). Plasma membrane $Ca^{2+}$-ATPases (PMCA) pump out cytoplasmic $Ca^{2+}$, and, PMCA2, one of four PMCA isoforms, has been found in spines using immuno-EM (Hillman et al., 1996; Stauffer et al., 1997). Also, two other PMCA isoforms, 2b and 4b, interact with PSD-95 family proteins (see below; De-Marco and Strehler, 2001). The cytoplasmic $Ca^{2+}$ is also sequestered into the SER by the sarco/endoplasmic reticulum $Ca^{2+}$-ATPase (SERCA; see figure 4.4), also present in spines (Majewska et al., 2000a).

**Actin and Associated Proteins**

Electron micrographs of spines show that spine heads are filled with a "fluffy" indistinct material (see figures 3.5 and 3.11). Indeed, this feature is a useful way to distinguish, in EM sections, spine profiles from their surrounding neuropil and particularly from dendritic shafts, rich in microtubules (Peters et al., 1991). This fluffy material represents actin filaments, broken during the fixation or staining procedure (Fifkova and Morales, 1992). Spines are therefore, to a first approximation, veritable "balls" of actin (figure 4.5). The organization of actin filaments can be preserved when they are decorated by myosin subfragments. With this technique, it was shown that actin filaments actually form a meshlike network in spine heads and interact with plasma membrane and postsynaptic density at their barbed ends, whereas, in spine necks, actin filaments form long bundles (Fifkova and Delay, 1982). Only 5% of the spine's actin is stable (Star et al., 2002), and treadmilling is assumed to occur, with polymerization at the barbed ends and depolymerization at pointed ends (Pollard and Borisy, 2003). As is generally true throughout cell biology, actin polymerization is indeed responsible for morphological plasticity (see chapter 6, Honkura et al., 2008).

Most neurons express two isoforms of actin, β- and γ-actin, both enriched in spines (Kaech et al., 1997). Polymerized actin (F-actin) in spines is particularly stable, in comparison to F-actin from other cellular compartments. For example, an actin polymerization blocker, cytochalasin D, does not depolymerize F-actin in spines even after 24 hours of treatment, whereas the same concentration readily disrupts F-actin in the cell body and dendritic shaft (Allison et al., 1998). However, another polymerization blocker, latrunculin A, can depolymerize F-actin effectively in spines (Allison et al., 1998).

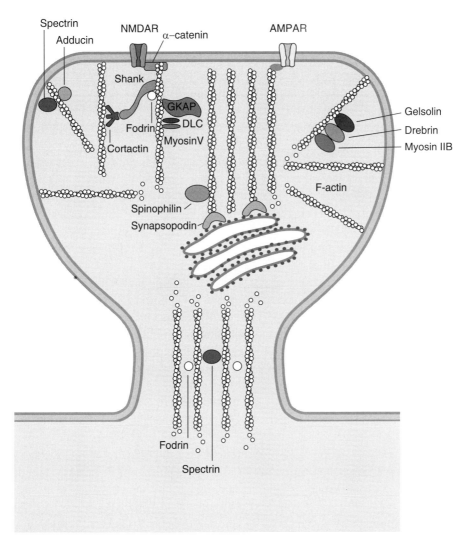

**Figure 4.5**
Actin and actin-binding proteins in dendritic spines. Actin monomers are represented by small open circles.

Spines also contain a variety of actin-associated proteins, including myosin, drebrin, α-actinin, fodrin, spectrin, adducin, spinophilin, synaptopodin, Arp 2/3, profiling, ADP/cofilin, gelsolin, neuroabin 1, SPAR, ABD-1, espin, IP2 kinase A, and cortactin (figure 4.5; see table 4.2; Ethell and Pasquale, 2005). Together with actin filaments, these proteins could play a role in functions such as vesicle and protein transport, regulation of spine morphology, or anchoring of membrane proteins. Interestingly, the removal of synaptopodin affects the spine apparatus and alters synaptic plasticity (Deller et al., 2003).

Two types of myosin heavy-chain subunits, myosin IIB (Cheng et al., 2000) and V (Walikonis et al., 2000), have been found in spines. Myosin V, which could act as a calcium sensor, interacts with GKAP through a light-chain subunit of myosin V, the dynein light chain (DLC), suggesting that the GKAP/DLC interaction may be involved in protein trafficking in the PSD-95 complex (Naisbitt et al., 2000). Myosin IIB can make a complex with actin, drebrin, and gelsolin. Drebrin regulates actomyosin interaction (Hayashi et al., 1996).

Two proteins, α-actinin and protein 4.1N, couple glutamate receptors to the actin cytoskeleton. α-Actinin binds to actin filaments and to the cytoplasmic tails of both NR1 and NR2B subunits (Wyszynski et al., 1997). This binding may be regulated by synaptic activity, since NR1/α-actinin binding is inhibited by $Ca^{2+}$/calmodulin (Wyszynski et al., 1997). Protein 4.1N contains spectrin-actin–binding domains (Walensky et al., 1999) and binds to a membrane proximal region of the GluR1 C-terminal (Shen et al., 2000). Two other actin-binding proteins, cortactin (Naisbitt et al., 1999) and α-fodrin (Bockers et al., 2001), bind to Shank and may connect NMDARs and mGluRs to the actin cytoskeleton through the PSD-95/GKAP/Shank/Homer complex.

As suggested by the multiple links between actin and glutamate receptors, the actin cytoskeleton could have important roles in anchoring glutamate receptors. Indeed, the complete depolymerization of F-actin in spines by latrunculin leads to a 40% decrease in the number of spines with NMDAR clusters or AMPAR clusters (Allison et al., 1998). Although the synaptic localization of NMDAR clusters becomes disrupted, NMDARs remain clustered in nonsynaptic sites. On the other hand, AMPARs disperse, suggesting that synaptic clustering of NMDAR and AMPAR depends on F-actin in different ways (Allison et al., 1998). Also, GluR1 is extractable with TritonX 100, but NR1 is not, suggesting that NMDAR tightly associates with the cytoskeleton, whereas AMPARs associate weakly (Allison et al., 1998). The association of NMDARs with PSD-95 and GKAP is not dependent on F-actin, whereas this protein complex is tightly associated with F-actin (Allison et al., 2000; Allison et al., 1998). The clustering of α-actinin, drebrin, and CaMKIIα (see below) in spines is F-actin–dependent, and these proteins are weakly associated with F-actin (Allison et al., 2000; Allison et al., 1998).

**Table 4.2**
Actin-binding proteins found in dendritic spines

**Myosin** (Miller et al., 1992; Cheng et al., 2000; Walikonis et al., 2000)
An actin-based motor protein. Two isoforms of myosin heavy-chain subunits, myosin IIB (Miller et al., 1992; Cheng et al., 2000) and V (Walikonis et al., 2000), are found in spines. Myosin IIB makes a complex with actin, drebrin, and gelsolin (Hayashi et al., 1996).

**DLC** (Naisbitt et al., 2000)
A light-chain subunit of microtubule-based motor, dynein, and myosin V. DLC interacts with GKAP (Naisbitt et al., 2000).

**Drebrin** (Hayashi et al., 1996)
Drebrin interacts with gelsolin and myosin IIB and modulates actomyosin interaction in vitro (Hayashi et al., 1996). Overexpression of drebrin makes spines longer (Hayashi and Shirao, 1999).

**Gelsolin**
A $Ca^{2+}$-sensitive actin-severing and capping protein (Kwiatkowski, 1999).

**α-actinin, Spectrin and Fodrin** (Ursitti et al., 2001; Wyszynski et al., 1997)
Actin-crosslinking proteins in spectrin family (Matsudaira, 1991). $Ca^{2+}$ inhibits actin-crosslinking ability. α-Actinin binds to the C terminal of both NR1 and NR2B subunits, and this binding may be inhibited by $Ca^{2+}$/calmodulin (Wyszynski et al., 1997). α-Fodrin binds to ankyrin repeats of Shank (Bockers et al., 2001).

**Protein 4.1N** (Walensky et al., 1999)
A brain isoform of protein 4.1 that contains spectrin-actin–binding domains (Hoover and Bryant, 2000); 4.1N binds to a membrane proximal region of the GluR1 C-terminal (Shen et al., 2000) and to a MAGUK protein, CASK (Biederer and Sudhof, 2001).

**Adducin** (Seidel et al., 1995)
Adducin binds to spectrin and recruits spectrin to the fast-growing end of F-actin (Matsuoka et al., 2000). This actin-related activity is regulated by $Ca^{2+}$/calmodulin and phosphorylation by PKA, PKC, and Rho kinase (Matsuoka et al., 1996; Matsuoka et al., 1998; Fukata et al., 1999).

**Spinophilin/Neurabin II** (Allen et al., 1997)
An actin binding protein with a PDZ domain. Spinophilin binds to PP1 and regulates PP1 activity (Allen et al., 1997; Satoh et al., 1998).

**Synaptopodin** (Mundel et al., 1997)
Synaptopodin is enriched in dendrites and spines, specifically around the spine apparatus in the spine neck (Deller et al., 2000).

**Cortactin** (Naisbitt et al., 1999)
An actin-binding protein that has a role in cortical actin assembly and membrane dynamics (Weed and Parsons, 2001). Cortactin binds to Shank (Naisbitt et al., 1999).

Many of these actin-binding proteins can be regulated by $Ca^{2+}$. For example, gelsolin is a $Ca^{2+}$-sensitive actin-severing and actin-capping protein (Kwiatkowski, 1999). Also, the actin-related activity of adducin is regulated by $Ca^{2+}$/calmodulin (Matsuoka et al., 1996). In addition, fodrin and spectrin can be degraded by a $Ca^{2+}$-dependent protease, calpain (Siman et al., 1984). These $Ca^{2+}$-dependent properties of actin-binding proteins might be important in regulating actin dynamics in spines. For instance, gelsolin is suggested to have an important role in activity-dependent regulation of actin turnover in spines (Star et al., 2002).

Finally, actin-binding proteins may regulate the formation and morphology of spines. For example, in spinophilin knockout mice, the spine density of pyramidal neurons was found to be abnormally high during development (Feng et al., 2000). Furthermore, the overexpresion of drebrin causes elongation of spines (Hayashi and Shirao, 1999).

**Other Cytoskeleton Proteins**

The existence of microtubules in spines is controversial. Microtubule-preserving techniques, including albumin-pretreatment, indicate that microtubules connect the spine apparatus to the PSD (Westrum et al., 1980). However, immunoelectron microscopy has detected β-tubulin only in the PSD, but not in the spine cytoplasm (Caceres et al., 1983). The presence of MAP2, a microtubule-associated protein, in spines is also controversial. Caceres et al. (1983) found strong immunoreactivity to MAP2 in the spine cytoplasm, whereas Bernhardt and Matus (1984) detected no immunoreactivity in spines and the PSD. Also, Kaech et al. (1997) showed the confinement of MAP2 to dendritic shafts using transfection of GFP-tagged MAP2.

Although intermediate filaments in spines have not been thoroughly studied, several neurofilament proteins have been found in the PSD (Walsh and Kuruc, 1992) and interact with GKAP (Hirao et al., 2000). In addition, a type IV intermediate filament protein, α-internexin, has been detected in spines (Benson et al., 1996; Suzuki et al., 1997).

**Adhesion Molecules**

Spines also contain a variety of cell-adhesion molecules, including N- and E-cadherin, cadherin-related neuronal receptor (CNR), integrins, neural cell adhesion molecule (NCAM), densin-180, neuroligin 1, and syndecan-2 (figure 4.6; table 4.3).

Like glutamate receptors, adhesion molecules are normally linked to the actin cytoskeleton. Cadherins interact with actin filaments through β-catenin and α-catenin

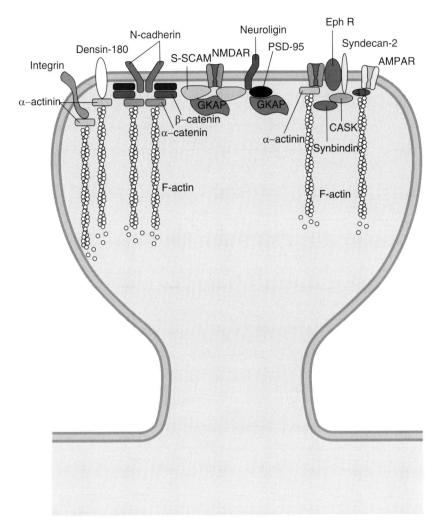

**Figure 4.6**
Cell adhesion molecules in dendritic spines.

**Table 4.3**
Adhesion molecules in dendritic spines

---

**N- and E-cadherins** (Beesley et al., 1995; Benson and Tanaka, 1998; Fannon and Colman, 1996; Uchida et al., 1996)
$Ca^{2+}$-dependent homophilic cell adhesion molecules. Their cytoplasmic regions are linked to actin filaments through β- and α-catenin (Takeichi, 1995).

**CNR** (Kohmura et al., 1998)
CNRs are products of 14 or 15 genes in mammals, but the proteins show a large variety, which might be produced by somatic DNA rearrangement or trans-splicing (Hamada and Yagi, 2001).

**Integrin** (Einheber et al., 1996; Nishimura et al., 1998; Schuster et al., 2001)
Heterodimers composed of combinations of α- and β-subunits that bind to the extracellular matrix. Integrins are linked to actin filaments through their binding to α-actinin and other actin-binding proteins (Geiger et al., 2001). Three subunits, α8 (Einheber et al., 1996), β8 (Nishimura et al., 1998), and β1 (Schuster et al., 2001) integrins, are found in spines.

**NCAM** (Persohn and Schachner, 1987; Persohn and Schachner, 1990)
A $Ca^{2+}$-dependent homophilic adhesion molecule, which has three splice variants: NCAM 120, 140, and 180. The extracellular region of NCAM can be glycosylated by polysialic acid (PSA), and the degree of polysialation has an effect on the adhesion property of NCAM and other adhesion molecules (Walsh and Doherty, 1997).

**Densin-180** (Apperson et al., 1996)
A transmembrane protein containing a PDZ domain (Apperson et al., 1996), which binds to α-actinin (Walikonis et al., 2001). Densin-180 also binds to CaMKII (Strack et al., 2000), and Densin-180, CaMKII, and α-actinin make a ternary complex (Walikonis et al., 2001). Densin-180 also binds to δ-catenin, which in turn binds to N-cadherin. δ-Catenin is enriched in spines (Izawa et al., 2002).

**Neuroligin** 1 (Song et al., 1999)
A ligand of β-neurexin (Ichtchenko et al., 1995). Neuroligin 1 and β-neurexin function as cell adhesion molecules in excitatory synapses (Song et al., 1999). Neuroligin 1 also intracellularly binds to PSD-95 (Irie et al., 1997) and S-SCAM (Hirao et al., 1998).

**Syndecan-2** (Hsueh et al., 1998)
A cell surface heparan sulfate proteoglycan. Its C-terminal binds to the PDZ domain of CASK (Hsueh et al., 1998). CASK colocalizes with Syndecan-2 in the PSD (Hsueh et al., 1998) and interacts with protein 4.1 and links syndecan-2 to the actin cytoskeleton (Biederer and Sudhof, 2001). The C-terminal of syndecan-2 binds to synbindin, which is structurally related to yeast proteins involved in vesicle transport (Ethell et al., 2000).

---

(Takeichi, 1995), and integrins (Geiger et al., 2001) and densin-180 (Walikonis et al., 2001) bind to α-actinin. Syndecan-2 (Hsueh et al., 1998) and neuroligin 1 (Hirao et al., 1998; Irie et al., 1997) are linked to actin filaments by binding to PDZ proteins, CASK (syndecan-2), PSD-95, and S-SCAM (neuroligin 1). Interestingly, neuroligin 1 may have a central role in presynaptic differentiation, since neuroligin 1 even when expressed in non-neuronal cells, triggers the formation of presynaptic structures on contacting axons (Scheiffele et al., 2000).

Syndecan-2 may also have an important role in spine development. Syndecan-2 accumulates on spines during the period of the morphological maturation of spines from filopodia, and the exogenous expression of syndecan-2 in immature neurons causes accelerated spine formation (Ethell and Yamaguchi, 1999).

N-cadherins (Tang et al., 1998), integrins (Bahr et al., 1997), and PSA-NCAM (Muller et al., 1996) may also be involved in synaptic plasticity. This is not surprising if one considers their roles in the interaction with presynaptic or extracellular components at the synaptic junctions. For example, N-cadherin seems localized in the adhesive structure surrounding the PSD in synaptic junctions (Beesley et al., 1995; Benson and Tanaka, 1998; Fannon and Colman, 1996; Uchida et al., 1996). ß-Catenin shows an activity-dependent redistribution (Murase et al., 2002), and the resulting change in cadherin adhesion may regulate synaptic function and spine morphology (Togashi et al., 2002).

## Kinases

Spines have a particularly rich complement of protein kinases. In particular, $Ca^{2+}$ calmodulin-dependent kinase II (CaMKII) is a major constituent of the PSD in spines (figure 4.7; Kelly et al., 1984; Kennedy et al., 1983; Ouimet et al., 1984), where it contributes more than 10% of the protein mass (Kelly and Cotman, 1978). In fact, there is so much CAMKII in the spines it could even play a structural role, in addition to its enzymatic functions, or perhaps as its main function (Erondu and Kenendy, 1985; Pi and Lisman, pers. comm.). CaMKII is a serine/threonine protein kinase and has two dominant isoforms, α and β, in the brain (Soderling, 2000). Binding of $Ca^{2+}$/calmodulin activates kinase activity and autophosphorylates Thr286 (Soderling, 2000). This $Ca^{2+}$-dependent activation of CaMKII induces targeting of CaMKII into the PSD through the binding of CaMKII to NMDARs (Leonard et al., 1999; Shen and Meyer, 1999; Strack and Colbran, 1998). CaMKII phosphorylates NR2B (Omkumar et al., 1996), and this phosphorylation inhibits the binding between CaMKII and NR2B (Strack et al., 2000). CaMKIIβ binds directly to F-actin, and may target CaMKIIα to synapses (Shen et al., 1998). Additionally, AMPARs may be regulated by CaMKII, since CaMKII phosphorylates GluR1 subunits and enhances their single-channel conductance (Barria et al., 1997; Derkach et al., 1999). Other CaMKII substrates include PSD95, SAP90, dynamin, and α-internexin (Yoshimura et al., 2000).

Protein kinase C (PKC), arguably the other most important kinase in the brain with CAMKII, is a $Ca^{2+}$-dependent serine/threonine kinase and is also present in the PSDs (figure 4.7; Wolf et al., 1986). Specifically, the α (Xia et al., 1999) and γ (Kose et al., 1990) isoforms of PKC are localized in spines. PKC binds to PICK1 and this complex may be transported to spines (Perez et al., 2001). Phosphorylation of GluR2 by PKC leads to dissociation of GluR2 from GRIP/ABP and binding of

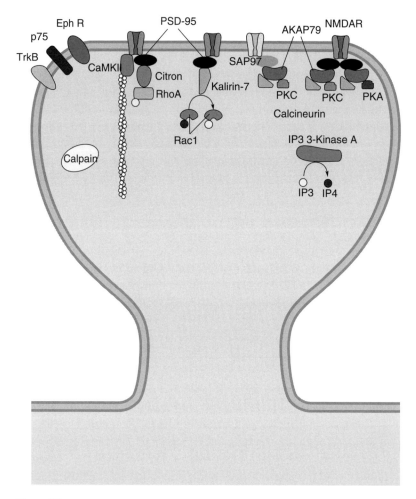

**Figure 4.7**
Protein kinases in dendritic spines.

PICK1 to GluR2 (Chung et al., 2000; Matsuda et al., 1999). PKC also phosphorylates adducin and regulates its actin-capping ability (Matsuoka et al., 1996; Matsuoka et al., 1998). In addition, PKC may regulate the distribution of NMDARs
(Fong et al., 2002; Lan et al., 2001) and the maintanence of spines through its target
MARCKS (myristoylated, alanine-rich C-kinase substrate (Calabrese et al., 2006).

Inositol 1,4,5-trisphosphate (IP3) 3-kinase A phosphorylates IP3 into inositol
1,3,4,5-tetrakisphosphate (IP4), which enhances the $Ca^{2+}$ entry through voltage-
gated $Ca^{2+}$ channels and the internal release from IP3 receptors (Irvine and Schell,

2001). IP3 kinase A is activated by its interaction with $Ca^{2+}$/calmodulin and through phosphorylation by CaMKII (Communi et al., 1997; Woodring and Garrison, 1997). IP3 kinase A binds to F-actin through N-terminal 66-amino acids, and this binding localizes the kinase to spines (figure 4.7; Schell et al., 2001).

Finally, the Eph receptors are a family of receptor tyrosine kinases that are found in the spine PSD (figure 4.7; Buchert et al., 1999; Torres et al., 1998). Many Eph-related proteins are present in spines and probably have significant functions (Ethell et al., 2001; Ethell and Pasquale, 2005). Ligand binding to a subtype of Eph, EphB receptors, induces a direct interaction of EphB with NMDARs in a kinase-independent manner, whereas EphB tyrosine kinase activity appears to be required for synapse formation (Dalva et al., 2000). EphB receptors phosphorylate syndecan-2, and this phosphorylation leads to an interaction between syndecan-2 and EphB. This phosphorylation seems crucial for syndecan-2 clustering and spine maturation (Ethell et al., 2001).

## Phosphatases

Several serine/threonine protein phosphatases have roles in synaptic transmission and plasticity (figure 4.8; Winder and Sweatt, 2001). Among them, two—protein phosphatase 1 (PP1) and calcineurin/protein phosphatase 2B—are found in spines (figure 4.8; Goto et al., 1986; Ouimet et al., 1995). The α and γ1 isoforms of PP1 are highly concentrated in spines (Ouimet et al., 1995). PP1 binds to spinophilin, and this binding regulates PP1 activity (Allen et al., 1997). PP1 also binds to a scaffold protein, Yotiao (Westphal et al., 1999). Yotiao in turn binds to the NR1 subunit of NMDAR (Lin et al., 1998) and to protein kinase A (PKA) (Westphal et al., 1999). This binding may enable PP1 and PKA to regulate NMDA receptor channel activity (Westphal et al., 1999). PP1 dephosphorylates CaMKII in the PSD (Shields et al., 1985; Strack et al., 1997), and this dephosphorylation may lead to dissociation of CaMKII from the PSD (Yoshimura et al., 1999).

Calcineurin is composed of a catalytic subunit and a regulatory subunit, and binding of $Ca^{2+}$/calmodulin on the catalytic subunit activates phosphatase activity (Klee et al., 1998). Calcineurin binds to AKAP79 (Coghlan et al., 1995), which also binds to PKA (Ndubuka et al., 1993) and PKC (Klauck et al., 1996). AKAP79 binds to PSD-95 and SAP97, and may target these kinases and phosphatase to glutamate receptor complexes (Colledge et al., 2000). AKAP79 is found in the spines, but not in the PSD (figure 4.8; Sik et al., 2000). Calcineurin also binds to an immunophilin, FKBP12. Calcineurin is targeted to the ryanodine and IP3 receptors through its association with FKBP, and may regulate $Ca^{2+}$ release from internal stores (figure 4.8; Snyder et al., 1998).

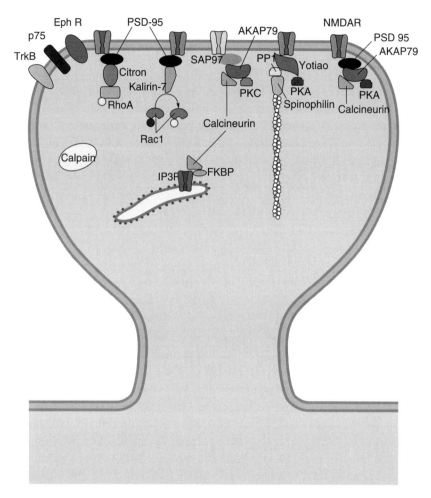

**Figure 4.8**
GTPases, protein phosphatases, and other proteins in dendritic spines.

## Neurotrophin Receptors

Spines also contain neurotrophin receptors, key molecules that, among other functions, link patterned neuronal activity to morphological changes during development. Two types of neurotrophin receptors are found in the PSD: TrkB and p75 (figure 4.8; Aoki et al., 2000; Dougherty and Milner, 1999; Drake et al., 1999; Wu et al., 1996). The neurotrophin BDNF is also found in the PSD (Aoki et al., 2000). TrkB is primarily a receptor for BDNF and NT-4, whereas p75NTR binds to all neurotrophins with similar affinity (Huang and Reichardt, 2001). Neurotrophins mediate synaptic plasticity in spine synapses (Kovalchuk et al., 2002). Also, neurotrophin signaling controls the morphology of spines. In cerebellar Purkinje cells, TrkB modulates spine density and morphology without any apparent effect on the parent dendrites (Shimada et al., 1998), whereas BDNF destabilizes spines and dendrites in cortical neurons (Horch et al., 1999).

**Rho GTPases and Related Proteins**

Rho GTPases are a family of proteins known to regulate the actin cytoskeleton in many cell types (Hall, 1994, 1998). RhoA and Rac1, the most well-characterized members of the Rho GTPase family, regulate spine density and morphology (see also chapter 6; Luo et al., 1996; Nakayama et al., 2000; Nakayama and Luo, 2000; Tashiro et al., 2000; Tashiro and Yuste, 2004, 2008). The presence of proteins interacting with RhoA and Rac1 in spines suggests that RhoA and Rac1 exist in spines (see figure 4.8). Kalirin-7 is a GDP/GTP exchange factor that activates Rac1. Kalirin-7 interacts with PSD-95, is localized in spines and regulates spine morphogenesis (Penzes et al., 2001). Also, citron, a downstream effector of RhoA, binds PSD-95 and is localized in spines in thalamus and cortex (Zhang et al., 1999). Other small GTPases and related proteins have been found in spines, among others: ARF3, cAMP-GEFII (RapGEF), GIT1 (ArfGAP), heterotrimeric G proteins, Kalirin (RhoGEF), PIKE-L (ArfGAP), Ras, SPAR (RapGAP), SynGAP (RasGAP), Rnd 1, intersectin, Beta PIX, oligophrenin, N-WASP, LIM kinases, and ROCK (Cheng et al., 2006; Ethell and Pasquale, 2005; Sheng and Hoogenraad, 2007). SPAR is downregulated by synaptic activity, and this can lead to changes in spine size, although this effect must be redundant because the KO has an apparently normal phenotype.

Rho GTPases play a major role in spinogenesis and spine motility, as will be discussed in chapter 6. Intriguingly, mutations in the Rho pathway regulators have been implicated in mental retardation syndromes in humans (Luo, 2000; Newey et al., 2005). Specifically, oligophrenin-1, a protein with GAP activities for Rho, Rac, and Cdc42, has been linked to nonsyndromic X-linked mental retardation (Billuart et al., 1998). Also, another locus encodes ARHGEF6, a GEF for Rho (Kutsche et al., 2000), and Pak3, a target of Rac (Allen et al., 1998). Finally, synaptojanin, a Rac1 effector, appears overexpressed in Down syndrome (Arai et al., 2002).

**Proteases**

A $Ca^{2+}$-dependent protease, calpain, is enriched in spines and the PSDs (figure 4.8; Perlmutter et al., 1988). Calpain can cleave a variety of proteins that exist in spines, including actin, spectrin, cortactin, NCAM, integrin, $Ca^{2+}$ channel, ryanodine receptor, and NMDAR (Chan and Mattson, 1999). Activation of NMDAR activates calpain and causes proteolysis of spectrins (Siman and Noszek, 1988). In addition, calpain degrades PSD-95 (Lu et al., 2000; Vinade et al., 2001) and GRIP (Lu et al., 2001) and may alter the structure of the PSD (Dosemeci and Reese, 1995; Lu et al., 2000; Vinade et al., 2001).

## Channels

Finally, we finish our tour of spine biochemistry discussing ion channels. Besides VGCC, a variety of active membrane conductances appears to exist in spines (figure 4.9). Specifically, voltage-dependent sodium channels are functionally active in spines (Araya et al., 2007), perhaps not surprising since they are present in the dendritic shafts (Stuart et al., 1997). In addition, there is both structural and functional evidence that different subtypes of potassium channels are located in spines, including SK2 (Lin et al., 2008; Lujan et al., 2009), GIRK (Jan et al., unpublished results; Chung et al., 2009), Kv4.2 (Kim et al., 2007), and probably also the nonselective cation channel HCN. Each of these channels could have a profound impact on spine physiology (see chapter 8).

## Functional Interpretation of the Molecular Structure of Spines

In a nutshell, spines are veritable nanomachines and appear to contain an enormous diversity of families of molecules, including membrane receptors and channels, molecular scaffolds, motor proteins, cell adhesion proteins, chaperones, cytoskeleton components, actin and actin-binding proteins, calcium homeostasis machinery, kinases and phosphatases, neurotrophin receptors, membrane trafficking factors, metabolic enzymes, and a particularly healthy assortment of actin-related proteins, including Rho-family GTPases. Among scores of different proteins belonging to all these families, some with particularly high stochiometry include CAM-kinase 2, PSD-95, SynGap, Shank, GKAP, NRS, Sap97, mGlurs, IRSp53, Homer, GluRs, and AKAP79 (Kennedy et al., 2005; Sheng and Hoogenraad, 2007; Tada and Sheng, 2006).

Why such an enormous molecular diversity? What is the purpose of this molecular richness? This molecular diversity could be key for the function and plasticity of the synapse and may endow it with unusual biochemical flexibility. Just from reading the spine molecular "laundry list," one could conclude that synapses must be very heavily regulated and must therefore be particularly key components for the nervous system to alter.

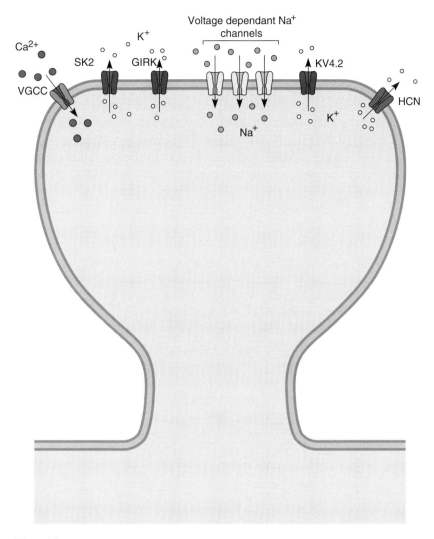

**Figure 4.9**
Membrane conductances in dendritic spines. K$^+$ ions are represented by small white circles, Na$^+$ by small dark circles and Ca$^{2+}$ ions by larger darker ones.

But given that dendrites are already endowed with many of these molecules, why duplicate all this cellular biochemistry in every spine? This indicates that the biochemistry of each synapse must be independently regulated, probably because synaptic strength must be controlled in an input-specific fashion. In fact, the biochemical independence could be one of the major functions of the spines: to provide a subcellular organization or isolation of the biochemical machinery of the synapse. Because essentially all spines have PSDs, perhaps the biochemical isolation of the PSD from the rest of the neuron could be key. Indeed, many of the proteins discussed, such as AMPAR (Nusser et al., 1998), Homer (Okabe et al., 2001a), and β-catenin (Murase et al., 2002) can differ from spine to spine and display activity-dependent redistribution into or out of spines.

It is also interesting to point out that all this biochemical diversity is crammed into a very small volume. Spines are so small (<1 fl), that it is difficult to imagine such a crowded and complex environment, to the point that some have argued that the PSD resembles a protein crystal (Kennedy, 2000). Spines could be one of the ultimate examples of miniaturization in biology. Indeed, as one would expect from a nanomachine, within spines there is evidence for both the existence of a small number of molecules, within each of the classes discussed, and precision in their location. For example, as explained earlier, the number of NMDARs or AMPARs on a given spine can be very small, down to single units (Nusser et al., 1998). Similarly, the number of VGCCs present on spines has been estimated to be as low as one (Sabatini and Svoboda, 2000). Moreover, in some cases, the position of the spine channels and receptors, particularly with respect to other molecular components of the spine, appears to be determined with extreme precision, as in the case of mGluR (Lujan et al., 1996). The more we discover about the molecular architecture of a spine, the more sophisticated and regulated spines appear to be. In future studies of spine structure and function, it appears necessary to achieve an equally high degree of precision as the spine molecular components show. It may not be far-fetched to argue that understanding the biochemical pathways present in spines may require a single-molecule level of probing and analysis (Mehta et al., 1999; Alcor et al., 2009; Triller, pers. comm.), together with detailed computational modeling of the spatiotemporal dynamics and kinetics of these molecules (Kennedy, 2000; Kennedy et al., 2005; Holcman and Triller, 2006).

This precision in synapse assembly, besides being difficult for investigators to disentangle, must be something quite difficult for the cell to achieve. Why undergo such an effort in miniaturization? This miniaturization supports the idea that spines are implementing a distributed connectivity and are essentially as small as possible. Since the number of glutamate receptors is already so low, it is difficult to imagine that spines could be made even smaller. With spines, nature is probably touching bottom.

In terms of the actual biochemical pathways present in spines, it is interesting to note the prominence of the actin biochemistry, since every molecular pathway we have discussed links directly with the actin cytoskeleton. Because actin is associated with cell movement, spines appear to be designed to move. The fact that spines lack tubulin also indicates that their structure is purposely not stable. The presence of actin in both developing and mature spines also suggests that this morphological plasticity must be important, not just in development, but also throughout the life of the animal. As is discussed in chapter 6, spines do move, and it will be pointed out that the purpose of this motility could be to enable them to efficiently connect with axons, exactly what one would need to maximize the connectivity and implement a distributed circuit. Moreover, the large number of actin-related proteins present in spines, together with the apparently sophisticated control of this actin biochemistry by the very many GTPases present in spines, indicates that the regulation of spine morphology is very sophisticated and must be essential for its function in the mature circuit. The idea that morphological changes in spines could mediate synaptic plasticity is the central hypothesis discussed in chapter 8.

Finally, when one considers the specific assortment of glutamate receptors spines have, it is interesting to note that spine synapses seem to have been built to be particularly slow in their electrical function properties. The calcium homeostasis biochemistry in spines is also on the slow side (see chapter 7). Thus, one could venture the hypothesis that there is something fundamentally slow about the function spines must be carrying out. As is argued in chapter 10, perhaps the reason spines are so slow is related to their fundamental role as integrators. Thus, in summary, considering the molecular architecture of a spine, if one were to attempt to functionally interpret this diversity, several threads emerge: miniaturization, independent regulation, motility, and temporally slow responses. In the remaining chapters, I will argue that these apparently disconnected threads are actually very directly linked and well matched to one another, when one considers the ultimate function of spines in the circuit.

# 5 Development

*Understanding how spines emerge during development could help us discern the function of spines in circuits and their role in neural plasticity. In Purkinje cells, spines can emerge in the complete absence of axonal terminals, so spinogenesis appears to be an intrinsic and cell-autonomous property of the cell. At the same time, neuronal activity can regulate the maintenance of some Purkinje cell spines.*

*On the other hand, in pyramidal neurons, axons and dendrites may interact to generate spines. Dendritic filopodia, generated in large numbers during synaptogenesis, could be precursors of many spines. Alternatively, spines could gradually emerge from the dendritic shafts. In any case, after a period of morphological plasticity during postnatal development, many spines are eliminated in a pruning stage, a process regulated by neural activity. The remaining spines are essentially preserved for the rest of the life of the animal. This stability of spines and their synapses could mediate the persistence of memories.*

*The developmental emergence of spines and filopodia suggests that their function is to facilitate synaptogenesis by acting as dendritic "arms" to contact neighboring axons. This, together with the straight course of most excitatory axons, could lead to an efficient method to implement a distributed connectivity matrix while minimizing the necessary wiring. Spinogenesis would therefore help to maximize circuit connectivity.*

How do spines originate during development? Answering this question could potentially shed light on the role of spines in the adult nervous system. In this chapter, I will discuss the development of spines in two types of neurons: cerebellar Purkinje cells and cortical pyramidal neurons. As I will argue, some features of spinogenesis may be intrinsic to the neuron and some could be extrinsic and activity-dependent. Indeed, Purkinje cells exemplify these two aspects of spine development: intrinsic, "hardwired" plan and an extrinsic, "plastic," and activity-dependent one. The development of spines in pyramidal neurons in the neocortex and hippocampus is less well understood, and the potential roles of dendritic filopodia in spinogenesis and of spinogenesis in the adult neocortex are subject to debate.

This chapter does not cover synaptogenesis. Since most spines are recipients of synaptic inputs (see chapter 3), synaptogenesis is potentially linked to spinogenesis. However, there are reasons why it is better to treat spinogenesis as its own separate topic. As will be explained below, the complete developmental program leading to the formation of mature spines can occur in the absence of axon terminals. Also, synaptogenesis, at least as understood traditionally, is a protracted phenomenon, taking days or even weeks to complete, whereas spines can arise in minutes (see chapter 6). Finally, how a synapse develops is a very large topic that merits its own focused review. For readers interested in synaptogenesis I recommend some past and recent reviews (Cline, 2005; Cotman and Nieto-Sampedro, 1984; Craig et al., 2006; Jacobson, 1991; Jontes and Smith, 2000; Purves and Lichtman, 1985; Ullian et al., 2004; Vaughn, 1989; Waites et al., 2005; Zhang and Benson, 2000; Ziv and Garner, 2001; Lu et al., 2009).

**Spinogenesis in Purkinje Cells**

**Parallel Fiber Spines: The Sotelo Model**

Besides having a stereotyped circuit, the mammalian cerebellum has a key advantage for developmental studies: it is not necessary for life. Indeed, removal of the entire cerebellum produces a variety of motor symptoms without affecting any vital function (Adams and Victor, 1985). Because of this, many natural mutations that affect the development of the cerebellum are not lethal and can be isolated. Moreover, many cerebellar mutants can be easily identified by deficits in motor coordination. These advantages have been well exploited, and have made possible a detailed analysis of many mutations affecting different neurons at different developmental stages. Some of these studies have helped address the issue of how spines first emerge, demonstrating that they can do so irrespective of the presence of axonal terminals (Sotelo, 1990). In the chicken-and-egg problem of whether spines emerge before or after the synapses, it seems that, at least for parallel fiber spines, spines not only can form before the axon terminals arrive, but they can even develop in the complete absence of axons. Indeed, as mentioned in chapter 3, even in mature circuits one can occasionally encounter apparently normal spines that lack axonal innervation (figures 3.7 and 3.8), suggesting the possibility that spines can develop independently of axonal terminals.

In fact, three distinct types of studies in which Purkinje cells grow in the absence of granule cells (figure 5.1) indicate that spinogenesis is intrinsic to the neuron, at least for Purkinje cells spines innervated by parallel fibers (Sotelo, 1990).

The first evidence comes from *weaver* mutant mice, in which granule cells, the presynaptic partners of the majority (~90%) of spines in the Purkinje cells, are absent

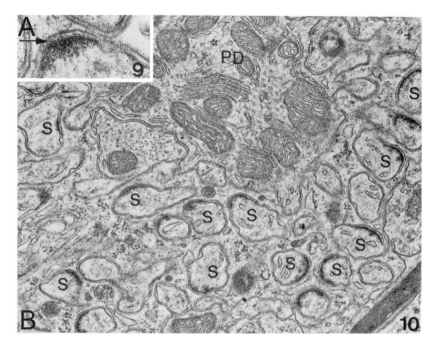

**Figure 5.1**
Dendritic spines without presynaptic input in mutant mice. (A) High-power electron micrograph of a non-synaptic spine from a mouse Purkinje cell dendrite. Note the PSD and the extracellular cleft (arrow) facing a glial membrane. (B) A Purkinje cell dendrite (PD) surrounded by numerous nonsynaptic spines (S) with normal-looking postsynaptic differentiations. Note the absence of axon terminals. Reprinted from Sotelo, 1975.

(Rakic and Sidman, 1973). In these animals, Purkinje cells develop abnormal and atrophic dendrites, which are, however, covered with spines. These spines actually appear quite normal, even to the point of having normal postsynaptic specializations ultrastructurally (Hirano and Dembitzer, 1973; Landis and Reese, 1977; Rakic and Sidman, 1973; Sotelo, 1975). A second line of evidence comes from *reeler* mutant mice, deficient in the production of the protein reelin (Caviness and Sidman, 1972; 1973). As a consequence of this deficiency, the migration of neuronal precursors in cerebellum is grossly disturbed. In many of these animals, a central region of the cerebellar cortex has a large number of ectopic Purkinje cells with no granule cells. Again, these Purkinje cells develop morphologically normal spines in the absence of their presynaptic partner (Mariani et al., 1975). Finally, X-irradiation of neonatal rats can selectively ablate granule cells, because of their delayed development with respect to Purkinje cells (Altman and Anderson, 1972). As in *weaver* and *reeler*, Purkinje cells in these animals develop morphologically normal spines at apparently normal densities (figures 5.1 and 5.2, Sotelo, 1977).

Wild Type                                                          Mutant

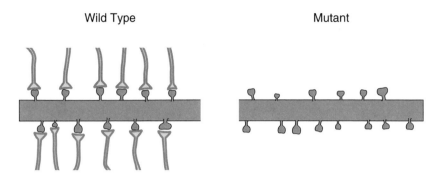

**Figure 5.2**
Illustration of the Sotelo experiments.

The normal developmental sequence of events in the cerebellar cortex is also in line with the implications from agranular mice. Indeed, spines in distal dendritic branches of Purkinje cells developed before they establish synaptic contacts with parallel fibers (Larramendi, 1969). Also, at early postnatal stages (P0–P12) "naked" spines without terminals can be encountered, whereas at later stages essentially all spines have a synapse (Altman and Bayer, 1997). It is possible that those "naked" spines lost a previously present terminal, since spines are resilient to the loss of parallel fibers (Rakic and Sidman, 1973). However, given the developmental sequence, this appears unlikely.

Therefore, evidence from both normal and mutant cerebelli suggests that the initial formation of parallel fiber spines on Purkinje cells does not depend on presynaptic axons, and that synaptogenesis occurs at a later stage, when incoming axons meet already formed spines (Sotelo, 1978). This is the Sotelo model, one of the three models of spine development I will discuss (figure 5.3). Spinogenesis thus appears to be in some cases an intrinsic property of the neuron. Somehow, each Purkinje cell "knows" how to build spines and probably also controls the density of spines intrinsically. In fact, the helical arrangement of spines along dendrites of Purkinje cells (figure 3.20; O'Brien and Unwin, 2006) is consistent with this intrinsic program. It is difficult to imagine how extracellular signals could instruct spines to precisely locate themselves along the dendrites forming helixes.

These results demonstrate that spines can arise in the absence of presynaptic partners, and that the developmental program that leads to the formation of a spine might be, for some classes of spines, cell-autonomous. Still, closer scrutiny could reveal some differences in spines that fail to make a synaptic contact. Indeed, given the importance reciprocal pre- and postsynaptic interactions have for synaptogenesis in the neuromuscular junction (Sanes and Lichtman, 1999), it seems unlikely that spines that lack presynaptic partners have normal postsynaptic specializations. For

Sotelo model

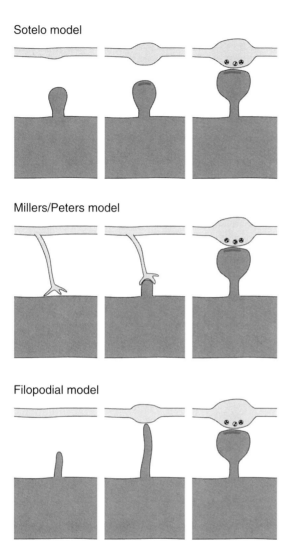

Millers/Peters model

Filopodial model

**Figure 5.3**
Three models for spinogenesis. Within each model, drawings represent sequential developmental stages. Axon terminals are on top (light gray) and dendrite on bottom (darker gray).

example, the development of purified cultures of Purkinje cells is aided by the addition of glial and granule cells, so presynaptic factors could help build a mature post-synaptic site (Baptista et al., 1994).

**Climbing Fibers: Spine Maintenance Can Be Controlled by Neuronal Activity**

As will be discussed extensively in chapters 6 and 8, spines are plastic. In fact, over a hundred years ago it was already suggested that changes in spines could underlie learning (Ramón y Cajal, 1891a, 1893, 1899c), and this still constitutes one of the major threads in contemporary research on spines (see chapter 8; Yuste and Bonhoeffer, 2001). The first observation of spine plasticity was actually made by Cajal himself. In a seminal observation, he noted that, in pyramidal neurons, the spine density was higher in early development than in adulthood, when the number of spines apparently decreased (Ramón y Cajal, 1899c). He inferred from this that the circuit somehow must rearrange itself by losing many connections. The initial proliferation of synapses located in spines, followed by a decline in their numbers, has been confirmed many times since (Rakic et al., 1986; Weiss and Pysh, 1978).

What controls this "pruning" of spines and their associated synapses? To shed light on this pruning, I will continue discussing Purkinje cells, this time concentrating on spines in the proximal region of their dendritic tree, mainly contacted by climbing fibers. Initially, Purkinje cells are innervated by a "nest" of multiple climbing fibers on the soma (Ramón y Cajal, 1904). These contacts are made on perisomatic spines (Larramendi, 1969; Laxson and King, 1983) and are electro-physiologically functional (Crepel et al., 1976; Crepel, 1971). Later in development, climbing fibers translocate to "thorns," large spines in proximal dendrites (Larramendi and Victor, 1967). Shortly afterwards, all but one of the climbing fibers is eliminated, resulting in the innervation of each Purkinje cell by a single climbing fiber (Crepel, 1971; Larramendi, 1969; Ramón y Cajal, 1904). These contacts are made on "spiny branchlets" (Palay and Chan-Palay, 1974). Because the number of climbing fibers in adult Purkinje cells is precisely one (not zero or more than one), the elimination of perisomatic spines, supernumerary climbing fibers, and "thorns" could be activity-dependent, involving the competition among different axonal afferents. The molecular mechanisms underlying this fascinating phenomenon, reminiscent of the formation of the neuromuscular junction (Sanes and Lichtman, 1999; Tello, 1907), are unclear.

Thus, the activity of climbing fibers could regulate spine formation in the proximal region of the Purkinje cell. But interestingly, climbing fiber activity also controls the parallel fiber spines in Purkinje cells. Lesioning the inferior olive, the nucleus that gives rises to the climbing fibers, produces supernumerary spines in the proximal Purkinje cell's dendrites (Sotelo et al., 1975). Thus, climbing fibers can repress spinogenesis, either through the release of neurotransmitters or through some other factor.

A separate experiment suggests that this repressive effect of climbing fibers depends on neuronal activity (Bravin et al., 1999). Blocking all neuronal activity by tetrodoxin (TTX) during development increases spine density in proximal dendrites of Purkinje cells by an order of magnitude. At the same time, the spine density in the distal dendritic tree, where most granule cells make their contacts, is unaffected (Cesa et al., 2003).

These data prove that neuronal activity is involved in suppressing spine formation in the proximal region of the dendritic tree, but not in distal spiny branches (Cesa and Strata, 2005). Since an inferior olive lesion results in similar increases in proximal spines, climbing fiber activity must be suppressing spine formation, either directly or indirectly. But it is also possible that the activity of Purkinje cells themselves, either spontaneous or evoked by climbing or parallel fibers, is crucial. These possibilities are not mutually exclusive. Indeed, data from *weaver* and *reeler* mice, in which Purkinje cells are deprived of granule cell inputs but the innervation by multiple climbing fibers persists (Crepel and Mariani, 1976), suggest that granule cell inputs can influence the fate of the more proximal, climbing fiber spines.

In conclusion, data from two populations of spines in Purkinje cells exemplify two different developmental plans: spines on distal dendrites are intrinsically generated and maintained regardless of the activity of the terminal and the neuron. On the other hand, spines on proximal dendrites, after being generated, perhaps also endogenously, are repressed by the activity of climbing fibers. These two types of spines define two developmentally, morphologically, and functionally different cellular compartments: proximal dendrites, innervated by climbing fibers and distal dendrites, receiving parallel fibers (Sotelo, 1978). Indeed, evidence from another mutant, the *staggerer* mouse, indicates that this compartmental distinction is actually recognized as such by the neuron. In *staggerer* the formation of spiny branchlets is selectively impaired, but proximal dendrites nevertheless develop with apparently normal spines, indicating that the *staggerer* gene has a specific effect on the proximal compartment.

## Potential Circuit Logic of Purkinje Cell Spines

The development plan of spinogenesis in Purkinje cells makes one wonder what the potential circuit function of their spines could be. The generation of spines that are recipients of parallel fiber input appears to be controlled very differently from that of climbing fiber spines. These two types of connections also mediate apparently opposite circuit functions: Whereas parallel fibers connect with as many Purkinje cells as possible, climbing fibers connect with only one. Moreover, in the adult circuit, climbing fibers end on dendritic branchlets, rather than on spines.

This difference in circuit function might be the ultimate reason underlying the two different developmental strategies for spinogenesis. The intracellular machinery of parallel fibers might build terminals at particular distances along the axon to make connections with Purkinje cells. The narrow dendritic tree of Purkinje cells and the orthogonal orientation of the granule cell axons make it almost impossible for a parallel fiber to contact a given Purkinje cell more than once. Purkinje cells, at the same time, might simply produce as many spines as possible to fill these orthogonal surfaces completely. It is then conceivable that the easiest way to achieve this would be by using some cell-autonomous, space-filling developmental algorithm (Berry and Bradley, 1976), and helixes could be an excellent solution to this problem (see figure 3.20). Therefore, spines may not serve just to connect with axons, but to enable the cell to connect only once with each axon. This strategy would help to distribute and fill, as completely as possible, the connectivity matrix of a circuit (see chapter 10).

Climbing fibers appear to follow an opposite circuit logic: In the proximal compartment, climbing fibers would initially be strongly attracted to Purkinje cells, avoiding other targets. But later, to ensure that each Purkinje cell is only innervated by at most one climbing fiber, activity-based competition rules could exist, resulting in a "winning" climbing fiber which would inhibit spinogenesis in the captured Purkinje cell, thus preventing other climbing fibers from regaining this territory. Because climbing fibers suppress spines in order to suppress innervation, one could argue that the function of spines might be to enhance innervation, as in the parallel fiber case.

To achieve a one-to-one match, a winner-take-all strategy may be used, as in the neuromuscular junction (Balice-Gordon and Lichtman, 1984; Sanes and Lichtman, 1999; Tello, 1907). At the same time, in contrast to the neuromuscular junction, additional rules must also operate in the cerebellum to prevent a climbing fiber from capturing more than one target. Perhaps the limiting number of neurotransmitter vesicles that a single inferior olivary axon can sustain limits climbing fibers from winning more than one "battle."

**Spinogenesis in Pyramidal Neurons**

Do these data from Purkinje cells apply to other spiny neurons? In cortical circuits, experiments that disrupt presynaptic axons without affecting postsynaptic cells are not as straightforward as they are in the cerebellum, as cortical manipulations fundamentally disrupt brain function. At the same time, transgenic and knockout animals are becoming increasingly useful for disentangling the role of pre- and postsynaptic structures (Verhage et al., 2000). In this discussion of pyramidal spinogenesis, I follow the distinction made earlier between an initial phase of spine emergence and a secondary maintenance period for spine development. As we will see, although there is clear evidence in cortical neurons for external regulation of spine generation and maintenance, it is possible that, just as in cerebellar cells, these extrinsic factors act on an underlying intrinsic developmental program that builds spines, as indicated by the fact that some pyramidal neurons have helical positioning of spines, yet also display differences in spine densities that could be generated by extrinsic factors (figures 3.19 and 3.20).

**Presynaptic Terminals Induce Spine Formation: The Miller-Peters Model**

In many, but not all mammalian species, spine formation in pyramidal neurons occurs after birth. In rat cortical pyramidal neurons, spinogenesis begins quite precisely in all layers by the middle of the first postnatal week (Miller, 1988). Spine density then increases during the next four weeks and is subsequently reduced with age (Miller, 1988), reflecting an initial overproduction and later elimination of synapses during early cortical development (see Rakic et al., 1986; Ramón y Cajal, 1899c, as examples from a large literature illustrating this effect).

During the initial spinogenesis, axonogenesis proceeds quite rapidly. In fact, axons from pyramidal neurons (the ones contacting most neocortical spines) develop slightly ahead of dendrites and spines, and axon extension occurs even before neuronal migration is complete (Miller, 1988). By the time spines emerge, axonal terminals are already formed. In adult neocortex, basically all spines have synapses, with generally one presynaptic terminal impinging on them (Arellano et al., 2007b, see chapter 3; Braitenberg and Schüz, 1998). The one-to-one matching between spines and terminals, as in the neuromuscular junction, could be seen as an indication that competitive mechanisms must be at play. At the same time, the few spines with no synapse lack a clear head and appear similar in morphologies to dendritic filopodia (figures 3.7, 3.8, 3.9; Arellano et al., 2007b).

In addition to a change in density, spines from pyramidal neurons undergo profound morphological rearrangements during postnatal development (Miller, 1988; Peters and Kaiserman-Abramof, 1970). Early in development, stubby spines lacking clear necks, are very common. In the mature circuit, thin or mushroom spines with more prominent necks and heads dominate (Miller and Peters, 1981), although a significant number of stubby spines are still present in adult cortices (Benavides-Piccione et al., 2002).

As an alternative to the Sotelo model, spine development in pyramidal cells could be related to synaptogenesis (figure 5.3, middle and bottom panels). In pyramidal cells, synapses on dendritic shafts are present during early developmental stages (Cotman et al., 1973; Crain et al., 1973; Juraska and Fifkova, 1979; Mates and Lund, 1983; Pokorny and Yamamoto, 1981; Schwartzkroin et al., 1982; Steward et al., 1988). During a first stage, synapses are on dendritic shafts, and there are also immature spines, recognized by their flocculent material. At a second stage, one detects many stubby spines, and the presynaptic region of the axon shows a swelling as synaptic vesicles accumulate. Finally, during a third stage, most spines are thin or mushroom-like, with a lollipop shape and a clear neck, and axonal terminals have well-developed varicosities. (Braitenberg and Schüz, 1998). To explain this, Miller and Peters proposed a three-stage model for spinogenesis in pyramidal neurons (figure 5.3, middle panel; Miller and Peters, 1981). A spine would appear in response to an axonal interaction and be drawn out by the axon terminal. Thus, when a spine grows, it would "grab" a preexisting shaft synapse and carry it along with it (figure 5.3; Miller-Peters model). Therefore, different from the Sotelo model, in which the terminal seems to play a minor role in spinogenesis, in the Miller-Peters model a spine is induced as a result of the effect of the terminal on the dendritic shaft. Similar ideas were proposed by others (Mates and Lund, 1983; Braitenberg and Schüz, 1998).

An objection to the Miller-Peters model arises from the fact that axonal trajectories through the neuropil are generally straight, and most axonal contacts are made *en passant* (Anderson and Martin, 2001). If axonal terminals were contacting dendritic shafts and "pulling out" spines, axons would be expected to have convoluted trajectories, at least during early development, something that has not been reported. At the same time, it is possible that the neuropil is more compact early in development, and that the subsequent interstitial growth of the neuropil could be the mechanism responsible for "pulling" spines away from shaft synapses, without altering the straight trajectories of axons.

Another problem with the Miller-Peters model is that the earliest synapses on dendritic shafts are found at very low densities (De Felipe et al., 1997), representing a very small proportion of the total number of synapses in the adult neuron. Even though they could indeed give rise to spines, most spines might develop differently.

A final objection could arise from the observation that spine helixes exist in pyramidal neurons (figure 3.20; Yuste et al., in prep.). If axons were responsible for inducing spines, it is hard to imagine how they could generate helical patterns.

**Role of Neuronal Activity on Pyramidal Neuron Spinogenesis**

Does neuronal activity influence the development of spines from pyramidal neurons? Do spines in pyramidal neurons behave like parallel fiber spines or more like climbing fiber spines from Purkinje cells? I will first focus on the role of sensory activity and then discuss the potential role for spontaneous activity.

An interesting and pertinent observation comes from comparative developmental studies. While some species (altricial), such as rats and mice, are born with relatively immature brains, others (precocious), are born with more developed brains. Indeed, in guinea pig, spinogenesis has already occurred by birth, and these animals are born with an essentially mature complement of spines and synapses (Schüz, 1981). This simple fact has an important implication, since it proves that, at least in some species, spinogenesis and synaptogenesis occur in the absence of environmental influences (Braitenberg and Schüz, 1998). Both processes therefore must be unrelated to sensory processing or learning.

In fact, in visual cortex, even in altricial species like rats or mice, a large proportion of spino- and synaptogenesis occurs before eye opening (Miller, 1988). Moreover, in all species examined, or in different individuals of the same species, there is less than one day offset in the overall time course of spino- and synaptogenesis (Jacobson, 1991). The only morphological event that actually correlates with eye opening apparently is the elongation of the spine neck (Miller and Peters, 1981), something quite interesting on its own, because the spine neck length could control synaptic strength (see chapters 9 and 10).

These data seems to indicate that sensory-evoked activity is not important for ontogenetic spinogenesis in pyramidal neurons, and even synaptic activity may not be important. However, the developing brain, also in utero, has robust patterns of spontaneous activity potentially important for circuit rearrangements (Katz and Shatz, 1996; Maffei and Galli-Resta, 1990; Shatz and Stryker, 1988). Therefore, it remains possible that spontaneous neuronal activity could be necessary for normal spinogenesis in pyramidal neurons. An ideal experiment to test the role of spontaneous activity on spinogenesis would be to block all activity, spontaneous or evoked, during uterine development. This was achieved in mice in the knockout of *munc18* (Verhage et al., 2000). This protein is necessary for transmitter release throughout the central and peripheral nervous systems (CNS and PNS), and mice that lack it surprisingly display apparently normal neocortical synapses and circuits at birth. Unfortunately, these mice die shortly after birth, before spinogenesis has taken place. Interestingly, massive apoptosis occurs in many regions of the nervous system (although apparently not in the cortex), suggesting that neurotransmitter release is necessary for neuronal survival throughout the CNS.

**Role of Neuronal Activity on Pyramidal Spine Maintenance**

The role of activity in the maintenance of connections, on the other hand, has been investigated extensively (Jacobson, 1991), though I will only touch on this issue as it relates to spinogenesis. As mentioned, spine density (and synapse density) appears to follow a stereotypical developmental pathway, with an initial overproduction followed by a reduction to a plateau level that then persists through adulthood (Jacobson, 1991; Purves and Lichtman, 1985; Rakic et al., 1986; Ramón y Cajal, 1899c). This pruning of spines is likely to reflect a similar pruning of synaptic inputs, thus representing a considerable reduction of connectivity in the developing brain, a reduction perhaps sculpted through learning rules or input competition (Katz and Shatz, 1996). After this overproduction stage, spine density can be affected by sensory deprivation or by experimental paradigms that modify synaptic activity (see chapter 8; Valverde, 1967, 1971; Engert and Bonhoeffer, 1999; Maletic-Savatic et al., 1999). These manipulations can generate not only reductions of spine density but also, in some cases, increases, implying that spinogenesis can occur at later stages in development as well.

Another interesting insight comes from recent molecular studies that indicate the Rho family of small GTPases is an important contributor to spinogenesis and spine loss (see chapter 6). Overexpression or suppression of these proteins results in the creation or elimination of novel spines in vivo and in vitro (Luo et al., 1996; Nakayama et al., 2000; Nakayama and Luo, 2000; Tashiro et al., 2000). Such "genetically engineered" spines can be produced not only in developing neurons, but also in mature cells (Tashiro et al., 2000). Moreover, spine density, size, and length are controlled by different members of the Rho family (Tashiro et al., 2000; see chapter 6). Existence of these artificially generated spines is therefore proof that even mature pyramidal neurons have the entire molecular complement necessary for extensive spinogenesis.

Finally, it is also worth mentioning that not only can spines appear and disappear, their basic morphology also appears to be continuously changing (see chapter 6; Dunaevsky et al., 1999; Fischer et al., 1998), in a manner that in some cases could also be controlled by activity (see chapter 8).

## Spine Stability and Spinogenesis in Mature Animals

The stability of neural circuits in adult nervous systems is an issue of basic importance for understanding brain function, yet it is still unknown whether the neuronal circuitry is constantly undergoing rewiring or whether, once developed, it constitutes a relatively stable network. Despite the importance of this question, technical limitations have made it difficult to address it.

For neuronal synapses in the peripheral nervous system (PNS), Purves and his colleagues have demonstrated substantial dendritic remodeling that reflects, at least in part, the rearrangement of synaptic connections (Purves and Hadley, 1985; Purves et al., 1986). These studies were initially performed in relatively young mice. Lichtman and colleagues in turn extended these studies to adult animals and specifically addressed the change in the rate of synaptic rearrangements over time (Gan et al., 2003). The authors used transgenic mice with sparsely fluorescently labeled axons to show that, in the submandibular ganglion, synaptic terminals undergo constant rearrangement during the first few weeks of life, whereas this rate of synaptic change was considerably decreased in older mice.

In the CNS, synaptic stability is still poorly understood, with most progress made in the neuromuscular junction (NMJ). Here, Lichtman and colleagues demonstrated that these structures are relatively stable over many months in the adult animal (Balice-Gordon and Lichtman, 1984; Sanes and Lichtman, 1999), whereas in developing animals the termination patterns of axons on the muscle fibers undergo substantial and constant remodeling (Walsh and Lichtman, 2003). These experiments, though a good starting point for what to expect in the dynamics of spine generation and retraction in the CNS, addressed *synaptic* stability and not the stability or generation of spines. The shortage of information on spinogenesis in vivo has been largely due to technical limitations. Until the advent of two-photon microscopy (Denk et al., 1990) it was basically impossible to image spines in living animals. The problem is that spines are so small (<1 μm in diameter and <1 fl in volume; Harris and Kater, 1994) that imaging them requires high light fluxes that are normally accompanied by photodamage in live preparations. Two-photon excitation (Denk et al., 1990) reduces this photodamage by triggering fluorescence excitation only at the focal point, avoiding out-of-focus excitation of the sample. In addition, two-photon excitation uses infrared light that enables imaging in highly scattering tissue such as brain slices (Denk et al., 1994). These two properties make two-photon microscopy particularly advantageous for imaging of living tissue, making it possible to investigate the generation of spines (and their disappearance) in the cerebral cortex in living animals (figure 5.4; Grutzendler et al., 2002; Holtmaat et al., 2005; Lendvai et al., 2000; Trachtenberg et al., 2002).

These more recent studies have used two-photon microscopy in transgenic mice, engineered to express fluorescent proteins in a subset of their neurons, to study spine stability or turnover in developing and adult animals (figure 5.4). Grutzendler and colleagues (2002) asked the simple yet crucial question of how stable spines are in the developing and adult visual cortex. They observed that the half-life of a spine in the adult is approximately 13 months, which is approximately the entire lifespan of the animal in the wild. These authors also report that during the mouse's adolescence the turnover rate is considerably higher, but, even during this phase, approximately 70% of the spines remain stable for at least a month (figure 5.4). Thus, the main message from this work is the remarkable stability of spines throughout life, including critical periods. Results from other groups have confirmed these important observations, highlighting the increasing stability of spines with the maturation of the nervous system (Holtmaat et al., 2005; 2006; 2008; Majewska and Sur, 2003; Majewska et al., 2006; Zuo et al., 2005; but see also Trachtenberg et al., 2002 for an opposite conclusion).

How does the morphological plasticity of spines early in development transition into their stability in mature circuits? A similar in vivo imaging study has documented a massive loss of spines during early postnatal development (Zuo et al., 2005), confirming past observations, of major developmental reductions in spine density (Rakic et al., 1986; Ramón y Cajal, 1899c; Weiss and Pysh, 1978). This study also revealed that this pruning is induced by neuronal activity, since sensory deprivation (whisker trimming) prevented it. A complementary study investigated cortical

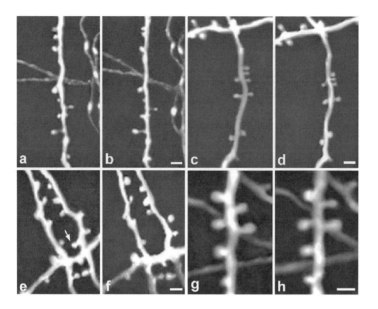

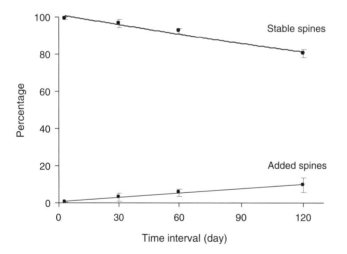

**Figure 5.4**
Long-term stability of dendritic spines in vivo. (a and b, c and d) Dendritic branches from adult mice imaged 3 days apart displaying the same spines at the same locations. (e and f, g and h) Repeated imaging of dendritic branches from younger animals (4 months old) imaged 2 months apart show small changes in spine number or location. Arrow points to an eliminated spine. (Bottom) Graph illustrating the evolution of the percentage of stable spines and new added ones during the life of the animal. Reprinted with permission from Grutzendler et al., 2002.

spinogenesis during postnatal development, altering the sensory input with a different paradigm (Trachtenberg et al., 2002). Trimming every other whisker on the snout of the animal increases the fraction of short-lived spines, as if the morphology were more plastic, in line with earlier experiments (Lendvai et al., 2000). Taken together, these studies suggest that, at least during postnatal development, the stability of spines can be modulated by sensory manipulations and therefore plastic adaptations in the cortex.

In conclusion, then, it is now possible to image spines in living animals, and even follow them over periods of weeks and months. This is a remarkable achievement, which will undoubtedly help considerably in our understanding of the roles of spines, and their appearance and disappearance, in the formation and plasticity of neural circuits.

These studies highlight a remarkable stability in spine shape and position in the adult, and a significant turnover of spines during the critical period of postnatal development, a turnover that is modulated by sensory inputs (figure 5.5). As Cajal envisioned, circuits become "crystalized" after a period of postnatal pruning and plasticity. Also, these imaging studies show that spinogenesis can occur in neocortical tissue in vivo, and that a small but potentially important proportion of spines in the mature circuit could be generated de novo. While, for example, new spines could potentially be used to implement novel learned associations between sensory stimuli, the substantial fraction of spines that are stable for many months could represent the basic mechanisms of storage of information by the brain.

**Dendritic Filopodia: Spine Precursors?**

As a final stop in our discussion of spinogenesis, I will consider dendritic filopodia and their stability. The reason for this special treatment is their potential role as spine precursors, particularly in pyramidal cells.

Cajal was probably the first to report the presence of long dendritic appendages in immature nervous systems. Although he did not name these protrusions, he noticed that their peculiar morphologies were distinct from spines, describing them as long and bending "appendages" that frequently changed directions and bifurcated. He concluded that these protrusions occur only transiently during development (Ramón y Cajal, 1934). The protrusions, now known as "filopodia," have since been found throughout the brain and spinal cord of vertebrates and invertebrates, as well as in pathological situations such as mental retardation (Marín-Padilla, 1972; Purpura, 1974). Nevertheless, they have not been extensively studied, since their presence in fixed material is not particularly abundant, perhaps a reflection of their great sensitivity to aldehyde fixation (see below).

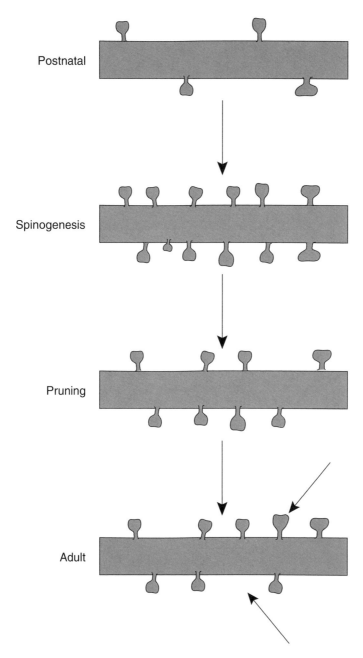

**Figure 5.5**
Model for spine emergence and stability during the lifetime of an animal. After an initial spinogenesis during development, most spines persist during the adulthood period, although some spines will be added or eliminated (arrows).

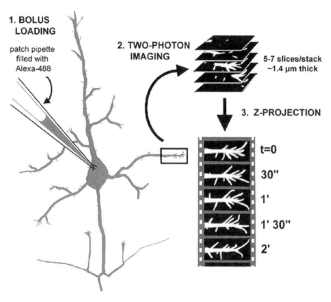

**Figure 5.6**
Time-lapse imaging of the motility of dendritic filopodia. Step 1: Neurons in brain slices are injected with a fluorescence dye, which diffuses quickly throughout the entire cell. Step 2: Selected dendrites are imaged with a two-photon microscope. Image stacks, each composed of several slices in the XY plane, are acquired quickly. Step 3: Using software, the individual slices for each time point are projected along the z-axis into a single image. Time-lapse movies of dendritic protrusions are generated. Reprinted from Portera-Calliau et al., 2003.

The introduction of imaging methods, on the other hand, has recently revealed the existence of filopodia on living samples and their great prevalence in developing tissue. In fact, time-lapse experiments of developing neurons have demonstrated that filopodia are strikingly motile, both in vivo and in vitro (figures 5.6 and 5.7). In living neurons, filopodia are longer and thinner than spines (measuring anywhere from 1 to 40 µm in length), and they branch and bend frequently (figure 5.7; Dailey and Smith, 1996; Fiala et al., 1998; Morest, 1969a, b).

Filopodia are part of a group of rather ubiquitous cellular specializations in many cells. These protrusions, first described in the early 1960s, were originally named pseudopods, though the term filopodia eventually won over (McClay, 1999). Dendritic filopodia resemble other types of filopodia in the nervous system, such as axonal growth cone filopodia, muscle cell filopodia (the so-called myopodia; Ritzenthaler and Chiba, 2003), and filopodia of glial cells (Asou et al., 1994; Cornell-Bell et al., 1992; Kachar et al., 1986). Moreover, they also are nearly identical to filopodia of nonneuronal cells (McClay, 1999). In fact, when dendritic and nonneuronal filopodia are examined side by side, the similarities between them are very striking.

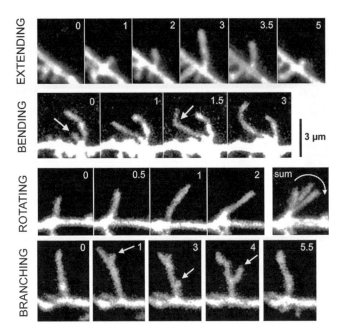

**Figure 5.7**
Motility of dendritic filopodia. Two-photon images from a time-lapse movie of a dendrite from a developing neocortical pyramidal neuron in a brain slice. Note the appearance and disappearance of filopodia and the diverse movement they display. Time in minutes. Reprinted with permission from Portera-Cailliau and Yuste, 2001.

Dendritic filopodia do not contain SER or a spine apparatus, and usually have a more homogeneous cytoplasm made up almost exclusively of actin filaments (Fiala et al., 1998). It is likely that a similar cytoskeletal apparatus generates filopodia in all cell types that express them. The lack of more robust structural components is probably responsible for the great lability of dendritic filopodia: they are very sensitive to fixatives. Moreover, filopodia are normally poorly impregnated with Golgi stains (Konur and Yuste, unpublished observations). In agreement with these problems to preserve and stain filopodia in fixed tissue, in histological preparations filopodia are seen at lower densities than those found in vivo (C. Portera-Cailliau and Yuste, unpublished observations).

The elongated shape of dendritic filopodia suggests an exploratory function in the extracellular space. Except for pathological circumstances (Marín-Padilla, 1972; Purpura, 1974), filopodia are rarely found on mature neurons, so their function is probably developmental. Unfortunately, no molecular marker has been found that can specifically label filopodia, so currently one has to rely on their morphological features to define them, like the presence of a thin, and particularly long stalk and lack of a distinct head (Dailey and Smith, 1996; Fiala et al., 1998). This constitutes a problem because the dynamic nature of spines and filopodia can confound this distinction (see chapter 6; Parnass et al., 2000).

## Filopodia in Purkinje Cells and the Vaughn Model

Hints to the potential function of filopodia might be gained from their developmental profile and distribution. Where and when do filopodia appear? Filopodia occur in most, or perhaps all, developing neurons. In Purkinje cells, two different types of filopodia have been described: *terminal* filopodia located near the distal tips of developing dendrites and *collateral* filopodia that occasionally emerge from dendritic shafts (Berry and Bradley, 1976; Laxson and King, 1983). The association of terminal filopodia with the tips of the dendrite suggests that they are involved in dendritic growth and branching, by interacting with the extracellular environment (Berry and Bradley, 1976; Laxson and King, 1983; Morest, 1969b). In this view, the final morphology of the dendrite would reflect the history of interactions of terminal filopodia with the environment. Which filopodium proceeds to form a terminal branch might then be determined by its success in making a synaptic contact. This idea was incorporated in Vaughn's "synaptotropic" hypothesis (figure 5.8), which states that filopodia (terminal filopodia in this case) serve to "catch" axons, and that synapses are first formed on the filopodia and then "passed down" to the dendritic shaft (Bradley and Berry, 1976; Vaughn et al., 1974; Vaughn, 1989).

Indeed, in developing spinal cord, approximately 70% of synaptic contacts are found on filopodia (Skoff and Hamburger, 1974; Vaughn et al., 1974). Nevertheless, reports conflict over whether in hippocampus and neocortex filopodia are preferential sites of early synaptogenesis (Fiala et al., 1998; Linke et al., 1994; De Felipe, unpublished observations). It is possible that filopodia do not have the prominent head of spines precisely because they lack synapses (figures 3.7, 3.8, and 3.9). Collateral filopodia, on the other hand, could have been "left behind" by the growth of the dendrite. They may represent the incipient growth of a new dendritic branch, or, as a hypothesis I will consider next, could be involved in spinogenesis or synaptogenesis (Berry and Bradley, 1976).

## Filopodia in Pyramidal Neurons: The Filopodial Model of Spinogenesis

In rat neocortical pyramidal neurons, filopodia of the collateral type are transient and occur mostly in P0–12 animals (Miller and Peters, 1981). They are very elongated and can be directly apposed to axons over their full length, although clear synapses between neocortical dendritic filopodia and axons have rarely been described. Neocortical filopodia often occur in groups, as if they emerged from particular hot spots of the dendrite, similar to filopodia of axons and other developing

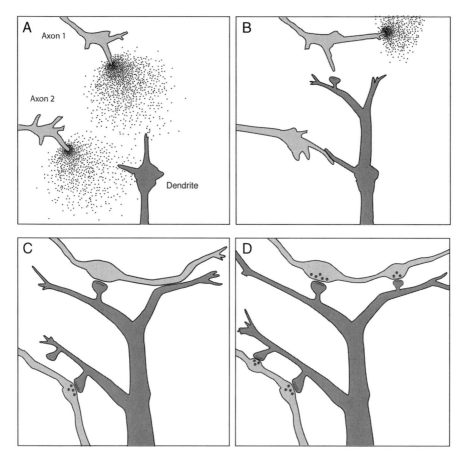

**Figure 5.8**
Vaughn model of synaptogenesis: role of filopodia in synaptogenesis and dendritic branching (based on Vaughn, 1989). (A) A dendritic growth cone at bottom right is growing in the vicinity of two axonal growth cones, which release a chemoattractant (for example, glutamate). (B) In response to this release, two dendritic filopodia emerge and are guided by a gradient in the concentration of the chemoattractant. (C) The axonal and dendritic filopodia interact closely and make initial synaptic contacts. (D) Synapses are established at sites originally defined by the initial contacts. Reprinted from Portera Cailliau and Yuste, 2001.

neurites (Portera-Cailliau et al., 2003; Tessier-Lavigne and Goodman, 1996; Wang and Macagno, 1997). In hippocampal CA1 pyramidal cells, the distribution of filopodia during development has been studied with ultrastructural techniques (Fiala et al., 1998). Two types of filopodia are described: an elongated type, similar to the "collateral" filopodia of Purkinje cells, and a sheetlike structure, more similar to a growth cone or a "terminal" filopodium. The authors characterized the first type and describe frequent presence of synapses, up to 20% of the total number of synapses on pyramidal neurons at this developmental stage. These dendritic filopodia sometimes contacted axonal filopodia. The authors interpreted their data as supporting Vaughn's hypothesis that filopodia contribute to synapse generation on the dendritic shaft.

More recently, a two-photon study of filopodia from living developing neocortical pyramidal neurons imaged their motility during early postnatal development in brain slices (P2–P12) (Portera-Cailliau et al., 2003). Based on differences in density, motility, length, and response to neural activity, the authors propose the existence of two populations of filopodia, one in growth cones and the other in shafts. While filopodia in growth cones, analogous to the terminal filopodia of Purkinje cells, could be involved in dendritic growth and branching in an activity-independent manner, shaft ("collateral") filopodia might be responsible for activity-dependent synaptogenesis and, in some cases, becoming spines (Dailey and Smith, 1996; Fiala et al., 1998; Ziv and Smith, 1996).

Indeed, the filopodial model is a third alternative model to spinogenesis, besides the Sotelo and Miller-Peters models (see figures 5.3 and 5.9). The first evidence for this was puslbished in two imaging studies from the Smith group, in which the dynamics of early dendritic protrusions of hippocampal pyramidal neurons were monitored in cultured brain slices (Dailey and Smith, 1996) and dissociated cultures (Ziv and Smith, 1996). Based on the developmental reduction of the motility and disappearance of elongated filopodia, and on the appearance of shorter spine protrusions with increasing developmental age, the authors proposed that dendritic filopodia become stabilized, turning into spines. They postulated the existence of a "protospine," an intermediate morphological structure representing the filopodia that becomes stabilized. The authors also speculated that, because most filopodia were very transient, only those that were successful at capturing an axonal terminal actually became stabilized. This could explain why protospines may be difficult to find. The function of dendritic filopodia, in these authors' view, is therefore to create a "virtual dendrite," that is, a volume around the perimeter of the dendritic shaft that can be explored in the search for axons and where potential axonal contacts can form. Similar ideas have been proposed independently for spines (Chklovskii et al., 2002; Peters and Kaiserman-Abramof, 1970; Swindale, 1981). Grabbing of axons by dendritic filopodia, presumably driven by actin networks or other motors, would

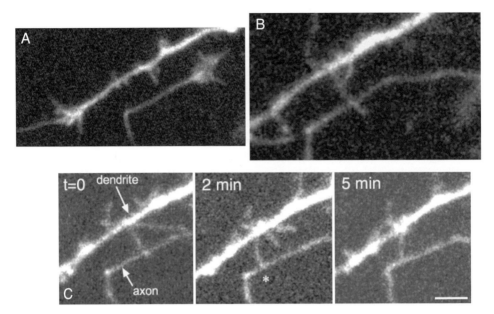

**Figure 5.9**
Potential synaptogenic interaction between a filopodia and an axon. (A) Image from a two-photon time lapse movie from a developing neocortical pyramidal neuron in which a growing dendrite (top) is passing next to a growing axon (bottom). A small dendritic filopodium has emerged from the middle of the dendritic shaft and is growing toward the axon. (B) Same field of view, a few minutes later. Note how the filopodium has reached the axon. (C) Subsequent images from same movie, showing how the filopodium retracts and remains attached to the axon (star). These interactions have been proposed to result in the formation of dendritic spines and excitatory synaptic contacts. Scale bar: 3 μm. Portera-Cailliau and Yuste, unpublished data.

then produce a spine, a structure that reflects the tension of the axonal pull on the dendritic membrane.

An alternative mechanism by which filopodia serve as precursors to spines was suggested by the ultrastructural studies of Fiala et al. (1998). In this model, the initial contact occurs between axonal and dendritic filopodia (figure 5.10). This arm-against-arm contact (Miller and Peters, 1981) could then persist, leading to the maturation of the dendritic spine and the retraction of the axonal filopodia. The Fiala and the Ziv-Smith versions of this model are similar, except for the involvement of axonal filopodia.

But are filopodia spine precursors? There is evidence for and against this hypothesis. In favor of a spine precursor role are imaging data documenting how filopodia become stabilized, at least for the duration of an imaging experiment (figure 5.9; Dailey and Smith, 1996; Maletic-Savatic et al., 1999; Parnass et al., 2000; Portera-Cailliau et al., 2003; Ziv and Smith, 1996), even though no ultrastructural confirma-

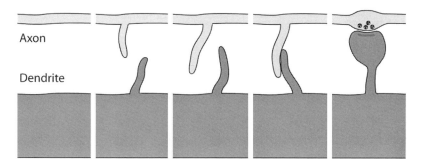

**Figure 5.10**
Filopodial arm-to-arm model. In this model, there are both axonal and dendritic filopodia, which find each other and establish incipient early contacts along their sides. These interactions result in the formation of a dendritic spine.

tion of postsynaptic specializations has been done in any of these cases. Also, a link appears to exist between filopodia and synaptogenesis (Vaughn, 1989), so it makes sense that they serve to create a virtual dendrite considering that one of the problems developing neurons face is the spatial sampling of axons (Chklovskii et al., 2002; Peters and Kaiserman-Abramof, 1970; Swindale, 1981). Furthermore, the very high numbers of filopodia (50,000 new filopodia/day in developing mouse neocortical neurons; see Portera-Cailliau et al., 2003), compared with the smaller number of spines present after spinogenesis (~2,000–10,000 total spines for these same cells, see Konur et al., 2003), could indicate that the sampling of potential axons by the dendrite is very extensive. In fact, it is difficult to believe that such major neuronal energy expenditure as producing and retracting thousands of filopodia per day is not related to synaptogenesis, which is arguably the most significant developmental stage these neurons are undergoing. Finally, an interesting piece of data that fits very well with a potential role of filopodia as axon detectors is the observation that collateral filopodia are attracted to glutamate, displaying fast extensions and movements toward sources of glutamate in the tissue (figures 5.11 and 5.12; Cornell-Bell et al., 1990; Portera-Cailliau et al., 2003; Zheng et al., 1994). This would make sense for a synaptogenic role, given that developing axons secrete neurotransmitter into their surroundings (O'Brien and Fischbach, 1986), providing a potential signal that the filopodia could detect.

At the same time, there are several pieces of evidence against the spine precursor hypothesis. First, the time course of the ontogenetic progression in spinogenesis—of shaft synapses turning into stubby and then mushroom spines (Miller and Peters, 1981)—appears incompatible with filopodia transforming into spines. Also, filopodia can occur in neurons that do not have spines once they mature (Mason, 1983; Wong et al., 1992), and they are even found in nonneural cells (Hall, 1994).

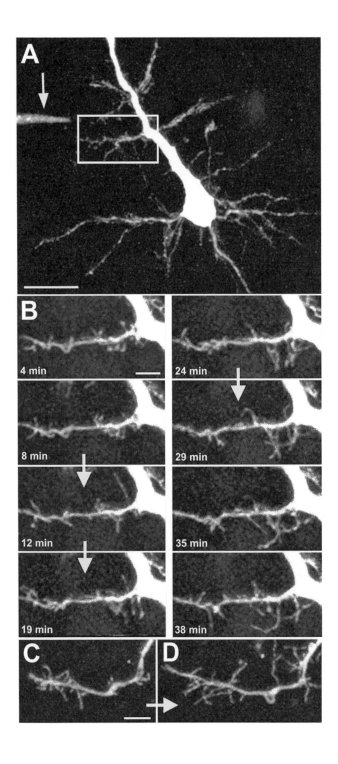

Further experimental work is necessary to clarify the fate of dendritic filopodia and their relation with spines. Ultrastructural studies of synaptogenesis in early filopodia are still scarce. But the simple yet important long-term imaging studies of developing dendrites and axons could solve this issue. In fact, imaging the interactions between filopodia and axonal terminals is becoming possible (Ahmari et al., 2000; Jontes et al., 2000; Vardinon-Friedman et al., 2000) and it should thus be feasible to document the function of dendritic filopodia, and also axonal filopodia, and their respective roles in spinogenesis.

As an alternative to the simultaneous imaging of pre- and postsynaptic partners, it is possible to detect the PSD, by labeling PSD95 with GFP, while simultaneously imaging the structure of the dendrite (Marrs et al., 2001; Okabe et al., 2001a; 2001b). Because a PSD is a hallmark of a mature synapse, imaging of PSDs is somewhat equivalent to imaging synaptic maturation, and one can thus correlate this maturation with the morphology of the dendrite and its processes. Indeed, in hippocampal cultures, Marrs et al. documented how mature spines (defined as morphological features and the presence of a cluster of PSD-95 labeling) can emerge from both the stabilization of dendritic filopodia and also, gradually, from dendritic shafts. Approximately half of the spines originated from filopodia, whereas the other half emerged from dendritic shafts (Marrs et al., 2001). Besides having different origins, these two populations of spines appeared otherwise similar. A similar mixture of filopodial and non-filopodial spinogenesis has been described in brain slices when spinogenesis is stimulated by rewarming after a prolonged cooling period (Kirov et al., 2004; Petrak et al., 2005).

Thus, these imaging data indicate that, in pyramidal neurons in vitro, both the Miller-Peters and the filopodial models of synaptogenesis might operate. But it is unclear which of these alternative mechanisms to generate spines is dominant in intact pyramidal neurons during development in vivo, since similar experiments to those of Marrs et al. have not been carried out. Favoring the Miller-Peters model, spines can reemerge after hibernation, apparently without a filopodial stage (Popov and Bocharova, 1992; Popov et al., 1992). On the other hand, when newborn hippocampal granule cells become incorporated into mature circuits, they generate filopodia whose tips are essentially always found in the vicinity of existing synaptic terminals (Toni et al., 2007), as if they were involved in generating new synaptic contacts. Also, in mature neocortex in vivo, newly emerging dendritic protrusions

Figure 5.11

Elongation of dendritic filopodia in response to glutamate application. (A) Low-magnification view of a layer pyramidal neuron. Arrow marks location of a pipette tip delivering glutamate. Scale bar: 20 μm. (B) Frames from the white box in (A). Images were acquired every 60 sec, and representative time points are shown. The white arrows separating certain frames represent the times when three puffs of glutamate were delivered. (C and D) Images before and after the application of the glutamate in a different dendrite. Note the appearance of longer filopodia. Scale bar: 5 μm. Reprinted from Portera-Calliau et al., 2003.

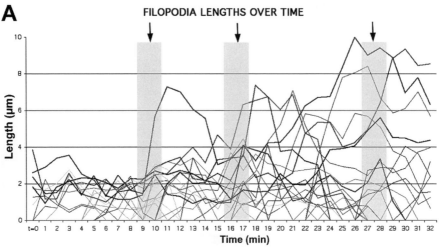

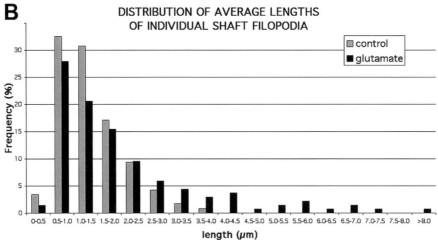

**Figure 5.12**
Emergence of filopodia after glutamate application. (A) Lengths of filopodia from the 40-min movie shown in figure 5.11. Black arrows and gray columns designate times when glutamate was delivered. Note that during the first 10 frames of the movie, filopodia lengths never surpass 4 μm, whereas after just two puffs of glutamate, a subset of filopodia have reached lengths well above 4 μm. The effect of glutamate is quite rapid as shown by the sudden increases (within 1 min) of some filopodia after individual puffs. (B) Distribution of filopodia lengths before and after glutamate application from five separate experiments. Gray histograms represent pooled data from filopodia analyzed before glutamate application, whereas black histograms represent data from filopodia analyzed after at least two puffs of glutamate. Note that glutamate generates a longer distribution of lengths. Reprinted from Portera-Calliau et al., 2003.

resemble filopodia and lack synapses (Knott et al., 2006), a result that would appear to be inconsistent with the Miller-Peters model. To definitely discern between these models in vivo, however, simultaneous imaging of pre- and postsynaptic structures during normal development, or at least of the spines and PSDs, seems to be necessary. Also, it could be useful to specifically block the motility or emergence of dendritic filopodia, perhaps by interfering with a selective Rho GTPase (Tashiro and Yuste, 2004), and document the consequences of this manipulation on the development of spines and synapses. These topics will be discussed in more detail in the next chapter, focusing on spine and filopodial motility.

## A Heterogeneity of Spines

As an aside from the thread of our discussion, it seems important to comment on the large diversity of spines and presumably also of synapses. In every one of the topics discussed, from developmental spinogenesis, spine maintenance in the adult, the role of presynaptic terminals and activity, the function of filopodia and the developmental origin of spines on pyramidal neurons, conflicting data emerge from the study of different cell types, or sometimes even the same class of neuron. As we have discussed, three models of spinogenesis have been proposed as a result of these data. One solution to this is to postulate that different populations of spines behave differently. Indeed, even in a single Purkinje cell there are two populations of spines with completely different dependencies on presynaptic innervation, and in pyramidal neurons spines may arise from either filopodia or shaft synapses. There are likely many classes of spines, and the "canonical" spine may not exist. This argument resonates well with the large heterogeneity of calcium compartmentalization (chapter 7; Yuste et al., 1999; 2000), receptor localization (chapter 3; Nusser et al., 1997; 1998) and morphological differences (chapter 3; Peters and Kaiserman-Abramof, 1970), found even among spines from of the same neuron. Understanding the heterogeneity of spines, with regard to not only their morphology, but also their functional roles in the circuits where they operate, is likely of great significance.

## Functional Interpretation of Spinogenesis

Taking this heterogeneity into account, can one summarize all the data on spinogenesis into a coherent picture, one that explains the life history of spines, from their first emergence to their permanence throughout the life of the animal? (figure 5.13). In the following section, I will attempt to reconcile most of the data in a single model, one that has intriguing implications for understanding the function of spines in mature

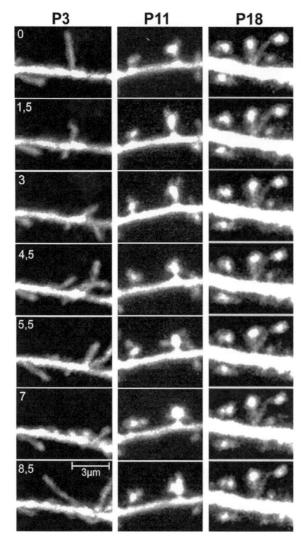

**Figure 5.13**
Development of spines: three stages. Representative time-lapse sequences from dendrites of mouse layer 5 pyramidal neurons at three postnatal ages. Note how at postnatal day 3 there are no spines yet dendritic filopodia emerge, are motile and dissapear. At P11 spines are present and have small fingerlike protusions that emerge from their heads and are motile. At P18, spine density is higher and spine motility is reduced. Numbers indicate time in minutes. Reprinted from Portera-Calliau et al., 2001.

circuits and the role of synaptic plasticity in the developing and mature CNS. This is a speculative model, since the examination of many of these topics is still incomplete.

The central idea, introduced in chapter 3, is that spines serve to enhance connectivity, and one could argue that Purkinje cells and pyramidal neurons cxcmplify two strategies to achieve the same exact final goal: to connect with as many axons as possible. For Purkinje neurons, the strategy seems clear: Since parallel fibers come in great packing densities at orthogonal trajectories, Purkinje cells would sprout spines intrinsically in three-dimensional helixes, to maximize the cross-section of their dendrites and generate a veritable "sieve." Then, with relatively minimal displacements (see chapter 6), Purkinje cells would rely on chance contact between parallel fibers and spines to establish synaptic contacts. This strategy would maximize the number of different inputs that a given Purkinje cell receives.

Pyramidal neurons, on the other hand, do not possess this two-dimensional fine sieve of dendrites, although they may have an intrinsic mechanism that builds a basic complement of spines, perhaps in helixes too. Moreover, input axons connecting to pyramidal neurons are not organized at perpendicular angles as are parallel fibers. Instead, pyramidal neurons have dendrites that cover roughly cylindrical volumes so they need to catch axons that course through that space. To maximize the opportunity of contacting an axon, it makes sense to use dendritic filopodia to enhance these encounters, a mechanism that Purkinje cells may not need. Filopodia that are successful in contacting axons would eventually give rise to spines. At the same time, some axons may find the dendritic shafts without need of filopodia, and those could represent a population of spines that emerge directly from shafts. Although the emergence of spines from dendritic shafts has been documented in vitro, where it appears quite significant, it is possible than in vivo they represent a small proportion of all spines, given that the shaft synapses in developing neurons are a very small proportion, compared to the final number of synapses.

As a consenquence of this model, regardless of whether pyramidal neurons develop from filopodia or from the existing synapses at the shafts, one would predict that the location of the synapse within the mature spine would be near its tip, as far away from the dendrite as possible. Although systematic analysis of the PSD position has not been done, it is interesting to note that, in most examples, the PSD is indeed located at the tip of the spine (see figures 3.5, 3.6, or 3.8, for example). For Purkinje cells, on the other hand, the synapse within spines may not necessarily be located at their tips, since the location would be determined by where parallel fibers happen to encounter the sieve of spines. Interestingly, at least from cursory observation of Purkinje cell spine reconstructions, PSD tip positioning does not seem to be as prominent as in pyramidal neurons (see chapter 6).

Without filopodia, pyramidal neurons may not achieve a rich connectivity, although they could still connect. And because these neurons spend large amounts of energy and time to sustain enormous numbers of filopodia and their motility during synaptogenesis, this implies that a rich synaptic matrix must be important for the ultimate function of the circuit. This may also explain why filopodia, once their job is done, essentially disappear after synaptogenesis; it also agrees with the fact that filopodia are thin and lack clear heads, since they have no synapses until they establish a synaptic contact and turn into spines with heads.

So in summary, both Purkinje cells and pyramidal neurons would then use spines to increase their synaptic input matrices and create a veritable *tabula rasa*, a network in which, ideally, all neurons could be interconnected (Kalisman et al., 2005). With Purkinje cells, this network would be essentially physically unaltered during the life of the animal, and synaptic plasticity would be responsible for fine-tuning this "network" (see chapter 10). Pyramidal neurons, on the other hand, might significantly modify this circuit, since activity-dependent learning rules appear responsible for a massive pruning during postnatal development. This pruning could then sculpt circuits that are efficiently matched to the computational tasks the particular cortical area needs to solve, and this would be reflected morphologically in the pruning of spines (Zuo et al., 2005). The spines that remain after this pruning phase would then be permanent for the rest of the animal's life, and carry out the skeleton of the essential computational algorithms of the circuit, perhaps being repositories of lifetime memories. In this view, the cortex would be a special type of *tabula rasa*, not a blank slate or an "empty cabinet where percepts accumulate" as Locke put it (Locke, 1669), but more like a "full slate" that is then pruned or sculpted into an essential circuit. Perhaps because of the multifaceted capabilities the cortex carries out, as a general type of circuit that must be specialized to be effective, this activity-dependent pruning could be essential for cortical circuits.

Therefore, the different types of spinogenesis in cerebellar and cortical circuits might be designed to optimally generate mature circuits with a particular wiring structure and a particular computational strategy. This model would predict that, if the basic developmental role of spines is to maximize connectivity, spines should be significantly plastic during this period of synaptogenesis, in order to interact more effectively with afferent axons. Indeed, spines and filopodia do move during development. Their motility is the subject of the next chapter.

# 6 Motility

*Spines have traditionally been considered stable structures, but live imaging techniques have demonstrated that they constantly change shape. Spine motility is intrinsic to the neuron, developmentally regulated and mediated by an actin-based cascade involving the Rho family of small GTPases. Synaptic transmission, intracellular calcium as well as dozens of other molecules can alter spine motility, although these effects are inconsistent across experiments, perhaps reflecting different responses according to the developmental stage of the synapse.*

*There appear to be two types of motility—neck elongation and head morphing— with different phenomenology and molecular mechanisms. Based on this, a two-step model of synaptogenesis is proposed: In a first stage, elongation of early protrusions could serve to transiently sample the surrounding neuropil, searching for axons. In a second stage, the wiggling movement of the spine head could reflect interactions with competing axonal terminals. Although the overall function of spine motility is still unclear, it could serve to facilitate synaptogenesis, allowing for more efficient circuit connectivity.*

In the discussion of spinogenesis, I suggested that the emergence of spines and filopodia could serve to effectively solve what could arguably be the major problem that the developing nervous system needs to tackle, which is how to connect axons and dendrites to form synapses. I raised the possibility that synaptogenesis would be most effective if spines and filopodia could move. In this chapter, I review studies that have demonstrated spine motility and address what its function could be. Discussing both spine and filopodial motility, their phenomenology and regulation, I arrive at the same conclusion as in the previous chapter: that motility serves to enhance synaptogenesis by enabling spines and filopodia to contact more axons. In this discussion, I continue to rely on data from cortical pyramidal neurons and cerebellar Purkinje cells, although the reader should be aware that similar phenomena have been documented in other preparations.

**Imaging Spine Motility: Phenomenology**

While looking at fixed speciments, Cajal imagined spines as being capable of movement, and suggested that this movement was controlled by neuronal activity. In fact, he wrote:

[S]ince it's very likely that such spines could be points where electrical charge or current is received, their retraction (which would then separate them from axons, with which they would be in contact) would give rise to the individualization or disconnection of the neurons. The state of activity would correspond, then, to the swelling and elongation of the spines, and the resting state (sleep or inactivity) to their retraction. (S. Ramón y Cajal, *Textura del Sistema Nervioso del Hombre y de los Vertebrados*, 1899, translated by the author)

Nevertheless, for many decades after Cajal, spines were assumed to be stable structures. This idea was challenged in 1982, when Crick proposed that spines move ("twitch") in response to synaptic stimulation (Crick, 1982). Based on the description of filamentous material in the spine head (Jones and Powell, 1969; Peters et al., 1976), Crick hypothesized that actin would be present in spines and endow them with motility. In fact, in an earlier study, Siekevitz and his colleagues had already biochemically identified actin at the PSD and proposed that spines move (Blomberg et al., 1977). The presence of actin in spines was confirmed by ultrastructural studies (Fifkova and Delay, 1982; Matus et al., 1982). Because of the universal correlation between morphological changes in cells and the actin cytoskeleton (Hall, 1994), spine motility because a real possibility.

Over the last 20 years the dynamics of the growth cone have been studied in great detail (Tessier-Lavigne and Goodman, 1996). However, it is only recently that similar experiments have been carried out on dendrites and their protrusions. The introduction of novel high-resolution imaging methods has enabled investigators to image spine morphologies and some aspects of their function in living neurons with unprecedented detail (figure 6.1). This was crucial since the proof that spines can move requires methods to follow the morphology of individual neurons over time. Such studies have confirmed that spine motility occurs in a wide variety of cell types, in vitro and in vivo. For the purpose of this discussion, under the term *motility* I group together many types of morphological changes, possibly combining phenomena with different mechanisms and function. In fact, to appreciate the richness of the phenomenon of spine motility I encourage the reader to view some of the movies that document spine motility (URLs are provided in following sections).

**Motility of Dendritic Filopodia**

As discussed in the previous chapter, in 1996, Dailey and Smith carried out a study demonstrating the dynamics of living dendritic protrusions with confocal time-lapse

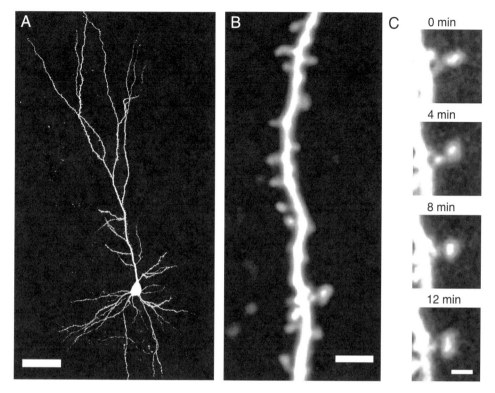

**Figure 6.1**
Imaging spine motility. (A) Two-photon image of a neocortical pyramidal cell transfected with EGFP. (B) High-magnification view of a segment of its dendritic tree. (C) Time-lapse images from the spine in the lower right of (B). Note how the spine is changing shape during the movie. Scale bars: (A) 50 μm; (B) 5 μm; (C) 2 μm. Tashiro and Yuste, unpublished data.

imaging. In hippocampal pyramidal cells in slice cultures, they observed widespread dendritic growth, retraction, and branching. Numerous filopodia appeared, disappeared and sometimes also gave rise to dendritic growth cones and new dendritic branches (figures 6.2 and 6.3).

The authors proposed a model of selective stabilization of synaptic contacts by which dendritic filopodia, after a period of active search for their presynaptic partners (Morest, 1969b), become *protospines*, that is, immature spines, and then finally spines (see figure 5.9). Ziv and Smith further pursued the idea that dendritic filopodia are direct precursors to spines, by imaging the interaction between filopodia and axons in dissociated cultures of hippocampal neurons (Ziv and Smith, 1996; http://www.neuron.org/cgi/content/full/17/1/91/DC1). Initially, cells had transient and dynamic filopodia, while later dendritic protrusions were long-lived and stable. These

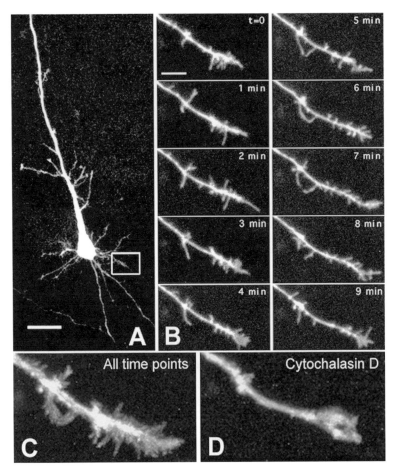

**Figure 6.2**
Motility of dendritic filopodia. (A), layer 5 pyramidal neuron from visual cortex of a P2 mouse imaged by
two-photon microscopy. Scale bar: 25 μm. (B) Time-lapse movie of box in (A). Numerous filopodia protrude in and out of the dendrite. Note that filopodia seem to be clustered at the dendrite tip (growth cone),
compared with those in the proximal shaft. Scale bar: 5 μm. (C) Collapsed view of all frames of the movies
shown above, displaying all existing filopodia throughout the 10-min imaging period. (D), Collapsed view
of all 20 frames from a 10-min movie of the same dendrite, 5 min after applying cytochalasin D, an actin
blocker that eliminates filopodia. Reprinted from Portera-Cailliau et al., 2003.

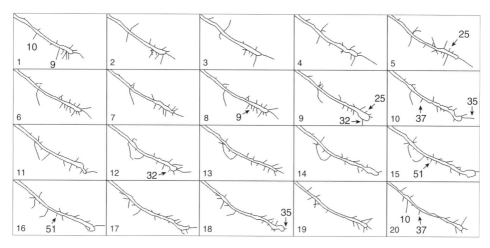

**Figure 6.3**
Analysis of filopodia motility. Skeleton representation of the movie shown in figure 6.3, tracing individual protrusions. A few representative filopodia are labeled; arrows point to the first and last frame in which those filopodia can be distinguished. Note the great dynamism of the filopodia. Reprinted from Portera-Cailliau et al., 2003.

studies, and many others since then, have proved that dendritic filopodia are highly motile, potentially serving an important role in the development of neuronal circuitry. This work raised the issue of whether similar motility would also occur in spines from more mature tissue.

## Spine Motility in Cultures and Slices

The picture of spines as largely stable changed forever in 1998, when Fischer et al. showed that spines from cultured neurons were continuously changing shape (Fischer et al., 1998). The authors investigated actin dynamics in dissociated hippocampal cultured neurons labeled by transfection of a GFP-actin fusion protein. GFP fluorescence was associated with protrusions that had spine shape and dimensions and displayed astonishing motility (http://www.neuron.org/cgi/content/full/20/5/847/DC1). These changes in shape in spines, on the order of a micrometer every few seconds, were smaller than those reported by the Smith group in filopodia, yet they were still large compared to the size of a synapse.

This report was met with skepticism, because the authors inferred morphological changes in spines from the rearrangements of the actin cytoskeleton. Because of this, it was theoretically possible that the "container" (the spine itself) might not change in morphology, whereas the "content" (the actin cytoskeleton) did. Also, spines in dissociated cultures, with less structural constraints, might move, whereas spines surrounded by neuropil might not (Edwards, 1998).

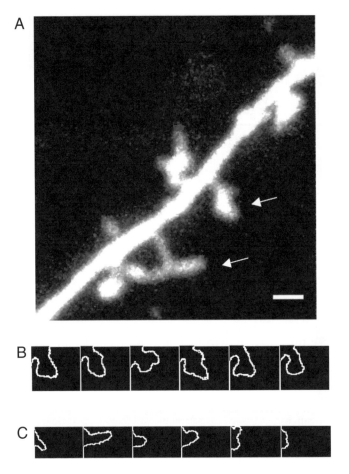

**Figure 6.4**
Analysis of spine motility. (A) Two-photon image of a P12 pyramidal neuron from mouse visual cortex, labeled with EGFP transfection. Diverse morphologies of dendritic protrusions can be observed. Scale bar: 1 µm. (B, C) Outlines of a spine (B) (upper arrow in A), and a filopodium (C) (lower arrow in A), shown at 2.5-min intervals. Reprinted from Konur and Yuste, 2004a.

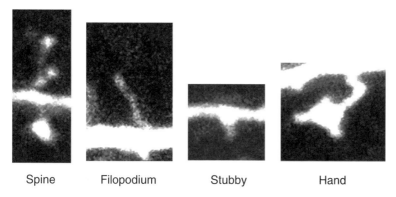

Spine    Filopodium    Stubby    Hand

**Figure 6.5**
Diverse morphologies of living spines. Reprinted from Konur and Yuste, 2004a.

These objections were dispelled by a study that reported rapid spine motility in acute and cultured brain slices from both cerebellum and cortex (figure 6.4; Dunaevsky et al., 1999). Using two-photon imaging of neurons biolistically transfected with soluble GFP, Dunaevsky et al. reported that spines also exhibited substantial morphological plasticity in brain slices (see http://www.pnas.org/cgi/content/full/96/23/13438/DC1). In fact, in living slices, spines displayed a large variety of morphologies that are constantly changing (figure 6.5).

For example, observed morphological changes of spines included their appearance and disappearance, elongation and retraction, growth of filopodial extensions from spine heads, "kissing" of neighboring spines, and "wiggling" or "morphing," that is, amorphous shape changes that more closely resemble the motility observed in dissociated cultures (Fischer et al., 1998). The observed movements were large in relation to the size of a synapse and were reduced in amplitude in more mature preparations. The demonstration that spine motility also occurred in brain slices was a step forward, but it was still possible that the slicing procedure or the concomitant deafferentation present in slices could have caused artifactual spine motility (Kirov et al., 1999). Moreover, analysis of these data revealed that, at least in developing preparations, the traditional classification of spines could represent snapshots from a constant state of morphological flux (figure 6.6; Parnass et al. 2000).

**Spine Motility in Vivo**

Does spine motility also occur in the intact nervous system? Evidence for this came from Lendvai et al., who observed the motility of spines of neurons in vivo. This study dispelled the criticism that spine motility in earlier studies was due to slicing or culturing conditions (Lendvai et al., 2000). From here, research has turned to the questions of what are the mechanisms and function of spine motility.

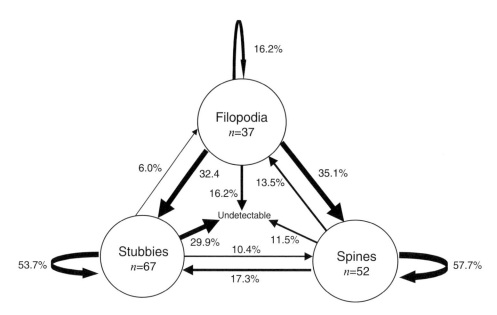

**Figure 6.6**
Morphological plasticity of spines and filopodia in developing pyramidal neurons. Each circle represents the population of protrusions categorized as filopodia, stubby, or thin spines at the beginning of the time-lapse sequences. Arrows point to the class in which those protrusions were categorized at the end of the 2-to 4-hour period. Thickness of line is proportional to the percentage of the initial protrusions that followed that fate. Reprinted from Parnass et al., 2000.

## Mechanisms and Regulation of Spine Motility

Understanding the molecular or physical mechanism that generates spine and filopodial motility could provide clues about their function. A first-order question is whether spines move by themselves or are pushed around by their extracellular environment. This question had a direct answer: Spine motility is intrinsic to the neuron. When one establishes whole-cell recording with a neuron, spine motility ceases (Majewska et al., 2000b). Whole-cell recording dializes the intracellular media and thus must interfere with the mechanisms responsible for spine motility. Something inside the neuron must make spines move.

### Actin Mediates Spine Motility

The original description of rapid movement of spines in acutely dissociated neuronal cultures was carried out using hippocampal neurons that expressed actin tagged with GFP (Fischer et al., 1998), and thus reflected rapid motility of the actin cytoskeleton inside spines (Blomberg et al., 1977; Fifkova and Delay, 1982; Matus et al., 1982). Indeed, bath application of cytochalasin D, a drug that interferes with actin polymer-

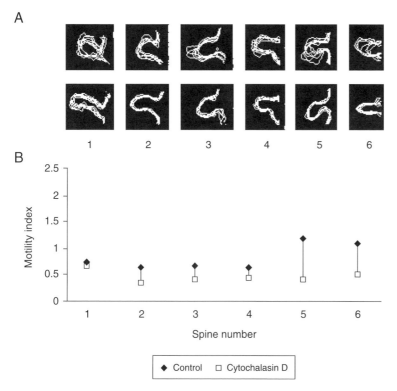

**Figure 6.7**
Spine morphology is actin-based. (A) Superimposed outlines of spines from a Purkinje cell, from time-lapse sequences before (top) and after (bottom) application of the actin polymerization blocker cytochalasin B. (B) The motility indexes of these spines (proportional to the changes in their projected area) are reduced by cytochalasin. Reprinted from Dunaevsky et al., 1999.

ization, blocked motility of spines (figure 6.7, Dunaevsky et al., 1999; Fischer et al., 1998) and of dendritic filopodia (figure 6.2; Portera-Cailliau and Yuste, 2001). This result demonstrates that actin polymerization is necessary; it also confirms that spine motility is not due to a random Brownian motion of intracellular particles, but to a specific biochemistry. Myosin motors could be involved in this phenomenon, given the presence of different isoforms of myosin in spines (see chapter 4), although results with myosin blockers have been inconclusive (Fischer et al., 1998; Tashiro and Yuste, unpublished observations).

**The Rho Signaling Network and Spines**

What are the biochemical cascades controlling actin polymerization? As discussed in chapter 4, the Rho family of small GTPases, a subgroup of the Ras superfamily of GTPases (Hall, 1998), are abundantly represented in spines. These proteins function as molecular switches that cycle between an inactive GDP-bound form and an active GTP-bound form. They were originally identified as regulators of the actin cytoskeleton in nonneuronal cells such as fibroblasts, in which they cause morphological changes such as growing (or retracting) filopodia and lamellipodia (Hall, 1998), so it is quite natural to think they could be involved in dendritic spine and filopodail motility. In fact, in mammalian neurons, some GTPases such as RhoA, Rac1, and Cdc42 play an important role in dendritic remodeling of *Xenopus* retinal ganglion cells (Ruchhoeft et al., 1999), tectal neurons (Li et al., 2000), and cultured neocortical neurons (Threadgill et al., 1997).

In the first study of the role of the Rho family on spines, Luo and coworkers engineered transgenic mice that expressed a constitutively active (CA) form of Rac1 (Rac1-CA) in cerebellar Purkinje cells and found that these cells had a large number of small, supranumerary spines (Luo et al., 1996). Thus, Rho GTPases must be involved in spinogenesis. The question of whether the Rho family is also involved in maintaining extant spines was addressed using biolistic transfection of rat hippocampal slice cultures at ages at which they had already developed spines (Nakayama et al., 2000). Rac1-CA again resulted in the overproduction of abnormal spines and membrane ruffles, whereas Rac1-DN (dominant negative) reduced spine density. These results therefore point at a key role of Rac1 in both the formation and maintenance of spines.

In further experiments, Tashiro et al. confirmed these results and in addition showed that RhoA-CA produced the opposite effect of Rac1, a reduced number of spines, even their complete elimination in some cells (figures 6.8 and 6.9; Tashiro et al., 2000). Rac and Rho also had differential effects on spine density and spine neck length: Whereas Rac promoted the development of new spines, Rho blocked their formation and maintenance as well as their elongation. A follow-up study demonstrated the role of the Rho family not only on spine morphogenesis but also on spine motility and stability (figure 6.10; Tashiro and Yuste, 2004). These data demonstrate that Rac1 and RhoA/Rho kinase pathways regulate different aspects of spine morphology, motility, and stability and presumably also different aspects of synaptic functions (figure 6.11). Moreover, two different types of spine motility—protrusive motility and wiggling/morphing—are differentially regulated by Rac1 and Rho kinase. These two types of spine motility may serve different functions in synaptogenesis and synapse maturation (see next section).

**Spine Motility with Synaptic Contact**
But, as we said in chapter 3, if all spines have a synapse, and spines now are constantly moving, do synapses become disconnected during spine motility? As mentioned, Cajal indeed imagined that neuronal activity would induce spine swelling, whereas inactivity their retraction (see above). What happens to the presynaptic terminal when the spine moves? Do presynaptic terminals also move?

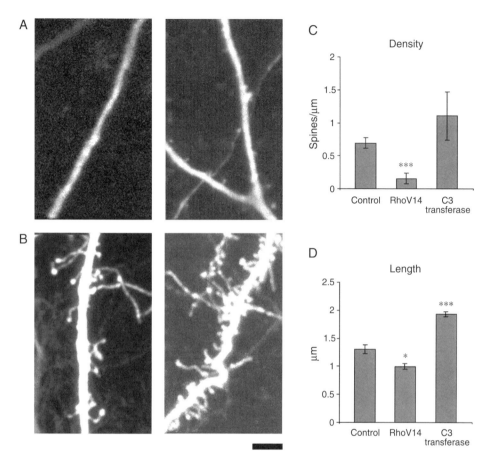

**Figure 6.8**
Effect of Rho on spine morphology. Effects of RhoA manipulations on spine density and length. (A) Dendritic segments from RhoAV14 (a constitutively active mutant)-transfected neurons. In many neurons, spines were undetectable (left) or existed at very low density (right). Most spines had short necks. (B) Dendritic segments from C3 transferase (Rho blocker)-transfected neurons. Spines are abundant and have longer necks. Some neurons have abnormally high spine density (right). Scale bars: 5 μm. Spine density (C) and length (D) in control, RhoV14-transfected, and C3 transferase-transfected neurons. Error bars are SEM. ***P < 0.001,*P < 0.05, t test. Modified from Tashiro et al. (2000).

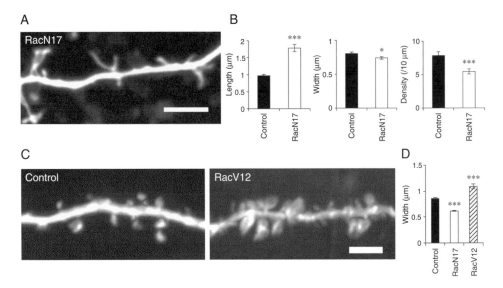

**Figure 6.9**
Effect of Rac on spine morphology. (A) Dendritic segment from neurons transfected with RacN17, a dominant negative form of Rac1. Scale bar: 5 μm. (B) Quantification of effect on spine length, width and density. (C) Dendritic segments from control and RacV12 (constitutive active)-transfected neurons. Scale bar: 3 μm. (D) Effect on spine head width. Error bars are SEM. ***P < 0.005, *P < 0.05, t test. Modified from Tashiro et al. (2000).

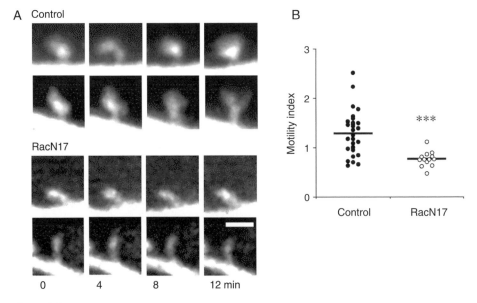

**Figure 6.10**
Effect of Rac on spine motility: blockade of Rac1 inhibits spine head motility. (A) Time-lapse images of spines in control and RacN17-transfected neurons. Scale bar: 1 μm. (B) Motility index of spines in control and RacN17-transfected neurons. Each circle represents single spines. Black bar represents mean values. ***P < 0.005, t test. From Tashiro et al., 2008.

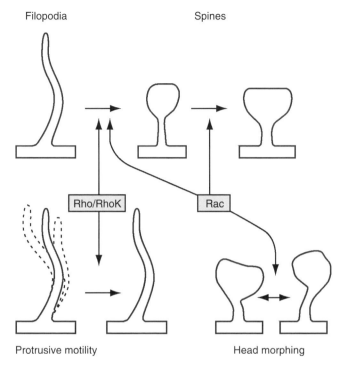

**Figure 6.11**
Regulation of spine morphology and motility by RhoA/Rho kinase and Rac1. Rac1 and RhoA/Rho kinase are involved in two different stages of spine morphogenesis: motility and stability. Both of them are required to transform long, filopodia-like protrusions into relatively stable, short spines and to maintain morphology of these short spines. Further, Rac1 promotes spine head growth and stabilization. RhoA/Rho kinase inhibits protrusive motility to convert dynamic filopodia into stable spines whereas Rac1 is essential in head morphing, which may be important in spine head growth and stabilization. Reprinted from Tashiro and Yuste, 2008.

Presynaptic terminals do not move significantly, or have very small displacements, on the order of the focus drift of the microscope (Deng and Dunaevsky, 2005; Tashiro and Yuste, unpublished observations). Moreover, simultaneous imaging of spines and presynaptic terminals reveals that, when spines appear clearly associated with a presynaptic terminal, they generally move around the space where the terminal is, but without significantly detaching itself from it (figure 6.12, plate 5; Konur and Yuste, 2004b). These light microscopy studies, however, have a spatial resolution limit, so it is difficult to ascertain if a synaptic contact between an opposing spine and terminal actually exists.

To tackle this issue, ultrastructural reconstructions can be made from spines that have been previously imaged, a difficult but necessary procedure (Dunaevsky et al., 2001). These reconstructions demonstrated that motile spines can have

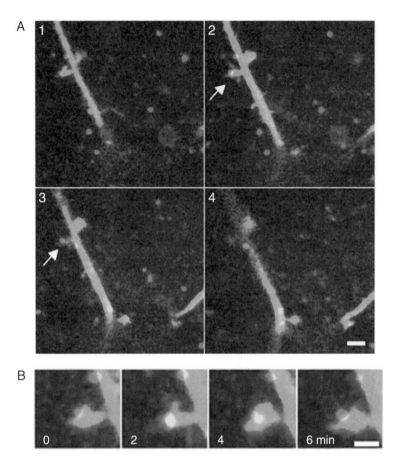

**Figure 6.12 (plate 5)**
Spine motility with synaptic contact. Acute hippocampal slices obtained from P7–P10 mice expressing GFP in a subset of CA1 pyramidal neurons. After selecting the dendrite of interest, a recording electrode is placed near the dendrite and stimulation electrode on its surface to stimulate Schaffer collaterals. FM 1–43 staining is used to image active presynaptic terminals. (A) Dual GFP (green = postsynaptic) and FM 1–43 (red = presynaptic) images of single z sections 0.7 μm apart. In the 2nd and 3rd frames, a potential contact can be identified between a hand-like spine and a FM 1–43-stained bouton (arrow). Scale bar: 2 μm. (B) Time sequence of projected dual images of this potential contact. Scale bar: 1 μm. Reprinted from Konur and Yuste, 2004b.

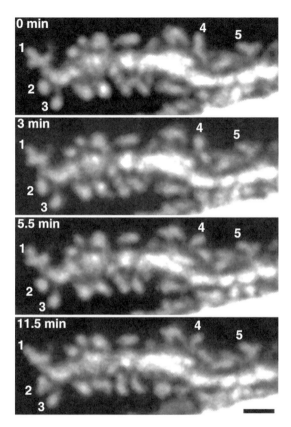

**Figure 6.13**
Spine motility with synaptic contact. Time-lapse two-photon images of a dendritic segment from an EGFP-transfected Purkinje cell. Notice the spontaneous motility of some of its spines. Time is indicated in minutes. Numbers indicate spines that were identified by electron microscopy in figure 6.14. Scale bar: 2 μm.

ultrastructurally confirmed presynaptic terminals (figures 6.13 and 6.14). Moreover, no significant difference in motility was found between spines that had or lacked a synapse. Thus, spines must move without losing their synaptic contact, if they have one already. Like a boat moored at a dock in wavy waters, spines might be attached flexibly at a terminal, and small displacements may not be strong enough to cause a detachment. This implies that within this partnership, if the presynaptic structure is stable, it is the postsynaptic one that must be the active agent, particularly when choosing among potential partners (see below).

### Role of Neurotransmitters in Spine Motility
The cytochalasin data mentioned proves that the actin-cytoskeleton plays a pivotal role in spine motility. But for actin-based spine motility to fulfill a functional purpose

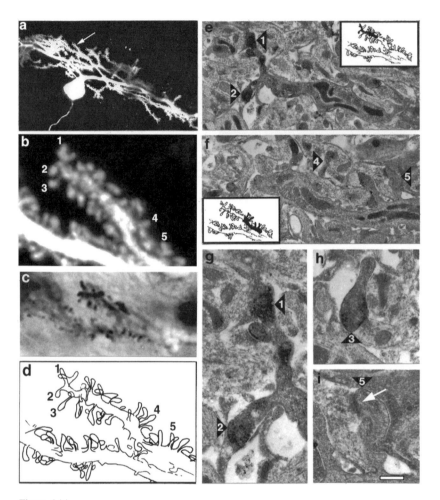

**Figure 6.14**
Spine motility with synaptic contact. Reconstruction of the dendrite imaged in figure 6.13 by electron microscopy. (a) Following live imaging, (b) slices were fixed and immunostained. After locating the imaged dendrite (c), serial thin sections (75 nm) were cut and processed for EM analysis. Imaged dendrites were reconstructed by tracing identified dendrites from electron micrographs of 20–40 serial thin sections. (d) Synaptic contacts were identified. In (b), numbers indicate some of the spines identified in EM (e–i) 1, not motile, no synapse; 2, motile, no synapse; 3, motile, with a synapse; 4, motile, with a synapse; 5, not motile, with a synapse. (e, f) Serial thin sections (shaded areas in insets are portion of dendrite in each panel). (g–i) High-power images of identified spines. 1, not motile, free; 2, motile, free; 3, motile, free; and 5, not motile, not free. Scale bar: 32 µm (a), 2.2 µm (b), 1 µm (e, f) and 450 nm (g–i). Reprinted from Dunaevsky et al., 2001.

in setting up and maintaining synaptic connections, it would need to be controlled by extracellular signals. Obvious candidates are neurotransmitters released by the presynaptic terminal.

Indeed, as discussed (figures 5.11 and 5.12), application of glutamate onto cultured neurons can result in rapid outgrowth of dendritic filopodia (Cornell-Bell et al., 1990; Portera-Cailliau et al., 2003; Zheng et al., 1994). In agreement with this, synaptically released glutamate can result in the growth of new filopodia-like structures (Maletic-Savatic et al., 1999) or spines (Engert and Bonhoeffer, 1999). This effect is apparently mediated by NMDA receptors, so one could argue that NMDAR stimulation can lead to filopodial extension. But, at the same time, bath application of NMDA or of "potentiation media," a combination of NMDA and potassium channel blockers, has no effect on spine motility in slices (Dunaevsky et al., 1999). Similarly, blockade of AMPARs, or even substituting sodium for choline to block action potential activity, had no detectable effect on spine motility. These results indicate that spine motility represents a very basic "housekeeping" cellular phenomenon, one that is relatively insensitive to external perturbations. By contrast, in neuronal cultures, bath application of AMPA can reduce spine motility (Fischer et al., 2000). Also, in cultures grown under conditions of reduced activity, glutamate stimulates the production of spines through an AMPAR-mediated pathway (McKinney et al., 1999). Therefore, the effect of glutamate on spine motility appears controversial, perhaps depending on the exact preparation and experimental conditions.

A potential solution to this controversy is suggested by data from the development of *axonal* mossy fiber filopodia (Tashiro et al., 2003), where glutamate appears to have different effects, depending on the exact developmental stage and the concentration tested. In a combined imaging and ultrastructural study, the authors found a correlation between the amount of motiliy and the proportion of free space around the filopodia (figure 6.15). This suggested the following hypothesis: In an early developmental step, immature filopodia could release glutamate, but, given that these filopodia would be essentially surrounded by empty neuropil, glutamate would then be quickly diluted to a low concentration (figure 6.16). In fact, low concentrations of glutamate, which activates high-affinity receptors, induces filopodial motility (Tashiro et al., 2003). This effect would therefore help axonal filopodia to move more and thus explore their environment and contact potential synaptic targets more effectively. In a second step, later in development, more mature filopodia would find a potential dendritic target. Since these filopodia would be now surrounded by dendritic structures, the glutamate they release would become more concentrated in the vicinity of the dendrite and would be able to activate low-affinity receptors, which would stop filopodial motility (Tashiro et al., 2003). The stabilized filopodia would then be prevented from growing further away and would become stable enough to form a synapse.

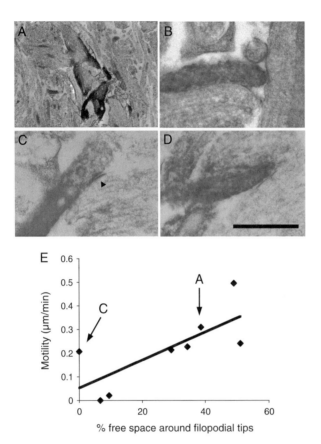

**Figure 6.15**
Motility of *axonal* filopodia is correlated with free extracellular space. (A) Mossy fiber axons of GFP-transfected hippocampal granule cells were immunostained by anti-GFP antibody and processed ultrastructurally. Dark staining represents an immunostained mossy fiber terminal. (B and C) Axonal filopodia with putative immature synapses (arrowhead) and contain synaptic vesicles. (D) A filopodium completely surrounded by neuropil. (E) Relation between filopodial motility and free extracellular space. Motility is plotted against the percent free space around filopodial tips. The points corresponding to filopodia shown in (A) and (C) are marked. Scale bars: 3 μm in (A) and 500 nm in (B)–(D). Modified from Tashiro and Yuste, 2004.

Motility induction

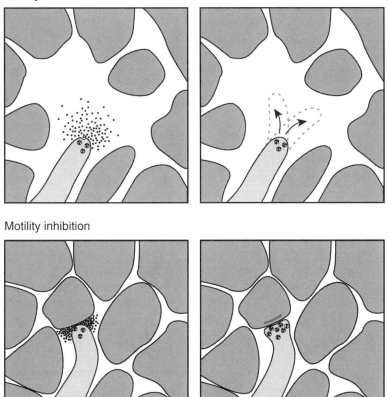

Motility inhibition

**Figure 6.16**
A two-step model of synaptogenesis of axonal filopodia. (Top) In the first step, immature filopodia release glutamate, which could stimulate high-affinity presynaptic glutamate receptors and, in turn, induces filopodial motility. In these immature filopodia without contacts, the induction of motility facilitates filopodia to explore their environment and contact potential synaptic targets. (Bottom) In a second step, more mature filopodia, which have a synaptic contact, release glutamate and activate low-affinity glutamate receptors such that filopodia are stabilized. The stabilized filopodia eventually form mature synapses. Modified from Tashiro et al., 2004.

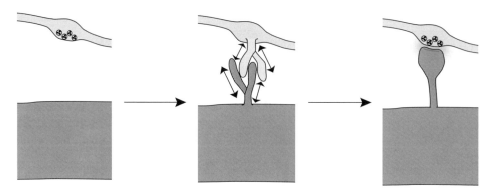

**Figure 6.17**
A two-step model of synaptogenesis of spines. In this model, the presynaptic release of glutamate induces an initial exploratory motility between dendritic and axonal filopodia (or dendritic filopodia and axonal terminals). In a second stage, further glutamate release actually prevents further motility and the dendritic filopodia is stabilized. These two stages could correspond to two different types of spine motility.

A similar model could be proposed for the regulation the motility of *dendritic* filopodia and spines by neurotronsmitter released from axons (figure 6.17). In a first step, the presynaptic terminal would secrete glutamate at lower concentrations (or it would become diluted due to the free extracellular space around the terminal) and stimulate high-affinity receptors that would promote the emergence and motility of axonal and dendritic filopodia. In a second stage, after initial contact has occurred, glutamate would act at higher concentrations (stimulating low-affinity receptors) and help stabilize developing synapses. Therefore, depending on the exact concentration of glutamate and the developmental stage of the sample, opposite results could be generated when one studies the effect of glutamate on spine or filopodial motility.

**Role of Calcium in Spine Motility**
As with glutamate, the role of calcium in regulating or mediating spine motility is controversial. For example, the number of spines from slices maintained in calcium-free solutions is higher than that those of slices in calcium-containing media (Kirov and Harris, 1999). This implies that a lower intracellular free calcium concentration ($[Ca^{2+}]_i$) could stimulate spinogenesis. By contrast, in other experiments, the application of calcium-free solution, the blockade of calcium channels, or the massive calcium influxes resulting from bath application of potassium chloride (KCl) did not appear to result in major changes in spine density, morphology, or motility (Dunaevsky et al., 1999). Finally, application of caffeine, which releases calcium from internal stores, apparently increases the size and the number of spines (Korkotian and Segal, 1999). Thus, after elevation of $[Ca^{2+}]_i$, increases, descreases, or unchanged spine densities all seem to occur under certain experimental conditions.

As in the case of glutamate, these contradictory results could be explained by a complex interaction between increases in calcium and changes in spine shape (compare with Kater et al., 1988), whereby small increases in calcium (or synaptic activity) produce spine retraction, intermediate-amplitude increases produce spine growth, and large-amplitude accumulations again lead to spine retraction (Harris, 1999; Matus, 2000; Segal and Andersen, 2000; Wong et al., 2000). It seems quite likely that the heterogeneity of effects, to a large extent, reflects different systems and experimental conditions, as well as heterogeneous spine populations or functional states of the spines.

### Other Pathways

Many other molecules have been reported to alter spine motility and morphology. The list includes steroid hormones (Woolley et al., 1990), volatile anesthetics (Kaech et al., 1999), cadherins (Takeichi, 1990), ephrins (Ethell et al., 2001), neurotrophins (Horch et al., 1999), actin-related molecules (Craig and Boudin, 2001; Luo, 2000; Rao and Craig, 2000), PSD proteins (Hering and Sheng, 2001), cocaine and amphetamines (Robinson and Kolb, 1999), and many others (Ethell and Pasquale, 2005). It seems that a multitude of molecules reaching from neurotransmitters to growth factors and from hormones to drugs of abuse seem to be intricately involved in spine morphology, and also spine dynamics. The experimental results are so varied and the number of molecules involved is so large that it is difficult to come up with a unifying hypothesis explaining all results. However, as mentioned in chapter 4, Rho family molecules interact with many of these pathways. For example, since Rho can be directly activated by p75 (Yamashita et al., 1999) and NMDA receptors (Li et al., 2000), the small GTPases of the Rho family might well be the central mechanism for the effects observed and, ultimately, could control spine and synaptic morphology.

### Potential Functions of Rapid Spine Motility

### Motility as a Cell-Biological Epiphenomenon

While spine motility is quite striking, it could be argued that, given that neurons are living structures, they should move, and it is the absence of motility that could be potentially unexpected. From this point of view, spine motility could be an epiphenomenon, a consequence of being alive, with no particular purpose for synaptic function. Indeed, the actin cytoskeleton fulfills many cell biological tasks, and spine motility may simply be a consequence of the dynamic nature of the actin networks. For example, in neurons, actin networks are involved in targeting and trafficking of receptors (Allison et al., 1998; Hirai, 2000; Wyszynski et al., 1997), and spine motility might simply be a consequence of these events, perhaps serving to enhance the diffusional mixing of molecules (Richards et al., 2004; Santamaria et al., 2006). Although this hypothesis cannot be ruled out, it is unlikely to be the sole function of the observed phenomena. Given that the typical spine movement per minute is an order of magnitude larger than the size of a synapse (Dunaevsky et al., 1999), and that the moving structure is exactly where the synapse is established, it is difficult to disregard potential functional consequences of spine motility. Indeed, growth of new spines, or changes in the spine neck length (see chapter 9), as well as physical changes in the width of the synaptic cleft (Liu et al., 1999), all figure prominently as potential mechanisms for changing synaptic efficacy (see chapter 8). Therefore, it seems likely that the processes that generate morphological dynamics in spines could also change synaptic transmission.

**Calcium Compartmentalization and Learning Rules**
An alternative hypothesis is that spine motility can control spine calcium dynamics and, through them, synaptic function and plasticity. As will be discussed in detail in the next chapter, spines compartmentalize calcium and can serve to biochemically isolate inputs, endowing them with independent calcium regulation (Koch and Zador, 1993; Wickens, 1988; Yuste et al., 2000). Several forms of synaptic plasticity require increases in calcium levels, and calcium compartmentalization is thought to be important for input specificity (Levy and Steward, 1979; Malenka et al., 1988; Wigstrom et al., 1986; but see Engert and Bonhoeffer, 1997). Therefore, spines could help to implement input-specific learning rules, and spine motility could serve to change these rules. Moreover, because diffusion through the spine neck scales with its length (Svoboda et al., 1996), the length of the spine neck could control the time constant of calcium compartmentalization, thereby determining the time constant of calcium-dependent synaptic learning rules (Majewska et al. 2000a and b; Holthoff et al., 2002b; but see Sabatini et al., 2002). Spine motility, and specifically that which involves changes in the morphologies of the spine necks, thus could serve to alter those time constants.

**Spine Motility and Critical Periods**
In every system it has been demonstrated that spine or filopodial motility decreases with increasing age of the animal (Dailey and Smith, 1996; Dunaevsky et al., 1999; Lendvai et al., 2000; Ziv and Smith, 1996). This regulation could be related to the heightened plasticity found during critical developmental periods. The reduction in spine motility might be related to the termination of critical periods, as spines may need to be motile to accomplish synaptic changes of the neural circuitry. Nevertheless, at least in the primary visual system of the mouse (Konur and Yuste, 2004a), it appears that motility is not regulated during the critical period, but decreases to a baseline level at around P14, two weeks before the critical period for monocular deprivation (~P25–30; figure 6.18, plate 6). Moreover, spine motility is decreased (rather than increased) by sensory input deprivation paradigms, manipulations that delay the critical period. These results rule out a major role for spine motility in critical periods and instead indicate that it could be related to an ealier event, one that actually occurs in the first two postnatal weeks: synaptogenesis.

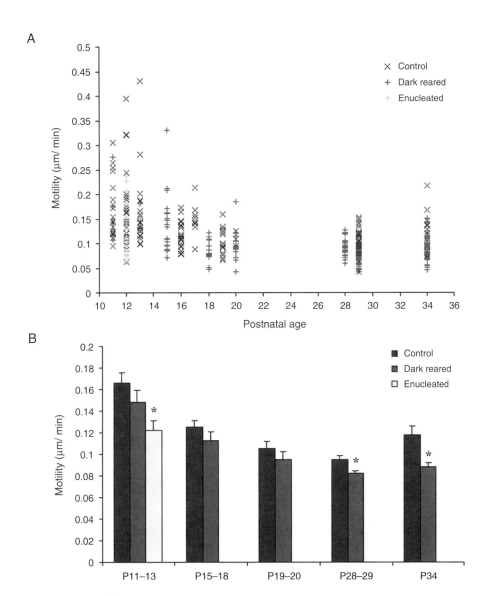

**Figure 6.18 (plate 6)**
Developmental regulation of spine motility in mouse primary visual cortex and effect of sensory deprivation. (A) In control animals, higher motility disappears after P14 and a baseline is then reached, well
before the critical period occurs (~P25–30). Dark-reared or enucleated animals follow a similar developmental trend and display a small reduction in motility. Each cross corresponds to data imaging spine motility in one neuron. (B) Mean motility in different age groups. Reprinted from Konur and Yuste, 2004a.

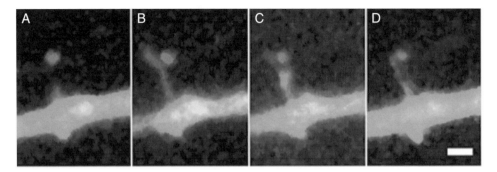

**Figure 6.19 (plate 7)**
Spine motility and potential synaptogenesis. (A–D) A highly motile postsynaptic filopodia (green) is interacting with a relatively nonmotile presynaptic bouton (red) and becomes stabilized. Reprinted from Konur and Yuste, 2004b. Scale bar: 1 μm.

### Spine Motility and Synaptogenesis

Continuing with the proposal made in the last chapter, I would argue that spine motility is intimately linked to synaptogenesis. Perhaps the strongest evidence for a functional role of spine motility in synaptogenesis is based on the direct observation of spines moving in the vicinity of axonal processes. In many of these cases, viewing of time-lapse sequences leaves little doubt that the dendrite must be playing a very active role in generating new synapses. One can often observe how a dendrite grows spines that shoot out toward an axon and appear to grab it, as if they wanted to make contact with it, presumably for the purpose of building a synapse (figure 6.19, plate 7). Indeed, the highest spine motility occurs at peak developmental stages for synaptogenesis (figure 6.18; Dunaevsky et al., 1999; Konur and Yuste, 2004a; Lendvai et al., 2000; Wong et al., 2000; Ziv and Smith, 1996). A better molecular understanding of the mechanisms of spine motility may soon enable direct testing of this hypothesis, for example, by examining the effect of modulating spine motility on critical period paradigms.

As discussed in chapter 5, hypotheses linking spines or filopodia to the formation of synaptic contacts have been put forward in various incarnations by different authors (Jontes et al., 2000; Peters and Kaiserman-Abramof, 1970; Ramón y Cajal, 1904; Saito et al., 1997; Swindale, 1981). The idea is that dendritic extensions such as spines or filopodia are convenient and efficacious means to connect basically straight wires like axons to a multitude of dendritic arbors (figure 6.20; for a different view see Anderson and Martin, 2001). This allows dendrites to contact axons not only in the immediate vicinity but also within reach of the spine, without the need for the axons (or dendrites) to run convoluted and tortuous paths. Moreover, it has been estimated that the presence of spines increases the number of potential contacts

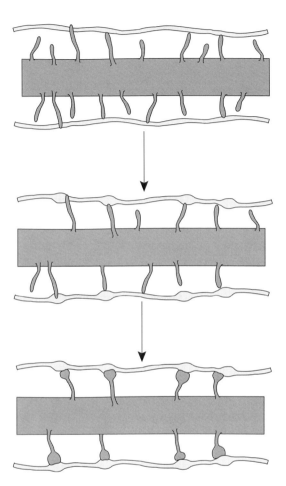

**Figure 6.20**
Spine motility and synaptogenesis: a model. (Top panel) Dendritic motility facilitates the initial contact between dendritic processes (dark grey) and axons (light grey). These contacts are later pruned and turned into mature synapses (bottom two panels). Spines thus help to minimize wiring by preventing the axon from having to run tortuous paths to form the necessary connections with the postsynaptic dendrites.

between axons and dendrites by approximately fourfold (Anderson and Martin, 2001; Stepanyants et al., 2002; Swindale, 1981). Therefore, spine motility would actually be necessary to take advantage of the space-filling strategy by the dendrite; if spines were not motile, under this model, their function would be severely hindered. Spine motility would be a very natural way to maximize this connectivity.

**Two Types of Motility: Elongation versus Morphing**
Can this model explain all data on spine motility? We have to acknowledge the heterogeneous phenomenology encompassed by the term *spine motility*. Observation of these data gives the impression that there are many types of spine motility, raising the possibility that there may be more than a single phenomenon. Indeed, phenomenological, developmental, and even molecular evidence differentiate at least two types of spine motility: the elongation of a protrusion and the wiggling or morphing of the spine head. Protusive motility of filopodia or spines is a relatively slow elongation and retraction that lasts a few seconds and is often observed at earlier developmental stages, typically before P10 in mouse neocortex (figure 6.19, for example; Konur and Yuste, 2004b). Protusive motility also seems to be specifically blocked by Rho/RhoK (Tashiro and Yuste, 2004). On the other hand, wiggling or morphing is a type of motility that is specific to spines and, when observed at higher magnification, it is generated by the movement of small filopodia-like protrusions emerging from the spine head (see figure 6.12b; Dunaevsky et al., 1999; Fischer et al., 1998). This type of motility occurs typically at later developmental stages (>P10 in mouse neocortex), is stimulated by Rac1, but not by by Rho (Tashiro and Yuste, 2004), and is the basis for the morphological description of spines as cup-shaped "hands" (figures 6.5 and 6.12; Roelandse et al., 2003).

**A Two-Step Model of Synaptogenesis**
How can we integrate both types of motility into a coherent picture of spine development and maturation? The two types of motility could reflect the life cycle of the synapse and correspond to the two developmental stages proposed above (figure 6.17). Filopodial or spine-protusive motility could serve to sample the surrounding neuropil, making perhaps initial contacts with potential presynaptic boutons and be ideally suited to maximize synaptogenesis, as discussed. But what about the wiggling/morphing type of motility? Why would a spine need to move, once it already has a synaptic contact, as shown above? At a later stage in development, spine motility, or more specifically, head morphing motility, could have a different function related to the maturation of the synapse. This idea derives from the one-to-one matching between synaptic terminal and spines mentioned in chapter 3. It appears that there are hardly any "naked" spines or terminals, and most spines have one synapse (see figure 1.3). Although spines can receive more than one synaptic contact, the second contact

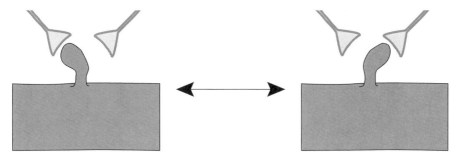

**Figure 6.21**
Spine motility could mediate synaptic competition. The morphing type of spine motility ("wiggling") could reflect the interactions of the spine with two axonal terminals competing to attract it.

is generally an inhibitory one. Therefore, each spine essentially receives a single excitatory synapse.

This relatively precise matching, with no empty spines or spines with more than one excitatory contact, cannot be due to chance. Although one could argue that both the Miller-Peters and filopodial spinogenesis will result in a one-to-one match, the Sotelo spinogenesis does not, so it is necessary to invoke a different mechanism. As in the neuromuscular junction, where Tello first pointed out this precise matiching between pre- and postsynaptic elements (Purves and Lichtman, 1985), one potential explanation for the matching is that it arises from a competitive mechanism, whereby different axons could compete for given spine and only a single terminal from the winning axon would remain (Sanes and Lichtman, 1999). Thus, during this competitive period, spines could "wiggle" and physically explore alternative terminals (figure 6.21).

Indeed, spines that have more than one nearby terminal in their vicinity move significantly more than those that have a single terminal (Konur and Yuste, 2004b). Inspection of the spine motility movies reveals many cases in which a spine head that is already touching a terminal, generates a small filopodial "finger" (also known as a "spinulus"), that interacts specifically with a second nearby terminal (figure 6.22, plate 8).

Thus, head morphing/wiggling could reflect the competition between different axons for a given spine. This model would predict that this synaptic competition for available spines exists during postnatal development and that, when it ceases, spine motility is greatly reduced.

The two-step model of synaptogenesis integrates ideas on spine development and motility. The two steps would correspond to two stages in the development of spines, their emergence and maturation, and they would be matched to the two types of

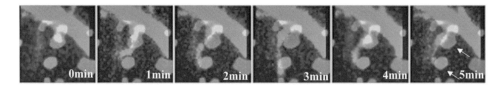

**Figure 6.22 (plate 8)**
Spine motility in the presence of neighboring synaptic terminals. Live imaging of a dendritic protrusion (green) superimposed on immunostained boutons (red). The base of the protrusion is in stable contact with an axonal bouton, whereas its filopodial tip (or spinule) transiently interacts with two nearby boutons. In the 4th frame, it overshoots to approach the second bouton. Reprinted from Konur and Yuste, 2004b.

motility one can observe. This model puts the focus of synaptogenesis on the postsynaptic structure, and agrees with the lack of motily observed by presynaptic terminals. The dendrite appears to be the active partner, the one that must choose between axons, not the other way around. Because spines often contain axons from similar types of neurons, it is unlikely that this choice is based on molecular differences, either on cell membranes or gradients of secreted molecules. Rather, it seems more natural that spines could choose their partner based on the activity of the presynaptic axon, just as it happens in the NMJ (Sanes and Lichtman, 1999). Terminals that release more glutamate, or whose spatial relationship with the spine generates an increased glutamate concentration, could first attract and then immobilize the spine, which otherwise could "wiggle" and send filopodia to search of higher glutamate concentrations. As in the NMJ, this competitive mechanism would prevent situations where a single axon could innervate too many spines, since the total amount of synaptic vesicles that it could synthesize would limit the number of terminals and vesicles per terminal, and, therefore, the number of "battles" that it could win. In the long term, such a strategy could normalize the average synaptic strength and guarantee the spread of connectivity.

**Functional Interpretation of Spine Motility**
In summary, spine and filopodial motility appears at the time in development when the neuron is engaged in synaptogenesis, so it makes logical sense to think that it could help mediate it. The structural role of spines in the circuits where they operate becomes quite clear: They are actually ideally designed to help fill the synaptic matrix of inputs of the neurons that have them. Moreover, different types of motility, occurring at different times in development, could be matched to first effectively maximize potential wiring, and then to spread out and normalize connectivity, reflecting two functions: connecting and choosing. This structural role of spines, given that axons are straight, could also have the advantage of minimizing the total

amount of wiring necessary for the circuit and thus represent an ideal optimization strategy (Chklovskii et al., 2002).

Continuing our journey in the next chapters, I will now turn our attention to more functional aspects of spines, examining their roles in calcium comparmentatlizaion, synaptic transmission and plasticity, and dendritic integration. As we will see, a compelling case can be made for the argument that spines appear designed to enhance the function of this distributed matrix of inputs and endow it with plastic and integrative properties.

# 7 Calcium

*Spines compartmentalize calcium, and this can generate input-specific synaptic plastic-ity. Calcium influx into spines is mediated by voltage-sensitive calcium channels, NMDA, and AMPA receptors. Calcium is also released from internal stores in spines. The endogenous calcium buffering in spines is weak and diffusional equilibration is rapid. Spine calcium decay kinetics are controlled by fast calcium pumps and slower diffusion through the spine neck. The variety of pathways that influence spine calcium dynamics provide a flexible regulation of this second messenger pathway. Finally, al-though spines generate input-specific calcium compartmentalization, input-specific cal-cium compartmentalization occurs also in neocortical interneurons without spines.*

As argued in chapter 1, because synapses can be made directly on dendritic shafts, spines must have additional functions besides merely receiving synaptic inputs. In particular, the peculiar morphology of spines, where a small ($<$1 µm in diameter) head is connected to the dendrite by a thin ($\sim$0.2 µm in diameter) neck, has sup-ported the notion that they are biochemical compartments and, specifically, that they serve to compartmentalize calcium (Holmes, 1990; Koch and Zador, 1993; Lis-man, 1989; Rall, 1974b; Shepherd, 1996; Wickens, 1988). As mentioned in chapter 4, this agrees with the finding that a significant fraction of the protein mass in a spine is CaM-kinase-2, an enzyme complex that acts as a calcium-activated molecular switch (Miller and Kennedy, 1985; 1986). In addition, calcium mediates input-specific forms of synaptic plasticity (Lynch et al., 1983; Malenka et al., 1989), so the regulation of calcium concentration in spines might be the key to their specific function.

In recent years, spine calcium dynamics have been measured for the first time. This has been possible because of the design of selective calcium indicators (Tsien, 1989) and the introduction of novel imaging techniques, such as digital cooled charged-couple-device (CCD) cameras (Connor, 1986), confocal (Fine et al., 1988), and two-photon microscopy (Denk et al., 1990). In addition, there have been important advances in the quantitative understanding of cellular calcium dynamics (Neher, 1998; Neher and Augustine, 1992; Tank et al., 1995). These data and analytical tools have confirmed the hypothesis that spines are calcium compartments (Bloodgood and Sabatini, 2007a; Hayashi and Majewska, 2005; Yuste and Denk, 1995; Yuste et al., 2000).

**Spine Calcium Influx: Parallel Pathways with Separate Functions?**

Imaging of calcium dynamics in spines started with the introduction of CCD cameras and ratiometric imaging (Guthrie et al., 1991; Müller and Connor, 1991). These studies, performed in dendrites from hippocampal pyramidal neurons in brain slices, demonstrated that measurements of calcium dynamics in living spines were feasible. An initial study showed that resting $[Ca^{2+}]_i$ levels in spines were the same as those in the dendrite, but that after synaptic stimulation, spines could reach higher $[Ca^{2+}]_i$ levels than their dendritic shafts (Müller and Connor, 1991). Weaker synaptic stimulation produced localized calcium accumulations in spines that were blocked by APV, an NMDA receptor antagonist, whereas stronger stimulation produced generalized accumulations throughout the dendritic tree and were unaffected by APV. Thus, individual spines could maintain a different $[Ca^{2+}]_i$ than the parent dendrite. These accumulations were mediated by an NMDA receptor-dependent influx pathway. In a second study, selective photodamage produced high calcium accumulations in dendrites and spines. While most spines faithfully followed dendritic $[Ca^{2+}]_i$, changes in some spines reportedly lagged or even preceded those of the dendrite (Guthrie et al., 1991).

These data were followed by confocal microscopy measurements showing that synaptically induced calcium influxes could occur in spines in the presence of the AMPA blocker CNQX (Alford et al., 1993) and somatic depolarization produced fast $[Ca^{2+}]_i$ accumulations in spines and adjacent dendrites (Jaffe et al., 1994). Higher calcium accumulations were measured in spines than in their dendrites, suggesting that these calcium accumulations were probably locally generated at the spine. Besides these evoked accumulations, spontaneous $[Ca^{2+}]_i$ increases were detected in dendrites and spines in cultured neocortical neurons (Murphy et al., 1994; 1995). These transients persisted in TTX, were blocked by APV, and were interpreted as the calcium signatures of miniature excitatory postsynaptic currents (mEPSCs) (Murphy et al., 1995). These transients, however, were not restricted to spines, involving small regions ($\sim$10 µm) of the dendrite (Murphy et al., 1994).

As explained in chapter 5, spines are so small ($<1$ µm in diameter and $<1$ fl in volume) that imaging them in live preparations is normally accompanied by photodamage. This technical problem was solved by the introduction of two-photon microscopy (Denk et al., 1990), which enabled, for the first time, systematic calcium imaging studies of living spines (figure 7.1).

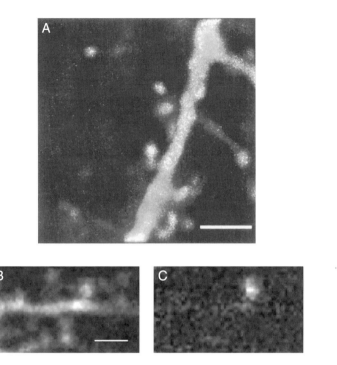

**Figure 7.1**
Spines compartmentalize calcium. (A) Two-photon imaging of spines from a living neocortical pyramidal neuron that has been injected with a calcium indicator. Reprinted from Holthoff et al., 2002b. Note the diversity of spine neck lengths. Scale bar: 5 μm. (B, C) Calcium accumulations in spines after synaptic stimulation. Two-photon images of a spine from a hippocampal pyramidal cell showing fluorescence intensity at rest (B) and the difference between subthreshold synaptic stimulation and rest (C), where white indicates pixels where $[Ca^{2+}]_i$ increased during the stimulation. Subthreshold synaptic stimulation produces calcium accumulation restricted to an individual spine. Scale bar: 2 μm. Reprinted from Yuste and Denk, 1995.

In the first two-photon calcium measurements of spines, three different functional regimes of calcium accumulation in spines of CA1 pyramidal neurons in slices were described (Yuste and Denk, 1995). While postsynaptic action potentials (APs) propagated through the dendritic tree and triggered generalized calcium accumulations in spines and dendrites, subthreshold synaptic stimulation produced $[Ca^{2+}]_i$ increases restricted to individual spines (figures 7.1 and 7.2). These localized $[Ca^{2+}]_i$ accumulations were stochastic, reflecting the stochastic nature of synaptic transmission, and could therefore be used to carry out "optical quantal analysis" of individual synapses, that is, physiologically study the effect of activating a single synaptic contact, whose location is known (figures 7.3 and 7.4, plate 9).

Moreover, in a third type of calcium accumulation, the temporal coincidence of APs and synaptic stimulation produced cooperative, "supralinear," calcium accumulations

A

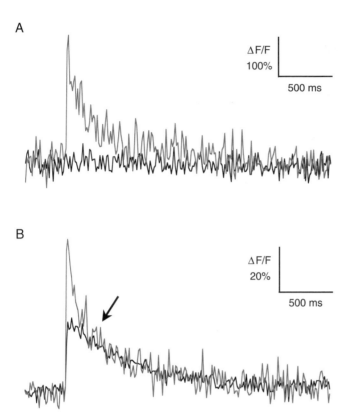

Figure 7.2
Two regimes of calcium accumulations in spines. (A) Two-photon measurements of calcium dynamics in a spine (gray) and adjacent dendrite (black) from a layer 5 pyramidal neuron under subthreshold synaptic stimulation. Note the fast onset and slow decay of the spine $[Ca^{2+}]_i$ transient, while the adjacent dendrite does not respond. (B) Calcium dynamics in response to a backpropagating action potential. Note how calcium accumulations now also occur in the dendrite. Reprinted with permission from Yuste et al., 2000.

(figure 7.5, plate 10; SY and AP). These very high $[Ca^{2+}]_i$ increases were restricted to the spine receiving the EPSP, with neighboring spines remained unaffected. A follow-up study examined the temporal properties of this supralinear accumulations, describing how they only happened if the synaptic stimulation was delivered before the backpropagating action potential (figure 7.6; Yuste et al., 1999). In other words, the presynaptic neuron has to fire before the postsynaptic one to trigger these large spine calcium accumulations.

Indeed, these three regimes have a direct functional interpretation: Since the EPSP is the input of the cell and the AP its output, their temporal pairing represents the coincidence, or temporal sequence, of input and output. Therefore, the supralinear

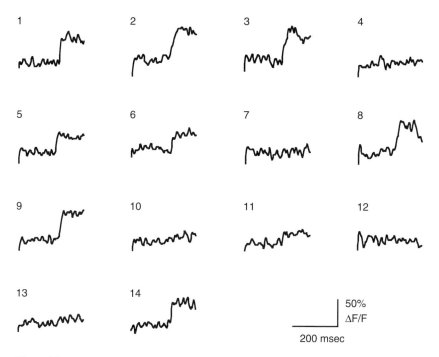

**Figure 7.3**
Stochastic calcium accumulations in spines after synaptic stimulation. Sequential calcium accumulations in a dendritic spine from a hippocampal pyramidal neuron in response to paired-pulse subthreshold synaptic stimulation (30-msec interval). Note how an identical stimulation protocol can elicit successes (traces 1, 2, 3, 5, 6, 8, 9, and 14) and failures (traces 4, 7, 10, 11, 12, and 13) in the calcium influx into spines and how approximately half of the stimuli result in a success. Responses measured in 2 mM $Ca^{2+}$ and 2 mM $Mg^{2+}$. Reprinted from Yuste et al., 1999.

calcium accumulations in spines is a biochemical event that signals the "coincidence detection," or "causality detection" of input and output, or cause and effect, exactly as the one postulated to mediate Hebbian or "spike timing dependent plasticity" plasticity (Ariens-Kapper et al., 1936; Hebb, 1949; Magee and Johnston, 1997; Markram et al., 1997b; Wigstrom et al., 1986; Zhang et al., 1998).

These experiments also provided evidence for the presence of voltage-sensitive calcium channels (VSCCs) in spines, both because of the speed of AP-induced calcium accumulation in spines and its blockade by the VSCC blocker $Ni^{2+}$ (Yuste and Denk, 1995; see chapter 4). Indeed, experiments used fluctuation analysis have been used to estimate the number of VSCCs in individual spines (Sabatini and Svoboda, 2000). The analysis of these data suggests that the number of active VSCCs is small (<10). Moreover, these channels apparently belonged to a different VSCC subtype than those in the parent dendrite, with a considerable heterogeneity in the composition of VSCCs from spine to spine (Bloodgood and Sabatini, 2007a).

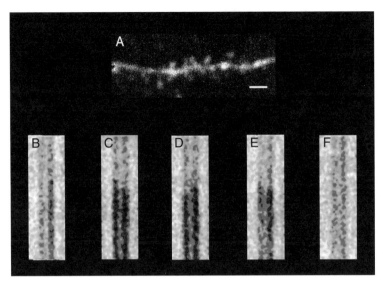

**Figure 7.4 (plate 9)**
Optical quantal analysis. (Top) Two-photon image of a dendrite from a CA1 pyramidal neuron. Approximately 16 spines can be detected, covering the surface of the dendrite. Scale bar: 2 µm. (Bottom) Five consecutive line scans of the fluorescent responses of two adjacent spines (those on the center top of the dendrite) to paired-pulse synaptic stimulation (30-ms interval). The line scan cuts through the heads of the two adjacent spines. In the pseudocolor scale, yellow is low $[Ca^{2+}]_i$, and blue is high $[Ca^{2+}]_i$. (B): the right spine responds alone to stimulation. (C) Both spines respond, but the left one responds slightly ahead of the right one. (D) The case is reversed, with the right spine responding ahead of the left one. (E) Both spines respond similarly. (F) They both fail. These data reveal the stochastic activation of two adjacent synapses. Reprinted with permission from Yuste et al., 2000.

Two-photon calcium measurements from spines were also performed in cerebellar Purkinje cells (Denk et al., 1995). In these neurons, EPSPs also caused calcium accumulations restricted to individual spines, whereas APs triggered calcium accumulations in the entire dendritic tree (Denk et al., 1995). Synaptically induced calcium accumulations were blocked by CNQX, as if they were mediated by calcium-permeable AMPA receptors (since there are practically no NMDARs in adult Purkinje cells). Indeed, in some, but not all, spines, calcium accumulations increased with hyperpolarization, as one would expect from a glutamate receptor–mediated calcium influx, operating under a stronger voltage gradient with hyperpolarization. This indicated that some spines had a predominantly VSCC-calcium influx, whereas other had a glutamate receptor–mediated calcium influx pathway. Thus, even on the same neuron there are populations of spines with different calcium influx mechanisms.

A complication of calcium imaging experiments is the fact that calcium indicators bind and buffer calcium, thus altering $[Ca^{2+}]_i$ amplitudes and dynamics (see below).

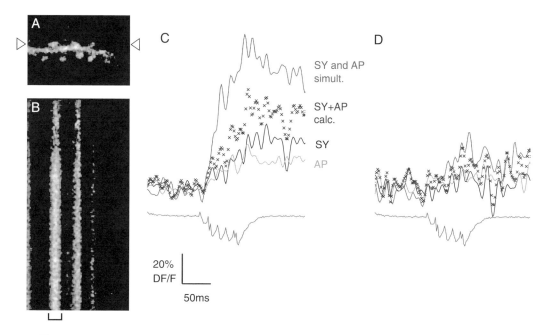

**Figure 7.5 (plate 10)**
Supralinear calcium accumulations in spines under temporal coincidence of excitatory postsynaptic potentials (EPSP) and action potentials (APs). (A) Fluorescence image of a dendrite from a hippocampal pyramidal neuron, field with a calcium indicator. (B) Line scan through three spines (shown between white arrowheads in A), during a train of five subthreshold synaptic stimulations. Note how the left spine displays an increase in fluorescence, corresponding to a large increase in calcium concentration. (C) Calcium accumulations in left spine under different experimental conditions: subthreshold EPSPs (SY), postsynaptic spikes (AP), and their simultaneous combination (SY+AP). Note how simultaneous application of the AP and the EPSPs produces a "supralinear" accumulation that is larger (red) than the arithmetic sum of the AP and ESPS independently (blue). Reprinted from Yuste and Denk, 1995. (D) Calcium dynamics in the neighboring spine, which does not receive the EPSP, do not display a supralinear accumulation. Unpublished results from Yuste and Denk.

In addition, these indicators are only selective at particular $[Ca^{2+}]_i$ concentrations, determined by their $K_d$. Indeed, all indicators used in the above mentioned studies have high affinity, distorting $[Ca^{2+}]_i$ dynamics and saturating at the $[Ca^{2+}]_i$ level reached in stimulated spines. These problems were circumvented in a study with the low-affinity indicator mag-Fura 5 to image calcium accumulations in CA1 spines (Petrozzino et al., 1995). Using CCD camera measurements, it was estimated that the $[Ca^{2+}]_i$ in spines under tetanic stimulation (condition presumably producing simultaneous APs and EPSPs) reached 20 to 40 μM, three orders of magnitude higher than the estimated resting $[Ca^{2+}]_i$ in these neurons. These high accumulations were blocked by APV. A different study also used high-affinity indicators to perform two-photon imaging of calcium accumulations generated by glutamate uncaging

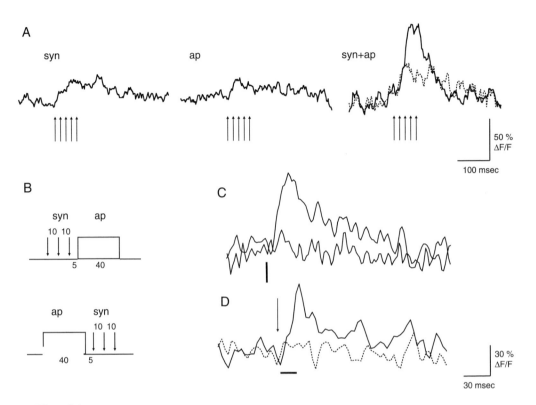

**Figure 7.6**
The supralinear calcium influx has a temporal dependency and is NMDA receptor dependent. (A) Supra-linear calcium accumulations in spines measured with a low-affinity calcium indicator. Panels show the flu-orescence intensity changes in a dendritic spine in response to a train of EPSPs (syn, left panel, arrow), five action potentials (ap, middle panel), and both simultaneously (syn+ap, right panel). Stippled line is the arithmetic sum of the responses to the EPSPs and action potentials. Note how the measured accumulation is larger than the expected sum. (B) Stimulation protocol used to test the temporal dependency of the supralinearity. Three EPSPs were generated before (top) or after (bottom) a postsynaptic depolarization that triggered action potentials. (C) The supralinearity has a temporal dependency. Fluorescence intensity changes in a spine in response to either EPSPs before (lower line) or after (higher line) the spike train. Note how only the first condition generates any significant calcium accumulations. (D) The supralinearity and its temporal dependency are blocked by MNDA receptor antagonists. Calcium accumulations in a den-dritic spine (synaptic first minus action potentials first) in control ACSF (solid line) and during perfusion of 100 APV (stippled line). Note how APV blocks any significant calcium supralinearity. Reprinted from Yuste et al., 1999.

(Noguchi et al., 2005). This study revealed that even the smallest spines cointain NMDARs.

The role of NMDA receptors mediating EPSP-induced calcium influxes and supralinear influxes that occurs with pairing of AP and EPSPs has been amply demonstrated. In CA1 spines, EPSP evoked calcium transients were blocked by APV (Emptage et al., 1999; Mainen et al., 1999; Pozzo-Miller et al., 1999; Yuste et al., 1999), and in one case (Emptage et al., 1999; but not in Kovalchuk et al., 2000) also blocked by internal-release antagonists. Interestingly, in two studies (Emptage et al., 1999; Yuste et al., 1999; but not in Kovalchuk et al., 2000), CNQX blocked EPSP evoked calcium transients, indicating that subthreshold stimulation of AMPA receptors may suffice to partially unblock NMDA receptors. As in Purkinje cells (Denk et al., 1995), a subpopulation of CA1 spines showed an APV-resistant influx pathway, which could be mediated by calcium-permeable AMPA receptors (Yuste et al., 1999). In addition, while APV blocked the supralinear calcium influx, VSCCs did not significantly contribute to EPSP-induced calcium accumulations, based on the lack of effect of "washing out" VSCCs (Yuste et al., 1999). In agreement with this, internal VSCCs antagonists did not block EPSP-induced calcium influxes into spines (Kovalchuk et al., 2000). Also, in layer 5 neurons, pairing of AP and EPSPs produced an APV-blockable, supralinear calcium accumulation when the AP followed the EPSP, whereas the response was sublinear in the reverse case (Koester and Sakmann, 1998). Supralinear calcium influxes, also blocked by APV, were also observed when APs were paired with glutamate uncaging on the dendrite (Schiller et al., 1998). More recent studies have examined these supralinear accumulations with more detail, in an attempt to biochemically disect the contributions that generate long-term potentiation or depression (Nevian and Sakmann, 2004; 2006).

In addition to these three regimes of calcium accumulations, spines can experience a fourth regime, under circumstances in which a segment of the dendrite is stimulated focally, either synaptically or by glutamate uncaging (Gasparini and Magee, 2006; Holthoff et al., 2004; Losonczy and Magee, 2006; Schiller et al., 2000). These stimuli generate local dendritic spikes that activate a small group of neighboring spines (figure 7.7, plate 11). These local spikes, mediated by the activation of NMDA receptors and VGCCs (Holthoff et al., 2004; Schiller et al., 2000), can trigger long-term depression (LTD) after a single stimulus (figure 7.8; Holthoff et al., 2004) and perhaps mediate branch-specific computations (Gasparini and Magee, 2006; Losonczy and Magee, 2006; Poirazi and Mel, 2001; see chapter 10).

## Calcium Release in Spines

In addition to calcium influx via the cell membrane described above, calcium is internally released by spines, most likely from their smooth endoplasmic reticulum (SER;

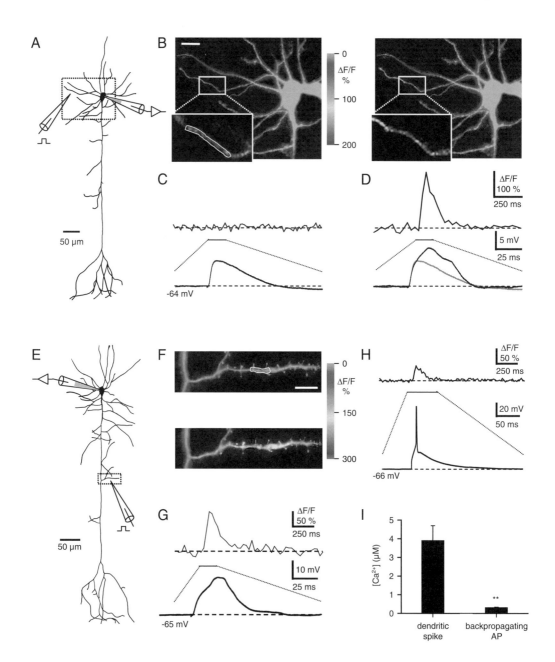

see chapter 3). Two types of receptors in the ER membrane, the ryanodine receptor (RyR) family and the inositol-1,4,5-triphosphate receptor (IP$_3$R) family, appear to control this process. Three different RyRs isoforms have been described: RyR$_1$ and RyR$_2$ were originally found in skeletal and heart muscle, where they are essential for excitation-contraction coupling (Marks et al., 1989). RyR$_3$ was actually first discovered in the brain and is predominantly expressed in CA1 neurons (Furuichi et al., 1994a). Nevertheless, the RyR$_2$ isoform is the most abundant one in the brain (Berridge, 1998). One known ligand of the RyR is calcium (Nabauer et al., 1989), hence, RyR-mediated internal release of calcium is also known as calcium-induced calcium release (CICR). The IP$_3$R family also comprises three isoforms called IP$_3$R$_{1-3}$, all expressed in the brain (Furuichi et al., 1994b).

A hint of the existence of functional intracellular calcium stores in dendrites came from the finding that synaptic stimulation of CA1 neurons induced dendritic calcium transients which were blocked by thapsigargin, a drug that inhibits the smooth ER calcium ATPase (SERCA) and depletes intracellular calcium stores (Alford et al., 1993). Subsequently, caffeine application, which induces RyR-mediated calcium release, was shown to produce calcium accumulations in spines of cultured hippocampal neurons (Korkotian and Segal, 1998). Thapsigargin and ryanodine blocked this caffeine-induced response.

Synaptic stimulation can also induce this fast form of internal release in spines. Data from cultured hippocampal slices indicated that synaptically-induced calcium transients in spines are blocked by CPA, another SERCA antagonist (Emptage et al., 1999). This implies that calcium accumulations entering the spine through NMDA receptors, but not through VSCCs, are subsequently amplified by internal release of calcium. However, in acute hippocampal slices, calcium transients in spines generated by synaptic stimulation were not blocked by CPA (Kovalchuk et al., 2000). It is possible that the discrepancies could be caused by different experimental conditions (cultured versus acute slices, microelectrodes versus patch pipettes), differences

**Figure 7.7 (plate 11)**
Local dendritic spikes. (A) Reconstruction of a layer 5 pyramidal neuron in mouse visual cortex. Whole-cell recording was obtained in current clamp mode, and the neuron was filled via the patch-pipette with a low-affinity calcium indicator and imaged with a confocal microscope. (B) Pseudo-color images of relative fluorescence changes in basal dendrites before and after dendritic spike initiation. Scale bar: 25 μm. (C) Weak synaptic stimulation evoked an EPSP (bottom trace), but no calcium accumulation (top trace). (D) Strong synaptic stimulation evoked local dendritic spike accompanied by a large calcium transient in the activated dendrite and a complex EPSP. (E) Reconstruction of another layer 5 pyramidal neuron in visual cortex. (F) Pseudo-color coded images of relative fluorescence changes in an apical dendritic branch before and after strong synaptic stimulation. Scale bar: 10 μm. (G) Strong synaptic stimulation evoked local dendritic spike accompanied by a large calcium transient in the activated dendrite and a complex EPSP. (H) Backpropagating action potential (AP) induced by somatic current injection evoked a significantly smaller dendritic calcium transient. (I): Comparison of dendritic calcium transient amplitudes evoked by local dendritic spikes and backpropagating APs. Reprinted from Holthoff et al., 2004.

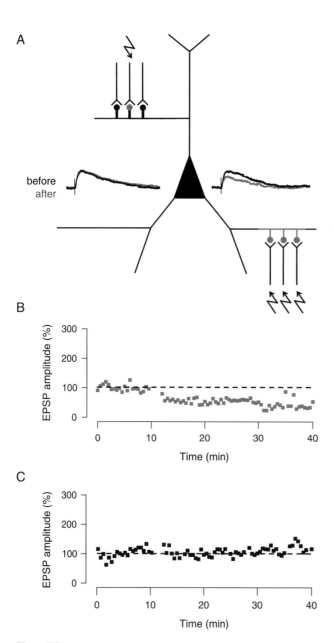

**Figure 7.8**
Local dendritic spikes induce input-specific long-term synaptic depression. (A) Experimental configuration. Two synaptic inputs, impinging different locations of the dendritic tree, were stimulated. The distance between the synaptic inputs was at least 500 μm. (B) The first input was stimulated to generate dendritic spikes, which induced LTD. (C) The control pathway, where dendritic spikes were not generated, did not show any significant change in synaptic transmission. Modified from Holthoff et al., 2004.

in loading of internal stores (Györke and Györke, 1998), or differences in spines tested, since the spine apparatus (Gray, 1959b), thought to be the morphological correlate for internal release, is not present in many spines (Colonnier, 1968).

A different mechanism of internal release in spines was demonstrated in Purkinje cells (Finch and Augustine, 1998; Takechi et al., 1998). In these neurons, high-frequency synaptic stimulation can induce IP3R-mediated release in single spines or in small spinodendritic compartments. These calcium dynamics show two distinct calcium increases: The first is fast and mediated by VSCCs whereas the second component, delayed by hundreds of milliseconds, is triggered by metabotropic glutamate receptor activation, and leads to production of IP3 and internal release. Thapsigargin blocks the second release events and also interestingly blocks LTD, indicating that internal release could be a biochemical trigger of long-term plasticity (Wang et al., 2000).

In principle, either type of release, the fast acting RyR-mediated or the delayed IP3 receptor–mediated, could serve as additional source for spine calcium, amplifying calcium signals and leading to very high and long-lasting calcium levels, which may mediate synaptic plasticity (Berridge, 1998; Lisman, 1989). Because the receptors involved in internal release show characteristic thresholds for activation, all-or-none calcium signaling could trasnform the spine into a biochemical switch (Berridge, 1998; Petersen et al., 1998).

## Calcium Buffering in Spines

Calcium-binding molecules in neurons essentially convert spatiotemporal patterns of calcium accumulations into enzymatic activity. But, by binding calcium, they also alter the calcium transients themselves. Calcium buffers can retard decay kinetics, shape diffusional profiles, and, depending on their saturation kinetics, they can also create complex temporal features. Moreover, nonequilibrium situations can also cause buffering profiles to change under different stimulation protocols (Markram et al., 1998; Neher, 1998). Although calcium buffers are key elements that control calcium dynamics, relatively few studies have focused on them.

Bovine chromaffin cells contained a low-affinity, immobile buffer with a capacity (i.e., the ratio of bound to free calcium ions) of 50 to 100 (Neher and Augustine, 1992). For comparison, the endogenous buffer capacity in crayfish presynaptic terminals was estimated to be around 600 (Tank et al., 1995). Low-mobility buffers of low capacity have been found in Aplysia axons (Gabso et al., 1997) and dendrites of pyramidal cells (Helmchen et al., 1996; Murthy et al., 2000). Meanwhile, somata of Purkinje cells have endogenous buffers whose capacity increased during development: While 6-day-old rats have an endogenous buffer capacity of 900, 15-day-old rats have capacities of about 2000 (Fierro and Llano, 1996). Purkinje cell dendrites also contain a mobile, high-affinity buffer and an immobile low-affinity buffer (Maeda et al., 1999). It is likely that the mobile buffer is calbindin, given that calbindin knockout mice show pronounced changes in their calcium dynamics (Airaksinen et al., 1997). The predominance of low-mobility, low-capacity buffers found in many systems implies that the measurement of calcium transients in spines must be highly influenced by high affinity calcium indicators.

The buffering capacity of spines has been estimated using two different experimental approaches. The first used different concentrations of calcium indicators of different affinities to backcalculate the physiological calcium buffer capacity in native situation, in the absence of exogeneous buffers (Sabatini et al., 2002). The second approach used fast measurements of calcium rises and decay times to fit the calcium dynamic equations for a single compartment and therefore solve the buffer capacity (figure 7.9; Cornelisse et al., 2007). In pyramidal neurons, both methods generate low estimates of spine buffer capacity (20–50), slightly below the dendritic buffer capacity (Helmchen et al., 1996; Cornelisse et al., 2007). These low numbers would imply that spines are endowed with fast calcium dynamics. Nevertheless, buffer capacities are difficult to estimate and these numbers could be artifactually low due to the washout of spines buffers during the whole-cell recording. Also, spines on different types of neurons, as well as spines within the same cell, could be heterogeneous in their buffering capacities and in their relative expression of different calcium buffers. In addition, the expression of buffers could be regulated by activity. Indeed, glutamate results in a fast, AMPA-mediated upregulation of calbindin in the cerebellum (Batini et al., 1993).

**Calcium Diffusion in Spines: Morphological Determinants**

As explained, the diffusion of calcium within a cell depends on the presence of buffers that can retard or enhance calcium diffusion. In oocyte extracts, calcium diffusion is faster at higher levels of $[Ca^{2+}]_i$, presumably as the binding sites of endogenous buffers become saturated (Allbritton et al., 1992). In fact, addition of exogenous mobile buffers can enhance calcium diffusion (Gabso et al., 1997). Because the endogenous buffer is relatively immobile, addition of Fura-2 increased the diffusion coefficient of calcium. Thus, experiments studying the spatial distribution of calcium may be additionally limited by the influence of the indicator on calcium diffusion.

The relatively slow diffusion of calcium in cytoplasm can cause steep spatial gradients across a cell. In large structures such as the soma, submembrane areas undergo fast, large increases in calcium, whereas increases in central areas are much slower and lower in amplitude (Eilers et al., 1995). Similar diffusional gradients for

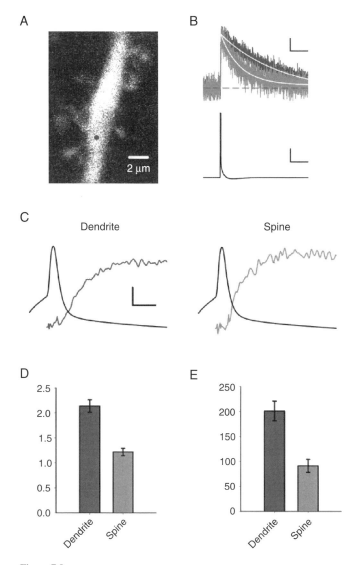

**Figure 7.9**
Fast imaging of spine calcium kinetics. (A) Image of a targeted spine and dendrite. The laser was succes-
sively parked on a spine and dendrite at the sites indicated by the black dots. (B) Calcium accumulations in
a spine (gray) and its parent dendrite (black) induced by a single AP evoked in the soma (lower panel).
White lines represent a monoexponential fit to the fluorescence decay. (C) Onsets: Same data displayed at
a faster time scale. (D) Summary data of all fluorescence rise time measurements evoked by a single AP
($n = 22$ for both spines and dendrites). (E) Summary data for decay time measurements. Scale bars: (B)
20% DF/F, 100 msec; (C) 20% DF/F, 4 msec. Reprinted from Cornelisse et al., 2007.

calcium have also been measured in dendrites (Holthoff et al., 2002b). These gradients are probably more prominent in the absence of mobile calcium indicator. The spine, however, is a small structure with an extremely high surface–to-volume ratio. The rise in $[Ca^{2+}]_i$ following an AP is faster than 2 msec (figure 7.9; Cornelisse et al., 2007; Yuste and Denk, 1995), indicating that diffusional equilibrium in the spine head can been attained very fast. Therefore, spatial gradients of $[Ca^{2+}]_i$ probably are not prominent within the spine head, although it is possible that co-localization of calcium channels and calcium sensors might allow high calcium concentrations to affect certain targets preferentially in a submsec temporal scale (Llinás et al., 1992; Naraghi and Neher, 1997). This scenario may explain how certain types of spine calcium accumulations, but not others, can activate SK channels, which need to bind calcium in order to open (Bloodgood and Sabatini, 2007b).

Although diffusion within the spine head is fast, and extrusion is also fast, diffusion between the spine and its parent dendrite can be quite slow, depending on the morphology of the spine neck, which could be as thin as 0.01 μm and also be filled with intracellular organelles (chapter 3). The diffusional barrier presented by the thin neck should, by itself, produce chemical compartmentalization (Holmes, 1990). Indeed, diffusion of fluorescein dextran across the spine neck depends directly on the length of the neck (Svoboda et al., 1996). Also, after caffeine application, long-necked spines have slower kinetics in refilling their internal stores of dendritic calcium (Korkotian and Segal, 1998; Volfovsky et al., 1999), suggesting that spine necks are barriers to the diffusion of calcium. Finally, the key role of the spine neck in controlling the time window of calcium compartmentalization in spines has been confirmed by measuring the time course of decays after AP-induced calcium entry into spines and of GFP diffusion from spines (Majewska et al., 2000a). The time scale of the fast decay component scaled linearly with the length of the spine neck, demonstrating how spine morphology determines calcium decay kinetics (Majewska et al., 2000a). Moreover, when the spine neck changes as a consequence of spine motility, the diffusional coupling is similarly affected (figures 7.10 and 7.11). All these results would appear to seal the case for the spine neck playing a key role in implementing calcium compartmentalization in the spines. At the same time, as we discuss next, these measurements have been performed with high affinity buffers, which can themselves diffuse, so one needs to calculate the calcium dynamics in the absence of these mobile buffers in order to make a better estimate of the actual spatiotemporal pattern of compartmentalization. Indeed, as we will see, other mechanisms such as local extrusion pathways also contribute, perhaps more importantly, to calcium compartmentalization in spines. Moreover, in cells without spines, and without any physical barried to calcium diffusion, extrusion mechanisms can generate calcium microcompartments with as much spatial restrictions as that present in spiny cells.

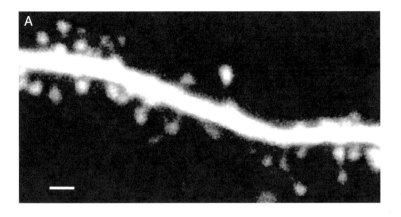

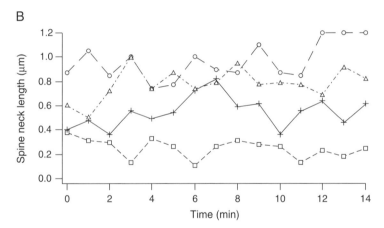

**Figure 7.10**
Spine motility can change the spine neck length. (A) Two-photon image of a dendrite from EGFP-transfected layer 2/3 pyramidal neuron during a time-lapse movie of its spine motility. (B) Analysis of the spine neck in four spines followed for a 15-min period. Note how spine necks elongate and retract as the spine moves. Scale bar: 1 μm. From Majewska et al., 2000b.

## Calcium Pumps in Spines: Local Extrusion Mechanisms

Just as the study of phosphatases was key to understanding the role of many kinases (Hunter, 1998), efflux pathways might prove as important as influx pathways for understanding spine calcium dynamics. In fact, many calcium pumps are expressed in the brain. PMCA2, a neuron-specific isoform of the plasma membrane calcium ATPase, exists in spine heads of cerebellar Purkinje cells (Stauffer et al., 1995). SERCA-2 mRNA is also found at high levels in cerebellum, hippocampus, and neo-cortex (Miller et al., 1991).

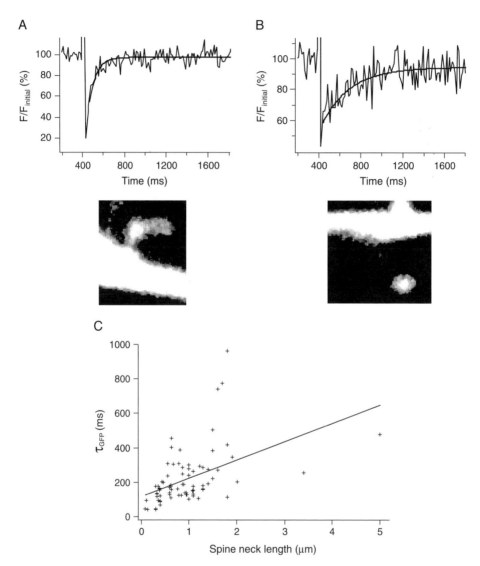

**Figure 7.11**
Diffusional coupling between spine and dendrite depends on the length of the spine neck. (A, B) Measurements of diffusional coupling between spine heads and dendrites, using fluorescence recovery after photobleaching (FRAP), in short- (A) and long- (B) necked spines, filled with GFP. (A, top) Fluorescence recovery curve of the spine shown in bottom panel, whose neck length is 0.4 μm. The fit shows a tGFP of 68 msec. (B, top) Similar measurement from a long-necked (1.5 μm) spine, with a tGFP of 275 msec. (C) Diffusional coupling between spine and dendrite is altered as spines elongate or retract. Relation between the change in fluorescent recovery time constant and the change in spine neck length. Notice the strong correlation between the two parameters. From Majewska et al., 2000b.

What controls the calcium decay kinetics in spines? In addition to diffusion of calcium through the spine neck, calcium pumps exist in spines and to contribute to the decay kinetics (Holthoff et al., 2002b; Majewska et al., 2000a; Sabatini et al., 2002). The presence of the SERCA pump in spines was initially suspected from the slowing of decay kinetics of calcium by CPA (Emptage et al., 1999; Kovalchuk et al., 2000) and the frequent undershoot of the spine versus dendritic $[Ca^{2+}]_i$, and the effect of CPA, on the fast decay kinetics, demonstrated that the pumps must be present in spines (Majewska et al., 2000a). The magnitude of these effects, however, varied from spine to spine (Majewska et al., 2000a). This heterogeneity suggests that individual spines can regulate the activity, and perhaps even the expression, of their pumps. Indeed, $Ca^{2+}$ influx can modulate the expression of PMCA isoforms (Guerini et al., 1999). In addition, the history of activity at a synapse could determine the loading of the intracellular calcium store and therefore affect the function of the SERCA pump.

### Role of Diffusion versus Extrusion Mechanisms

Spines therefore have two pathways that control calcium decay kinetics: pump-mediated extrusion (to the extracellular media or into the SER) and diffusion into the dendrite (figure 7.12). Most researchers agree that extrusional pathways are probably dominant in unperturbed spines (Holthoff et al., 2002b; Sabatini et al., 2002), but a lively debate has focused on whether diffusional pathways are at all important. It has been argued that the relatively low buffering capacity for calcium in spines would speed up spine kinetics and make extrusion more dominant and diffusion through the spine neck negligible (Sabatini et al., 2002). At the same time, one should keep in mind that although most experiments are performed with single stimulus, in physiological conditions, trains of synaptic inputs are likely to be more common and could generated long-lasting calcium influxes in spines (Holthoff et al., 2002a). These larger calcium accumulations could saturate calcium pumps (Scheuss et al., 2006). Moreover, given the heterogeneity among spines, diffusion could even dominate extrusion mechanisms in some spines (Holthoff et al., 2002b; Majewska et al., 2000a), so it is likely that the diffusional pathways, though perhaps weaker than extrusion overall, are not negligible (Holthoff et al., 2002a). For example, in stubby spines, which lack a neck and can constitute a significant proportion of spines, even in adult preparations (Benavides-Piccione et al., 2002), the contribution of diffusion is likely to be quite significant. Finally, in recent measures of calcium compartmentalization after glutamate uncaging, in the absence of significant indicator buffering, diffusional pathways, and therefore the morphology of the spine neck, appear to play an important role in controling spine calcium dynamics (Hayashi and Majewska, 2005; Matsuzaki et al., 2004; Noguchi et al., 2005).

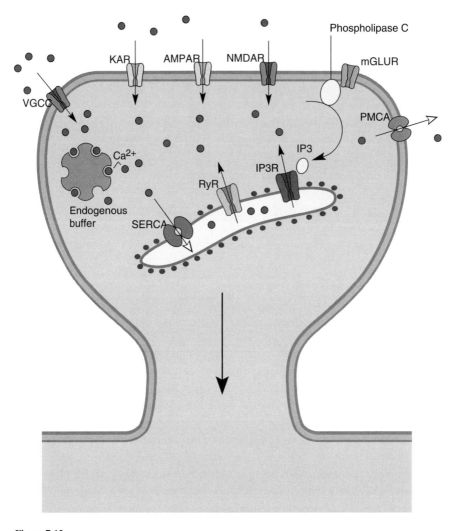

**Figure 7.12**
Calcium dynamics in spines. Closed arrows depict influx of calcium into the spine while open arrows show calcium efflux pathways. Influx can occur through NMDA channels, voltage-sensitive calcium channels (VSCCs), and calcium-permeable AMPA receptors. Calcium can also enter the cytoplasm from internal stores through ryanodine or receptor-dependent mechanism or through IP3Rs, engaged by the activation of metabotropic glutamate receptors. In the cytoplasm, calcium can bind to calcium buffers whose kinetics and affinities alter calcium dynamics. Calcium then leaves the spine by extrusion mechanisms such as the plasma membrane calcium ATPase (PMCA), which pumps calcium into the extracellular space, or the SERCA pump, which sequesters calcium into the intracellular calcium store. Calcium may also dissipate by diffusing through the thin spine neck into the adjacent dendrite.

Pyramidal neuron dendrite                          Basket cell dendrite

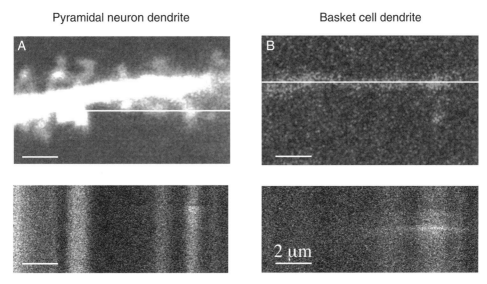

**Figure 7.13**
Calcium compartmentalization in spiny and aspiny neurons. (A) Calcium compartmentalization in spiny
neurons. (Top) Two-photon image of a dendrite from a pyramidal neuron filled with a calcium indicator.
(Bottom) Line scan through the line illustrated in (A), during subthreshold synaptic stimulation. Note how
there is an increase in fluorescence (corresponding to an increase in calcium concentration) that is selective
to the spine in the right part of the image. Reprinted from Skeberdis et al., 2006. See also figures 7.1 and
7.2. (B) Calcium compartmentalization in nonspiny neurons. (Top) Two-photon image of a dendrite from
a neocortical fast spiking interneuron, filled with a calcium indicator. Bottom, line scan placed through
dendritic segment from above, during subthreshold synaptic stimulation. Note the resulting localized calcium accumulation. Vertical scales: 400 ms. Reprinted from Goldberg et al., 2003a.

## Calcium Compartmentalization in Aspiny Dendrites

A final note on the discussion of the mechanism of calcium comparmentalization in
spines comes, rather surprisingly, from studies of aspiny interneurons (Goldberg
et al., 2003a; Soler-Llavina and Sabatini, 2006). As explained, spines receive excitatory synapses and serve as calcium compartments, which appear necessary for input-
specific synaptic plasticity. At the same time, dendrites of GABAergic interneurons,
and other cells in the brain, have few or no spines and thus do not possess a clear
morphological basis for synapse-specific compartmentalization. Activation of single
synapses on aspiny dendrites of neocortical interneurons creates highly localized
calcium microdomains, often restricted to less than 1 μm of dendritic space (figure
7.13). The absence of any morphological basis for this compartmentalization was
confirmed with ultrastructural reconstruction of imaged dendrites (figure 7.14,
plate 12). These calcium microdomains are dependent on the fast kinetics of calcium-permeable (CP) AMPA receptors and fast local extrusion via the $Na^+/Ca^{2+}$

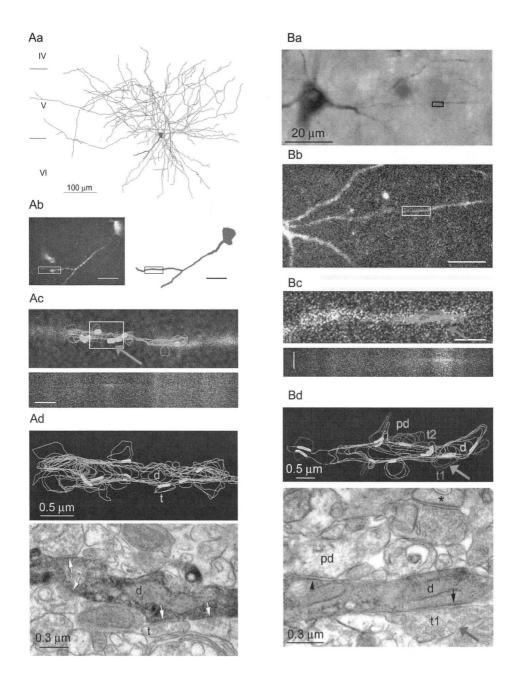

exchanger. Therefore, the diffusional isolation caused by the spine neck is not necessary to generate a calcium compartment, as long as the extrusional pathways are fast (figure 7.15). Also, because aspiny dendrites throughout the CNS express CP-AMPA receptors, it is possible that CP-AMPA receptors, together with $Na^+/Ca^{2+}$ exchangers, mediate a spine-free mechanism of input-specific calcium compartmentalization. Therefore, in principle, diffusional isolation and morphological features such as the spine neck are not strictly necessary to generate a calcium compartment. Although these data do not negate that spines can compartmentalize calcium, they call into question the idea that the only function of spines is to generate calcium compartments.

**Calcium in Spines: A Functional Interpretation**

In summary, it is clear that spines compartmentalize calcium under different functional regimes. With subthreshold EPSPs, elevated $[Ca^{2+}]_i$ can be restricted to individual spines, in fact, to the spine receiving the synaptic input (figure 7.2; Denk et al., 1995; Emptage et al., 1999; Koester and Sakmann, 1998; Kovalchuk et al., 2000; Müller and Connor, 1991; Yuste and Denk, 1995). Also, even under APs, when calcium influxes occur simultaneously in spines and dendrites, many spines experience substantially higher calcium accumulations than their parent dendrites during a short window of time (figure 7.2; Koester and Sakmann, 1998; Majewska et al., 2000a; Yuste and Denk, 1995). Finally, under simultaneous (or temporally consecutive) EPSPs and APs, individual spines sustain highly elevated levels of $[Ca^{2+}]_i$ (figures 7.5 and 7.6; Koester and Sakmann, 1998; Petrozzino et al., 1995; Yuste and Denk, 1995; Yuste et al., 1999) and these extremely high accumulations do not spread to their parent dendrites or neighboring spines (figure 7.5; Yuste and Denk, unpublished). Although with some small disagreements concerning the effect of CNQX

**Figure 7.14 (plate 12)**
Calcium compartmentalization in aspiny neurons does not result from morphological diffusional boundaries. Ultrastructural reconstructions of imaged dendrites in an experiment similar to figure 7.13B. (Aa) Biocytin reconstruction of neocortical layer 5 fast spiking interneuron. Dendrites, orange; axon, black. Red dendritic segment represents region of interest in (Ab). (Ab) Two-photon z projection of imaged region of interest of the neuron, field with a calcium indicator, left, and corresponding region from the cell reconstruction, right. Boxes indicate the dendritic segment selected for line scan imaging and for EM reconstruction. Scale bar: 20 μm. (Ac) (Top) Horizontal dendrite of interest with the cartoon of the serial EM reconstruction overlay at the precisely realigned section. (Bottom) Line scan through dendrite reveals the evoked single synaptic calcium signal. Note how its position appeared aligned to the synapse, as indicated by the red arrow in the cartoon. (Ad, top) Cartoon detail of the serial reconstruction. Dendrite (d) is labeled in green, and terminals (t) in white. The terminal labeled by the "t" corresponds to the terminal of interest in Ac. (Bottom) The electron micrograph focusing on the site aligned to the microdomain; arrows indicate synapses. (B) Data from a different neuron, laid out as in (A). (Bb) Scale bar: 20 μm. (Bc) top, scale bar: 2 μm; bottom, scale bar: 400 ms. (Bc–Bd) Red arrow points to a candidate synapse aligned with the microdomain. Reprinted from Goldberg et al., 2003a.

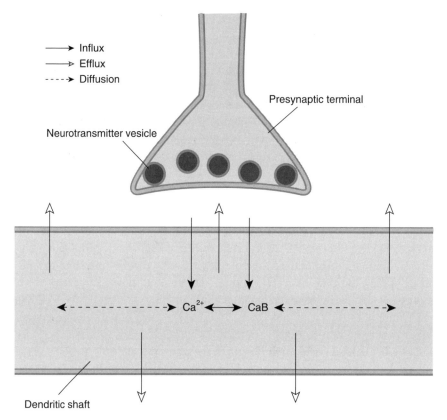

**Figure 7.15**
Calcium dynamics in nonspiny neurons. The spatiotemporal evolution of calcium compartmentalization results from the interactions between the effect of fixed and mobile buffers, the kinetics of calcium influx and efflux, and the dendrite radius.

and release blockers, perhaps due to different experimental methods, these studies paint a consistent picture of the calcium influx mechanisms into spines, confirming that spines are calcium compartments that can detect the temporal relation between input (EPSPs) and output (AP) of the neurons using NMDA receptors, and transform them into different calcium dynamics. In addition, as a spin-off from these experiments, the visualization of the activation of individual synapses (optical quantal analysis) has become feasible (Emptage et al., 1999; Mainen et al., 1999; Yuste and Denk, 1995; Yuste et al., 1999; see figures 7.3 and 7.4).

   Calcium compartmentalization in spines likely results from a combination of morphological and physiological determinants. While the thin spine neck restricts diffusional coupling of dextrans (Svoboda et al., 1996), proteins (Majewska et al., 2000b), and even calcium (Holthoff et al., 2002b; Majewska et al., 2000a), local influx and extrusion mechanisms probably play a dominant role in restricting and locally controlling spine calcium dynamics (Denk et al., 1995; Emptage et al., 1999; Holthoff et al., 2002b; Koester and Sakmann, 1998; Kovalchuk et al., 2000; Majewska et al., 2000a; Sabatini et al., 2002; Yuste and Denk, 1995). Indeed, local extrusion by itself can generate calcium microcompartments in aspiny cells (figure 7.13).

What is the purpose of calcium compartmentalization in spines? The exquisite sensitivity of spine $[Ca^{2+}]_i$ to the timing of input or output of the cell (Koester and Sakmann, 1998; Yuste and Denk, 1995) strongly suggests that spine $[Ca^{2+}]_i$ dynamics are involved in computational tasks. In fact, the pairing of input and output that generates the supralinear $[Ca^{2+}]_i$ increases in spines drives synapse-specific LTP (or spike-timing dependent plasticity) in a variety of systems in vitro and in vivo (Magee and Johnston, 1997; Markram et al., 1997b; Wigstrom et al., 1986; Zhang et al., 1998). This LTP is synapse specific and blocked by calcium chelators (Lynch et al., 1983; Malenka et al., 1989). As in the cricket auditory system (Sobel and Tank, 1994), the computational variable, in this case the synapse-specific change in synaptic weight (i.e., the term $dw_{ij}$ of the learning rule in a neural network; Hopfield, 1982), could be physically implemented as the concentration or dynamics of a chemical species such as calcium (see chapters 8 and 10). In the case of spines, then, calcium compartmentalization would restrict plasticity to individual inputs and thus implement local learning rules.

The morphological determinants of calcium compartmentalization suggest that spines might compartmentalize other ions, such as sodium or protons, second messengers such as IP3 or cAMP, signaling enzymes such as small GTPases or calmodulin, mRNA of different types, small proteins, such as Ras (Yasuda et al., 2006), or even voltage (Rall, 1974b). In fact, recent imaging experiments go beyond calcium, describing the rich dynamics of this spatially dependent biochemistry in spine (Lee et al., 2009; Murakoshi et al., 2008).

An additional lesson learned is that spines have multiple mechanisms for calcium influx and removal. There are at least five independent pathways that contribute to calcium accumulations in spines: VSCCs, NMDA receptors, calcium-permeable AMPA receptors, IP3 receptors, and Ryanodine receptors. Also, extrusion is controlled by at least two pathways—SERCA pumps and diffusion through the spine neck—although other pathways (PMCA and exchangers in particular) are likely to be effective. Even if we strictly consider spines as individual calcium compartments, these data reveal that spines are not simple structures, but have a rich diversity of mechanisms that affect their calcium dynamics. The purpose of such diversity is probably to sustain independent regulation of $[Ca^{2+}]_i$. Each pathway may subserve a particular function, and different mechanisms could produce different spatiotemporal $[Ca^{2+}]_i$ dynamics. Evidence for this idea includes the data showing that APs specifically increase spine $[Ca^{2+}]_i$ through VSCCs, whereas EPSPs mediate calcium

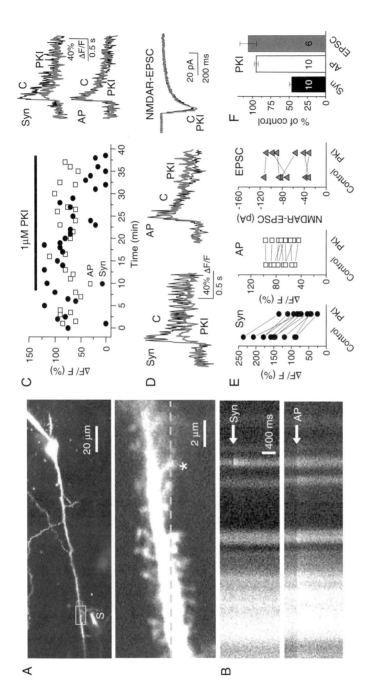

**Figure 7.16**
Modulation of spine calcium influx by protein kinase A. (A) Two-photon image of a CA1 pyramidal neuron filled with a calcium indicator. The rectangle indicates a portion of the apical dendrite (enlarged below) adjacent to the stimulating electrode (S); the asterisk indicates a spine in which synaptically evoked calcium accumulations were observed. Line scans (shown in B) were performed along the trajectory indicated by the horizontal dashed line. (B) Calcium accumulations induced by subthreshold synaptic stimulation (Syn, top), or a backpropagating action potential (AP, bottom). Calcium accumulations in several additional spines and the dendritic shaft. (C) Representative experiment in which Syn and AP calcium accumulations were evoked alternately and plotted as a function of time. On right, representative calcium transients (expressed as fractional change in fluorescence DF/F) before and after the application of the inhibitor PKI(14–22) calcium transients in control cells were stable for up to 50 min. (D–F) Calcium transients and NMDAR-mediated EPSCs recorded from the same CA1 pyramidal cells. (D) Sample traces from a representative experiment in CNQX (C, control; PKI, after 30 min in PKI(14–22)). (E) Summary data of the calcium accumulations (Syn, AP) and NMDAR-EPSCs in control conditions and after PKI(14–22) for each individual experiment. (F) Summary bar graph of the normalized responses (numbers indicate the total number of independent experiments). Reprinted from Skeberdis et al., 2006.

influx through glutamate receptors (Denk et al., 1995; Emptage et al., 1999; Koester and Sakmann, 1998; Kovalchuk et al., 2000; Yuste and Denk, 1995). Moreover, even a single pathway, such as the NMDARs calcium influx, can be differently regulated in spines according to their exact subunit composition (NR2A vs NR2B) (Sobczyk et al., 2005). As a dramatic example of the functional regulation of these calcium pathways, the state of the NMDAR PKA-dependent phosphorylation can shut off this main pathway of calcium influx into spines (figure 7.16; Skeberdis et al., 2006). Thus, the spine can modulate quite well its calcium dynamics according to the biochemical state of the cell. A similar functional regulation, with different functional regimes engaging distinct pathways, is conceivable for different extrusion mechanisms.

A final conclusion, already mentioned in past chapters, is that spines are quite heterogeneous. As the reader can appreciate, even in a small dendritic region of a single cell type, like the CA1 pyramidal neuron, heterogeneity holds for spine morphologies (Harris and Stevens, 1989), receptor composition (Nusser et al., 1998), and calcium influx and efflux mechanisms (Majewska et al., 2000a; Yuste et al., 1999; Denk et al., 1995). Additionally, as I have discussed in chapter 6, morphological changes in spines can be observed in rapid (<1 minute) time scales (Dunaevsky et al., 1999; Fischer et al., 1998), implying that the diffusional clearance mechanisms in spines can change quickly (figures 7.10 and 7.11). What is the purpose of this heterogeneity? As the correlation between spine size and presynaptic terminal parameters indicates (chapter 3), this diversity could match the diversity of synaptic inputs spines receive. The fact that functional spine diversity is found even in the molecular region of Purkinje cells (Denk et al., 1995), where spines receive a relatively pure input, suggests that factors other than the nature of the input might be at play. Perhaps spine diversity could also reflect the life history of a spine, particularly if spine-specific learning rules regulate spine structure (see chapter 8) or locally control the proteins present in spines.

# 8 Plasticity

*The search for morphological correlates of learning has constituted a central question in neuroscience. One dominant hypothesis for a mechanism for learning in the brain is that spines implement input-specific long-term synaptic plasticity, because of their calcium compartmentalization. From many studies in this field, I focus on the link between spine plasticity and hippocampal long-term potentiation (LTP), the most widely studied cellular model of learning. Ultrastructural and imaging studies have reported changes in spines after LTP, such as enlargements of the spine head and shortenings of the spine neck. These changes can help explain the increased synaptic strength. Although increased spinogenesis can occur after synaptic stimulation, it is unlikely to contribute to LTP. The correlation between spine morphological changes and input-specific forms of synaptic plasticity, together with the long-term structural stability of spines in the adult CNS, supports the idea that spines can implement learning rules. In this scenario, after a critical period of postnatal development with major structural plasticity and synaptic pruning, the nervous system would become hardwired. In the adult CNS, most plasticity would result from increases or decreases in synaptic strength, rather than from the generation of new connections or loss of existing ones.*

After several chapters highlighting different aspects of the spine biology, we arrive at the discussion of the relation between changes in spines and learning. In fact, the search for the mechanisms underlying learning in the brain spans more than a century. Cajal speculated that learning required growth of neuronal processes, rather than the addition of new neurons (Ramón y Cajal, 1893). In fact, in one of the few recordings of Cajal's original voice, he states that "if we do not have the possibility of increasing our neuron number, we are blessed instead with the privilege of altering, ramifying and complicating the neuronal arbors, which, like telegraph wires, can combine up to the infinity the reflex associations and created ideas" (Cajal's original voice recording from TVE documentary *Las Mariposas del Alma*, translated by the author).

As an alternative idea, recapitulating an earlier suggestion from Spencer (1862), Tanzi (1893) argued that it was not actual neuronal growth, but changes in existing connections that might underlie storage of memories in the brain. Both ideas were later incorporated into a unified proposal by Hebb in his landmark book, where he suggested that alterations in synaptic strength, as well as formation of novel synapses, could mediate memory storage (Hebb, 1949).

**Morphological Plasticity of Spines**

Over many decades, many experimental or behavioral conditions have been associated with changes in spine morphology. In fact, this is such a large literature that it sometimes seems that pretty much anything that alters the function of the nervous system can produce changes in spines. Given the tight link between spine morphology and synaptic function, this may not be so surprising.

From this vast literature, I will highlight only some particularly relevant studies, and then discuss in detail the manipulations that give rise to LTP, because it is perhaps the most studied form of synaptic plasticicity and also exemplifies an archetypical learning rule. I will not discuss the molecular mechanisms associated with morphological changes in spines, a topic partly covered already in chapters 4 and 6.

With some exceptions, studies that have investigated morphological changes in spines after an experimental manipulation indicate that increases of neural activity generate more spines. For example, light deprivation in mice causes a reversible reduction in the number of spines in pyramidal neurons from primary visual cortex (Globus and Scheibel, 1967; Valverde, 1967, 1971). The opposite alteration, visual stimulation, increases spine density (Parnavelas et al., 1973). Other environmental manipulations, such as rearing animals in complex environments, can alter spine morphology (Greenough and Volkmar, 1973); so does social isolation (Connor and Diamond, 1982) and even space flight (Belichenko and Krasnov, 1991). Spine size reduction has been reported after the first orientation flight in honeybees (Brandon and Coss, 1982). In birds, plastic changes in spine morphologies are observed during postnatal development (Rausch and Scheich, 1982), after imprinting with light (Bradley and Horn, 1979) and in association with learning tasks involving pecking (Patel et al., 1988). Finally, squirrels lose 40% of their spines during hibernation, and recover them in a few hours after arousal from hibernation (Popov and Bocharova, 1992; Popov et al., 1992).

Alterations in spine form and number after changes in neuronal activity have also been observed in vitro. In fact, pyramidal neurons in dissociated cultures (Boyer et al., 1998; Papa et al., 1995; Papa and Segal, 1996) as well as in brain slices (Kirov et al., 1999) have increased spine densities, compared with pyramidal neurons in vivo, confirming the idea that neurons could adjust their spine number according to their environment (see chapter 5). Pharmacological manipulations also influence spine morphology and number. In slices, stimulation of AMPA receptors is needed to maintain spines, whereas blocking AMPA receptors reduces the number of spines (McKinney et al., 1999). On the other hand, synaptic blockade with high $Mg^{2+}$ and low $Ca^{2+}$ increases both spine number and size (Kirov and Harris, 1999). In cultured neurons, disinhibition with bicuculline (Papa and Segal, 1996) as well as stimulation of internal calcium release increase the number and size of spines (Korkotian and Segal, 1999).

As discussed in chapter 5, spines (and synapses) are first generated, and later reduced in number, during normal development and aging (Rakic et al., 1986; Ramón y Cajal, 1904). In fact, even during the estrous cycle, large numbers of spines are produced in the hippocampus and later eliminated in substantial numbers (Woolley and McEwen, 1994). Finally, many diseases such as dementia (Mehraein et al., 1975), mental retardation (Purpura, 1974), Down syndrome (Marín-Padilla, 1972), irradiation sickness (Brizzee et al., 1980), malnutrition (Salas, 1980), fragile X syndrome (Wisniewski et al., 1991), and epilepsy (Multani et al., 1994) produce abnormalities in spine densities or morphologies.

## Long-Term Potentiation as a Cellular Model for Memory

From the preceding brief exposition, it is clear that spine morphologies are quite plastic and could indeed be involved causally in the mechanisms the brain uses to adapt to new environmental situations or store new information. At the same time, the manipulations described above are likely to produce global changes in brain function, making it difficult to disentangle the role of spines in any given part of the brain in these processes. A more focused approach is therefore necessary, one in which the experimental manipulation is relatively clean-cut and the region of the brain involved in the changes has been clearly identify.

One of the key regions involved in learning and memory behaviors in the mammalian brain is the hippocampal formation. An important milestone in this field occurred in 1973, when it was discovered that brief tetanic stimulation produced a long-lasting form of synaptic plasticity, LTP, which can last for days in the mammalian hippocampus (Bliss and Lømo, 1973). Thus, the brief and repeated stimulation of a synaptic pathway leads to its persistent enhancement. Interestingly, the involvement of the hippocampal formation in memory was established by clinical data indicating that lesions of this structure in humans produce anterograde amnesia (Milner, 1966). Since this time, many laboratories have studied LTP as a cellular model for information storage in the brain, and it is fair to say that hippocampal LTP is the main hypothesis to explain how the brain might store information (for a collection of reviews, see Baudry and Davis, 1996). In fact, just as LTP could be a cellular model of learning, long-term depression (LTD) is often cited as a potential cellular model of forgetting (Bear and Abraham, 1996). So, one could also focus on how the brain forgets, rather than learns, and how that relates to morphological changes in spines. Finally, recent research is pointing out that LTP and LTD are just two aspects of a more general, temporally dependent learning rule, often described as "spike timing dependent plasticity" (STDP), where the potentiation or depression crucially depends on the temporal relation between the synaptic input and spike output (Markram et al., 1997b). Therefore, many of the LTP experiments that will be reviewed in the following sections could be in principle be understood as sampling one single point, out of a larger temporal structure of this learning rule.

I should mention that, although the relation of LTP to learning is not universally accepted (see Mayford et al. 1996 in favor and Zamanillo et al. 1999 against it), it is a widely used and helpful paradigm for long-term synaptic plasticity in a central synapse. LTP, furthermore, nicely relates to neural network theories of brain function, because it implements a local learning rule, an essential element for associative neuronal networks (Hebb, 1949; Hopfield, 1982), which ensures many of the computational features that make neural networks so attractive (Rolls and Treves, 1998).

A recent flurry of work, much of it using novel imaging techniques and time-lapse recordings, has added important information with regard to the role of morphological changes of spines in LTP (Alvarez and Sabatini, 2007; Bourne and Harris, 2008). In addition, the relation between morphological and functional parameters of the spine is clear: The volume of the spine-head is directly proportional to the number of postsynaptic receptors (Nusser et al., 1998) and to the presynaptic number of docked vesicles (see chapter 3; Schikorski and Stevens, 1999). Also, the length of the spine neck controls the time constant of calcium diffusion from spines and electrically filters the synaptic potential (see chapters 7 and 9; Araya et al., 2007; Majewska et al., 2000a, b; Yuste et al., 2000). This implies that the morphology of a spine directly reflects its function, making it particularly relevant to investigate morphological changes of spines during synaptic plasticity.

**Ultrastructural Studies of Spines after LTP**

Even when examining a relatively focused question such as the relation between LTP and spines, the number of studies is very large with often contradictory results, making it difficult to be thorough and impossible to agree with every proposal. To help our review of this topic, I focus only on LTP or synaptic stimulation experiments from mammalian hippocampus and, briefly, on LTD in this discussion.

As we will see, the relation between LTP and spine morphological plasticity appears as a relatively straightforward issue, with few and clear-cut possibilities: LTP could either give rise to new spines or to changes in the morphology of existing spines. Nevertheless, published results are controversial, with studies claiming one or another possibility, both, or neither.

## Spine Morphological Changes after LTP

Although long-lasting potentiation of the myotatic reflex in the mammalian spinal cord was already described by Eccles and McIntyre in 1953 (Eccles and McIntyre, 1953), it was the report by Lømo and Bliss of LTP in the monosynaptic connections between the perforant pathway and the granule cells in the dentate gyrus of the hippocampus that triggered enormous interest in the investigation of the morphological consequences of long-term synaptic enhancement in the CNS (figure 8.1; Lømo, 1970; Bliss and Lømo, 1973).

Some of the earliest studies on the effect of hippocampal LTP on the morphology of spines were carried out by Van Harrefeld and Fifkova (1975), with a similar experimental protocol to that of Bliss and Lømo. By using a rapid freeze-substitution electron microscopy, which largely preserves spine morphology, the authors compared spines from granule cells in the distal region of the dentate gyrus (the region that receives perforant pathway inputs) with those in the proximal region, devoid of such inputs, in stimulated and unstimulated tissue. In control animals, distal spines had on average 13% larger head areas than proximal spines, but that difference increased to 53% in stimulated animals. This effect was present as early as 2 minutes after stimulation and lasted at least 60 minutes, indicating that, like the synaptic enhancement produced by LTP, the increased volume was immediately produced by the tetanization and was long lasting. The authors proposed that the increase in head volume was produced by swelling caused by the uptake of electrolytes. To further explore the relation between synaptic stimulation and spine swelling, in a second study the same authors carried out a temporal characterization of the effect, extending their observation time up to 23 hours (Fifkova and Van Harrefeld, 1977). Again, they observed an increased volume of spines from stimulated animals compared to controls. This increase was significant at all times tested (2 minutes to 23 hours), although it was largest (39%) 10 to 60 minutes after the stimulation. As a further control, no systematic differences were observed in the proximal spines between stimulated and control animals.

The effect of tetanic stimulation on the size of the spine neck was specifically examined by Fifkova and Anderson (1981). Again, this study found an increase in the volume of the spine head in distal spines after tetanic stimulation. In addition, they found major increases (up to 42%) in the width of the spine neck, as well as shortenings (as much as 31%) of its length. These changes were, again, specific to distal spines and were present for as long as 90 minutes after the stimulation.

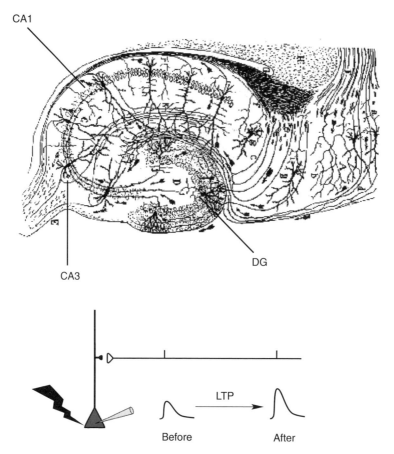

**Figure 8.1**
Hippocampal long-term potentiation (LTP). (Top) Drawing of the hippocampal circuit, labeling the trynaptic pathway from the dentate gyrus (DG), to the CA3 field, to the CA1 field. Modified from Cajal. (Bottom) LTP experiment. The response of a neuron to the stimulation of one of its inputs (top axon) increases after LTP.

These initial studies painted a consistent picture of the effects of tetanizing the perforant pathway: The spine heads in the distal region of the dentate gyrus become larger, while the spine necks become shorter, yet wider (figure 8.2). Although these studies did not confirm electrophysiologically the LTP presumably produced by the stimulation protocols, or proved that the spines analyzed were the ones that had been tetanized, the anatomical changes were long lasting and restricted to distal spines receiving perforant path inputs, just as one would predict from the properties of LTP. Fifkova proposed that the enlargement of the spine head was in fact a result of the synapse's increased size, and that its ultimate stabilization might be mediated by the mobilization of actin caused by local increases in $[Ca^{2+}]_i$ (Fifkova, 1985).

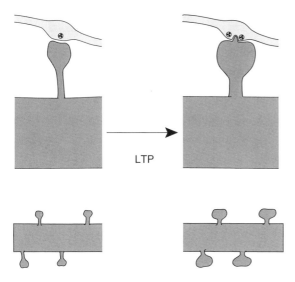

**Figure 8.2**
LTP induces changes in spine morphologies. Fifkova results: LTP results in larger spine heads, and shorter and wider spine necks.

Similar conclusions to the Fifkova studies were drawn by Desmond and Levy from a series of combined electrophysiological/ultrastructural experiments (Desmond and Levy, 1983; 1986a; 1986b; 1988; Levy, 1985). They again used the rat perforant pathway/dentate gyrus as the model system and combined field potential recordings and quantitative EM to search for changes in size and number of synapses after LTP. In these studies, two different stimulation protocols were used: either a short burst of stimuli or a more distributed protocol with the same number of electrical shocks but spread out over time. Anatomical changes occurred following the two forms of conditioning, with up to 48% increases in the density in concave spines, but described a concomitant 23% decrease in the number of nonconcave spine profiles (Desmond and Levy, 1983; 1986a). Concave spine profiles, in their nomenclature, correspond to the population of larger spines that have spinules or U-shaped profiles (perforated spines), thus they essentially described an increase in larger spines and a decrease in smaller ones.

These changes were more pronounced in the middle third of the molecular layers, the dentate gyrus region that was stimulated by their more medial electrode placement in the perforant pathway. Although increases in the shaft synapses were initially observed (Desmond and Levy, 1983), in their later studies Desmond and Levy failed to detect significant changes in the total density of shaft or spine synapses (Desmond and Levy, 1986a).

These observations were further extended in a quantitative study of the size of the postsynaptic densities (PSD), in which the total PSD surface area per unit volume in the larger, concave spines increased significantly, whereas the PSD area of the smaller, nonconcave ones decreased (Desmond and Levy, 1986b). In addition, the mean PSD length increased significantly across all spine profiles in stimulated animals and persisted for at least 60 minutes. In a later study, the authors found concomitant changes in the presynaptic terminals (Desmond and Levy, 1988).

While these data demonstrated increases in spine size after LTP but, at the same time, other groups provided evidence for increases in spine number (see below). This prompted Desmond and Levy to consider the possibility of an increase in the number of synapses in the dentate gyrus (Desmond and Levy, 1990). The authors used the presence of two morphological markers of synaptogenesis—polyribosomes and multiple synaptic contacts—and found statistically significant *decreases*, rather than increases, in their incidence after LTP, arguing for a modification of existing synapses, rather than de novo synaptogenesis. This result was extended to somatic ribosomes in a later publication from the same group, indicating that LTP is associated with increased protein synthesis (Wenzel et al., 1993).

In conclusion, the Fifkova and Desmond/Levy studies proposed a scenario with an interconversion of spine shapes during LTP, without addition of new synapses (figure 8.2). Smaller spines become larger, and this is mirrored by increases in the size of the synaptic surface area and shortening and widening of the spine neck. In agreement with Tanzi's early suggestion, these data argued for the hypothesis that the change in the function of the brain after repeated stimulation protocols results not from the addition of new synapses or spines but from the morphological and physiological modification of existing ones. As we will see later, these results have been confirmed in more recent experiments, imaging living spines during LTP.

**Effects of LTP on Synapse Localization**

In their studies, Fifkova et al. did not establish whether the stimulation protocols used indeed produced long-lasting synaptic plasticity. To address this, Lynch's laboratory undertook several studies combining electrophysiological recordings with EM, examining the morphological effects of synaptic plasticity (Lee et al., 1979a, 1979b, 1980). These experiments were carried out stimulating the Schaffer collateral pathway in vivo (Lee et al., 1979b, 1980) or in vitro (Lee et al., 1979a). Instead of examining LTP in the dentate gyrus, they focused on the CA1 region of the hippocampus. The authors used ultrathin EM sections to compare the effects of low-frequency stimulation, which did not produce any long-lasting potentiation, with high-frequency stimulation, which produced LTP. After both in vivo and in vitro stimulation, the authors found a 33 to 50% increase in synaptic contacts on dendritic shafts in high-frequency–stimulated animals. No significant differences were found in the number

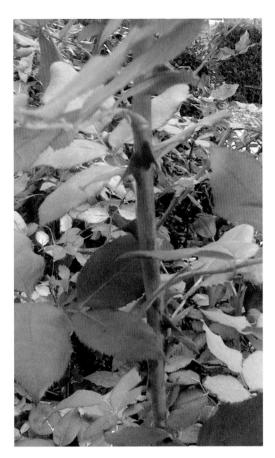

**Plate 1 (Figure 2.3)**
Spines in a rose bush. Suggested by J. De Felipe.

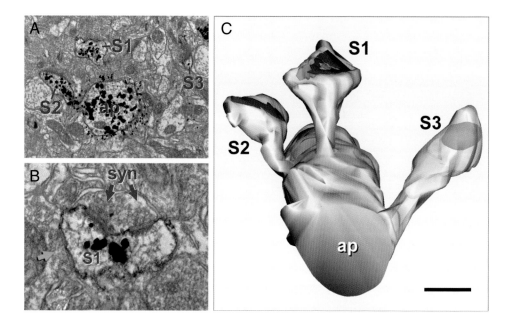

**Plate 2 (Figure 3.6)**
Inhibitory synapse on spine. (A) Ultrastructural section through the head of two spines from an apical dendrite of a mouse neocortical pyramidal neuron. (B) Detail of the asymmetrical synapse (syn) on one of
them; note the perforated PSD, the synaptic cleft and the presynaptic terminal with rounded vesicles.
This spine also established a symmetrical synapse (green arrow, left membrane). (C) Three-dimensional
reconstruction of the same segment, displaying three spines (S1–3); the rendering has been slightly shifted
down to show the synaptic junctions and S3 is partially transparent to show the location of the PSD. S1
has an inhibitory synaptic contact (green), in addition to an excitatory one (red). Scale bar: 0.6 μm.
Reprinted from Arellano et al., 2007a.

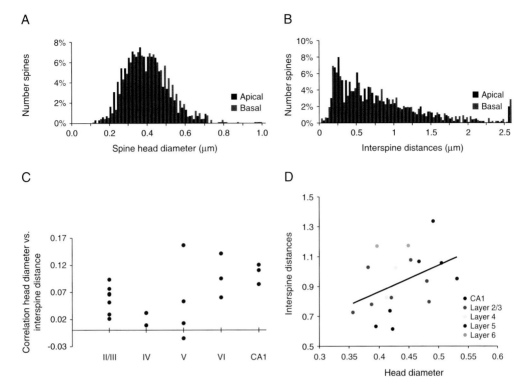

**Plate 3 (Figure 3.18)**
Distribution of spine sizes and densities in pyramidal neurons and correlations between spine size and densities. (A) Apical (black) and basal (red) dendritic spine head diameter histogram of a layer 2/3 pyramidal neuron. Histogram is normalized such that total amount of apical and basal head diameter values adds up to 100% each. Distributions are approximately normal. (B) Apical (black) and basal (red) interspine distance histogram. Distribution is highly skewed. (C) Analysis of spine head diameters and interspine distances. The correlation coefficients between interspine distances and spine head diameters plotted with respect to the layer that the cell belongs to. In 18 out of 19 cells a positive correlation is observed. (D) Average spine head diameter plotted against its average interspine distance. Reprinted from Konur et al., 2003.

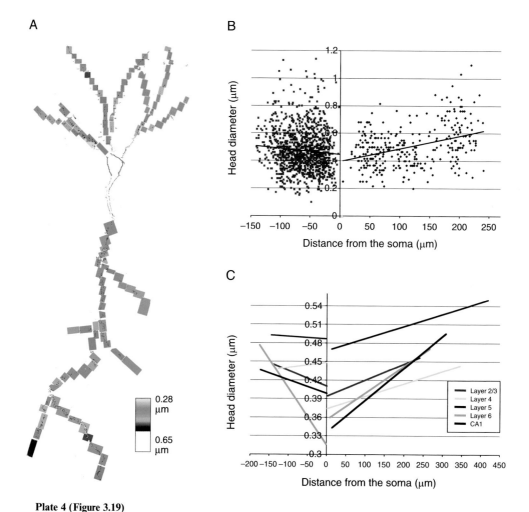

**Plate 4 (Figure 3.19)**
Spine size increases in distal dendrites. (A) Topographical distribution of spine head diameters along a CA1 pyramidal neuron. Each dendritic segment is color coded according to the average head diameter of the spines within that segment. The color scale shows the corresponding values. Bluer hues correspond to larger heads whereas yellowish hues signify smaller heads. Note blue regions at the distal apical dendrite in the stratum lacunosum-moleculare region. (B) Measurement of spine head diameter as a function of distance from the soma from this CA1 neuron. Note how spines become larger in the distal apical dendritic tree (blue). (C) Average relations for CA1 cells and neocortical pyramidal neurons from different layers. Reprinted from Konur et al., 2003.

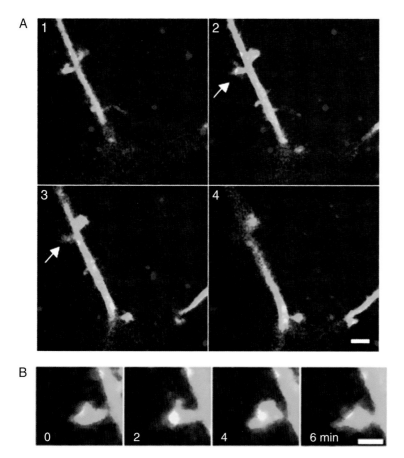

**Plate 5 (Figure 6.12)**
Spine motility with synaptic contact. Acute hippocampal slices from P7–P10 mice expressing GFP in a subset of CA1 pyramidal neurons. FM 1–43 staining is used to image active presynaptic terminals. (A) Dual GFP (green = postsynaptic) and FM 1–43 (red = presynaptic) images of single z sections 0.7 μm apart. In the 2nd and 3rd frames, a potential contact can be identified between a hand-like spine and a FM 1–43-stained bouton (arrow). Scale bar: 2 μm. (B) Time sequence of projected dual images of this potential contact. Scale bar: 1 μm. Reprinted from Konur and Yuste, 2004b.

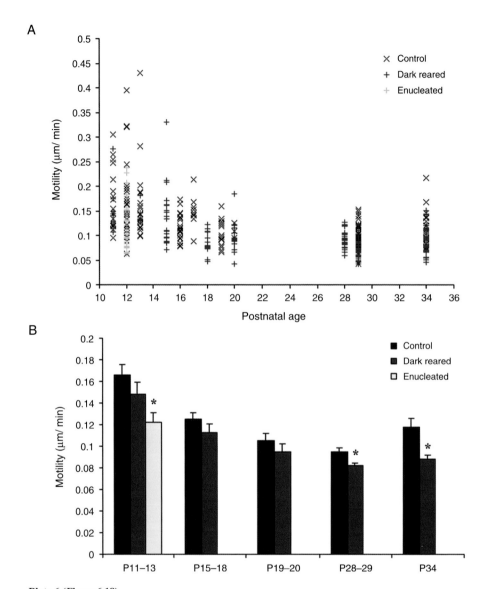

**Plate 6 (Figure 6.18)**
Developmental regulation of spine motility in mouse primary visual cortex and effect of sensory deprivation. (A) In control animals, higher motility disappears after P14 and a baseline is then reached, well before the critical period occurs (~P25–30). Dark-reared or enucleated animals follow a similar developmental trend and display a small reduction in motility. Each cross corresponds to data imaging spine motility in one neuron. (B) Mean motility in different age groups. Reprinted from Konur and Yuste, 2004a.

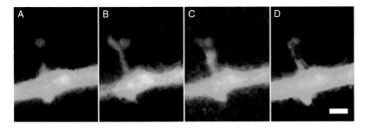

**Plate 7 (Figure 6.19)**
Spine motility and potential synaptogenesis. (A–D) A highly motile postsynaptic filopodia (green) is interacting with a relatively nonmotile presynaptic bouton (red) and becomes stabilized. Reprinted from Konur and Yuste, 2004b. Scale bar: 1 μm.

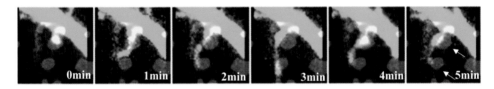

**Plate 8 (Figure 6.22)**
Spine motility with neighboring synaptic terminals. Live imaging of a dendritic spine (green) and presynaptic boutons (red). The spine moves while touching two boutons (arrows). In the 4th frame, it approaches another bouton. Scale bar: 1 μm. Reprinted from Konur and Yuste, 2004b.

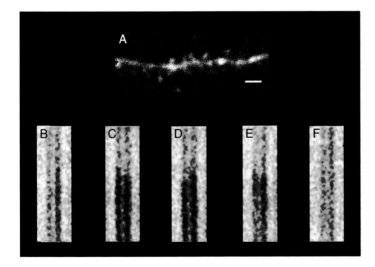

**Plate 9 (Figure 7.4)**
Optical quantal analysis. (Top) Two-photon image of a dendrite from a CA1 pyramidal neuron. Approximately 16 spines can be detected, covering the surface of the dendrite. Scale bar: 2 μm. (Bottom) Five consecutive line scans of the fluorescent responses of two adjacent spines (those on the center top of the dendrite) to paired-pulse synaptic stimulation (30-ms interval). The line scan cuts through the heads of the two adjacent spines. In the pseudocolor scale, yellow is low $[Ca^{2+}]_i$, and blue is high $[Ca^{2+}]_i$. (B): the right spine responds alone to stimulation. (C) Both spines respond, but the left one responds slightly ahead of the right one. (D) The case is reversed, with the right spine responding ahead of the left one. (E) Both spines respond similarly. (F) They both fail. These data reveal the stochastic activation of two adjacent synapses. Reprinted with permission from Yuste et al., 2000.

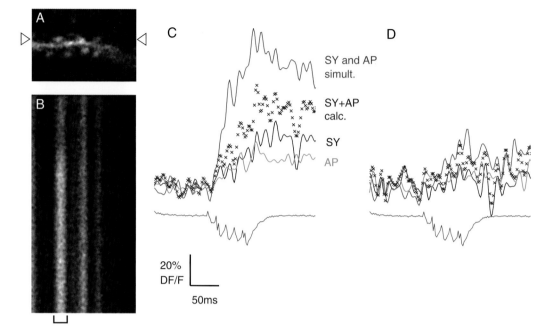

**Plate 10 (Figure 7.5)**
Supralinear calcium accumulations in spines under temporal coincidence of excitatory postsynaptic potentials (EPSP) and action potentials (APs). (A) Fluorescence image of a dendrite from a hippocampal pyramidal neuron, field with a calcium indicator. (B) Line scan through three spines (shown between white arrowheads in A), during a train of five subthreshold synaptic stimulations. Note how the left spine displays an increase in fluorescence, corresponding to a large increase in calcium concentration. (C) Calcium accumulations in left spine under different experimental conditions: subthreshold EPSPs (SY), postsynaptic spikes (AP), and their simultaneous combination (SY+AP). Note how simultaneous application of the AP and the EPSPs produces a "supralinear" accumulation that is larger (red) than the arithmetic sum of the AP and ESPS independently (blue). Reprinted from Yuste and Denk, 1995. (D) Calcium dynamics in the neighboring spine do not display a supralinear accumulation. Unpublished results from Yuste and Denk.

**Plate 11 (Figure 7.7)** ▶
Local dendritic spikes. (A) Drawing of a layer 5 pyramidal neuron in mouse visual cortex. Whole-cell recording was obtained in current clamp mode, and the neuron was filled via the patch-pipette with a low-affinity calcium indicator and imaged with a confocal microscope. (B) Pseudo-color images of relative fluorescence changes in basal dendrites before and after dendritic spike initiation. Scale bar: 25 μm. (C) Weak synaptic stimulation evoked an EPSP (bottom trace), but no calcium accumulation (top trace). (D) Strong synaptic stimulation evoked local dendritic spike accompanied by a large calcium transient in the activated dendrite and a complex EPSP. (E) Drawing of another layer 5 pyramidal neuron in visual cortex. (F) Pseudo-color coded images of relative fluorescence changes in an apical dendritic branch before and after strong synaptic stimulation. Scale bar: 10 μm. (G) Strong synaptic stimulation evoked local dendritic spike accompanied by a large calcium transient in the activated dendrite and a complex EPSP. (H) Back-propagating action potential (AP) induced by somatic current injection evoked a significantly smaller dendritic calcium transient. (I): Comparison of dendritic calcium transient amplitudes evoked by local dendritic spikes and backpropagating APs. Reprinted from Holthoff et al., 2004.

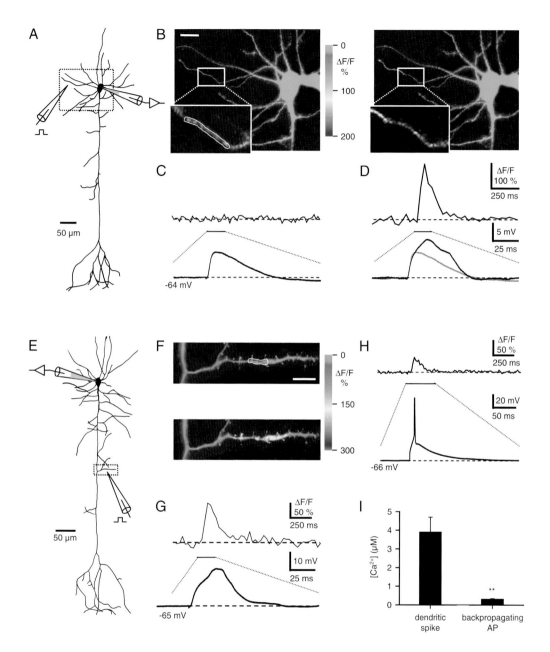

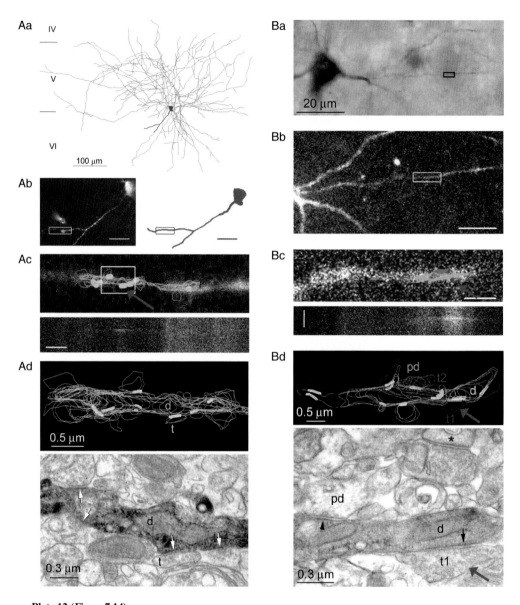

**Plate 12 (Figure 7.14)**
Calcium compartmentalization in aspiny neurons does not result from morphological diffusional boundaries. Ultrastructural reconstructions of imaged dendrites in an experiment similar to figure 7.13B. (Aa) Biocytin reconstruction of neocortical layer 5 fast spiking interneuron. Dendrites, orange; axon, black. Red
dendritic segment represents region of interest in (Ab). (Ab) Two-photon z projection of imaged region of
interest of the neuron, field with a calcium indicator, left, and corresponding region from the cell reconstruction, right. Boxes indicate the dendritic segment selected for line scan imaging and for EM reconstruction. Scale bar: 20 μm. (Ac) (Top) Horizontal dendrite of interest with the cartoon of the serial EM
reconstruction overlay at the precisely realigned section. (Bottom) Line scan through dendrite reveals the
evoked single synaptic calcium signal. Note how its position appeared aligned to the synapse, as indicated

**Plate 12 (Figure 7.14)** (continued)

by the red arrow in the cartoon. (Ad, top) Cartoon detail of the serial reconstruction. Dendrite (d) is labeled in green, and terminals (t) in white. The terminal labeled by the ''t'' corresponds to the terminal of interest in Ac. (Bottom) The electron micrograph focusing on the site aligned to the microdomain; arrows indicate synapses. (B) Data from a different neuron, laid out as in (A). (Bb) Scale bar: 20 μm. (Bc) top, scale bar: 2 μm; bottom, scale bar: 400 ms. (Bc–Bd) Red arrow points to a candidate synapse aligned with the microdomain. Reprinted from Goldberg et al., 2003a.

**Plate 13 (Figure 9.2)**

Active models of spines. (A) Amplification of EPSP by spines. Single-spine model with high sodium channel densities ($\sim$7000 mS/cm$^2$) can elicit localized AP responses in the spine (red) but not in the dendrite (black). Note that in order for this to occur, spine neck resistances need to be high ($>$100 MΩ) to provide sufficient electrical decoupling. (B) Moderately higher sodium channel densities ($\sim$200 mS/cm$^2$) globally in many spines can increase the efficacy of backpropagation. (Black) AP at soma; (blue) AP seen in apical dendrite 200 μm away, with weakly active spines ($G_{Na}$ = 40 mS/cm$^2$); (red) AP seen in apical dendrite with active spines ($G_{Na}$ = 200 mS/cm$^2$). Modulation of backpropagation does not require extensive electrical decoupling of spines. (C) The peak voltage response to a backpropagating action potential, represented by a color code. Backpropagation when Na channel densities in spines are relatively low (110 mS cm22) exhibits decremental invasion of the apical tree (left); with only moderately higher densities in spines (200 mS cm22), a backpropagating action potential is now able to invade the dendritic tree fully (right). Reprinted with permission from Tsay and Yuste, 2004.

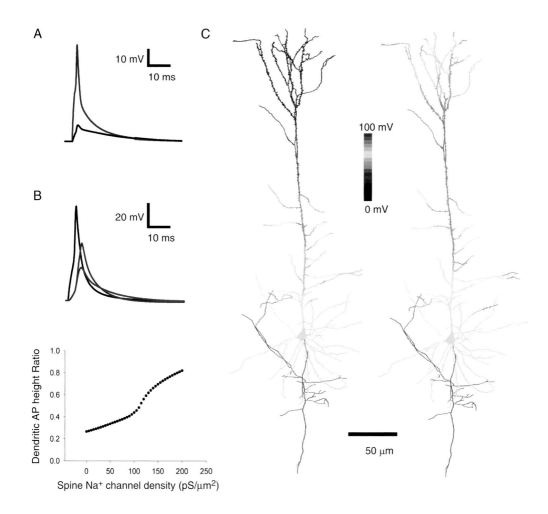

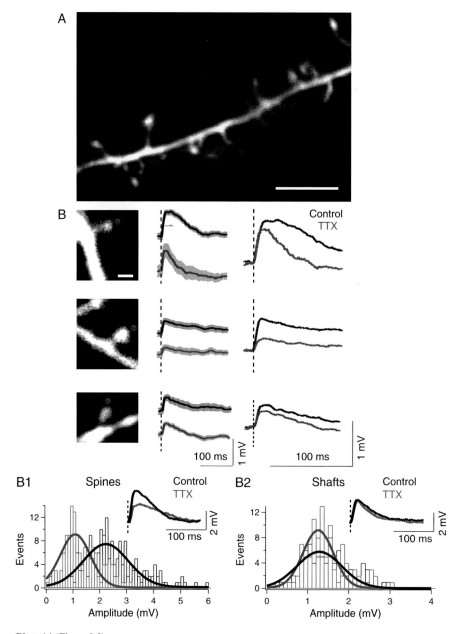

**Plate 14 (Figure 9.3)**
Spine sodium channels amplify spine potentials. The sodium channel blocker TTX reduces spine uncaging potentials. (A) Dendrite from a layer 5 pyramidal neuron, filled with a fluorescent indicator, whose spines where stimulated with two-photon glutamate uncaging. Scale bar: 5 μm. (B) Spine uncaging experiments. (Left) Red dots indicate site of laser uncaging. (Center) Uncaging potentials under control conditions (black traces) and in TTX (red traces). Dashed line is time of uncaging onset. Thicker traces are average of 10–15 depolarizations, and shaded areas illustrate SEM. (Right) Superimposition of average uncaging potentials. Note how TTX attenuates spine uncaging potentials. Scale bar: 1 μm. (B) Histogram of all individual uncaging potentials on spines (B1) and shafts (B2) in control and TTX. Note a shift toward smaller potentials caused by TTX in distribution of spine, but not shaft potentials, indicating that the TTX effect is specific to spines. Reprinted from Araya et al., 2007.

of synapses on spines, length of the spine PSDs, area of spines, width of spine necks, or length of the PSDs on the dendritic shafts. Nevertheless, in the potentiated group the authors found a reduction in the variance of several morphological features of the spines.

These studies did not confirm the swelling of spines or shortening of spine necks described by Fifkova and coworkers, showing instead an effect of LTP on the number of spines. A similar study was carried out by Chang and Greenough (1984). The authors also used hippocampal brain slices and ultrastructural analysis to compare the effects on CA1 spines of different protocols of stimulation, including high-frequency stimulation that produced LTP, high-frequency stimulation that did not produce LTP, low-frequency stimulation, and synaptic inactivation by high-$Mg^{2+}$ and low-$Ca^{2+}$ ACSF. After LTP, the authors found significant increases in the number of short, stubby spines and shaft synapses, with no detectable differences in the total number of spines or perforated synapses. Also, statistical reductions were observed in average spine perimeter, contact length, and the percentage of cup-shaped synapses (i.e., concave), although no significant changes were encountered in spine head area, bouton area, PSD length, spine neck width or length, and number of presynaptic vesicles. These authors concluded that LTP increased the synaptic innervation of interneurons, although they raised the possibility that it also induced the transition from shaft–to-spine synapses in CA1 pyramidal cells. These two effects would explain the increased number of synapses on dendritic shafts and stubby spines. They proposed that LTP produced a change in spine shape, where typical cup-shaped spines are transformed into a flatter spine profile with reduced spine perimeter and contact length.

**Increased Spinogenesis after LTP**

In the studies discussed so far the authors had reported rather small changes in spine number, spine shape, or geometry of the postsynaptic density. Andersen and co-workers were the first to report large increases in the number of spines, as well as rather dramatic changes in spine shape. The initial studies (Trommald et al., 1990) involved inducing LTP in the dentate gyrus. Serial reconstructions of EM material showed a doubling in spine number, changes in the diameter of the spine neck, and an increase in so-called bifurcated spines (figure 8.3). These structures are hypothesized to result from a splitting of a single synapse, first into a larger and supposedly more effective "perforated synapse" (Peters and Kaiserman-Abramof, 1969) and then into two synapses on different spine heads residing on a single spine trunk. Since perforated synapses could be particularly effective synapses, the observation of increased numbers of bifurcated spines naturally explained an increased synaptic efficacy. A later study by the same authors (Trommald et al., 1996) elaborated on these initial findings and found also an increased spine density and bifurcated spines.

Unstimulated                                    Stimulated

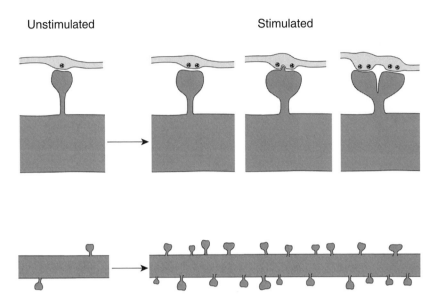

**Figure 8.3**
LTP induces new spines. According to this model, LTP results in the splitting of existing spines or appearance of new ones. After LTP, more spines are found.

The overall density of spines increased by about 30% while the number of bifurcated spines even rose by a factor of 3. The authors reported no statistically significant changes in the dimensions of the spines (Trommald et al., 1996).

The same authors later used confocal microscopy instead of electron microscopy to further investigate morphological correlates of synaptic plasticity (Moser et al., 1994). This allowed them to analyze more spines and have a better statistical sample to detect small changes. In these new studies, plastic changes were not induced by electrical stimulation but by an altered sensory environment. The assumption in this work is that the enriched sensory environment stimulated learning and thus LTP, but it was not know if these behavioral manipulations actually induced LTP. Instead of the dentate gyrus, morphological changes were assessed in the CA1 region of the hippocampus. Rats were housed either alone or in pairs in plastic cages and the experimental group was allowed to explore an environment with multiple platforms containing interesting items such as wooden blocks, branches, paper bags, and leaves placed on them. Although the animals who had the exploratory experience, on one hand, showed a better performance of behavioral tasks like the Morris water maze, they also showed a small but significant increase in spine density, with all other measured parameters being unaffected. The enhanced spine density occurred only on basal dendrites and not on apical dendrites (Moser et al., 1997).

## Unaltered Spine Shapes and Numbers

Harris and coworkers (Sorra and Harris, 1998) also tested whether tetanus-induced LTP would also result in an enhanced number of synapses in the CA1 region. They used an unbiased volume sampling procedure to detect possible changes in spine density or in the geometrical parameters of preexisting spines. In line with other investigators (Chang and Greenough, 1984; Lee et al., 1980; and others) they found no changes in absolute spine number. This contrasts with the findings by Andersen et al. (1980), who observed that in the dentate gyrus in vivo such changes occur. Two major differences between these studies could contribute to this contradiction: (1) The brain area investigated was different in the different studies (dentate gyrus versus CA1 region), and (2) the Sorra and Harris study was performed in slices whereas the others were performed in vivo. In this respect, a follow-up study (Kirov et al., 1999) is interesting and worrisome at the same time: These authors found that tissue that was prepared as hippocampal slice after one hour showed roughly twice the number of spines than "native" perfusion fixed tissue. A similar result had been reported earlier in somatic spines from granule cells from the dentate gyrus after slicing (Wenzel et al., 1994). Therefore, a possible explanation for the lack of changes in the CA1 region of slices is that so much spinogenesis had occurred after the initial preparation that additional changes were not possible any more. In fact, as with hibernating squirrels (Popov and Bocharova, 1992; Popov et al., 1992), the chilling and rewarming of brain slices appears to trigger the dissapearance and reappearance of spines (Bourne et al., 2007a; Kirov et al., 2004). Finally, in yet another study, Andersen's group replicated the study of Sorra and Harris showing that after 4 hours of LTP no net increase in spine number was observed in the CA1 of hippocampal slices, although they verified that the enriched environment causes spinogenesis (Andersen and Soleng, 1998).

From all these studies, it was clear that online observation of potential morphological in living samples would be a major technical improvement for detecting potential changes. It would obviate the requirement to rely on comparisons of large samples of experimental and control tissue and enabled the use of the temporal correlation of observed morphological changes with the experimental manipulations as a sensitive measure to detect causality. In fact, certain kinds of morphological changes are only detectable by online observation. For example, statistical methods have no way of excluding that an overall null change of spine density is actually caused by some new spines forming as a consequence of LTP and that this net gain of spines in the potentiated region is compensated by loss of spines elsewhere. In addition, another important drawback of studies on fixed tissue is that they all rely on comparison of different population of cells from different animals. Therefore time-lapse imaging of *living* tissue is clearly an important step forward in investigating morphological changes after LTP.

## Live Imaging Studies of Living Tissue during LTP

Hosokawa et al. (1992, 1995) pioneered in imaging living spines during synaptic plasticity. They used confocal microscopy of hippocampal slices in which individual CA1 pyramidal cells were stained by a DiI-microdrop technique. Synaptic potentiation was induced by chemical LTP, produced by application of a superfusion solution containing elevated $Ca^{2+}$, reduced $Mg^{2+}$, and tetraethylammonium (TEA). The reason for choosing this kind of LTP induction is to cause potentiation in as many synapses as possible. The authors observed that a subpopulation of small spines became longer and there was an increased range of angular displacement of spines in the potentiated tissue. All other parameters showed no significant changes. In particular, the appearance of completely new spines was a rare (and statistically insignificant) event. Hosokawa et al. concluded that LTP did not lead to increase spinogenesis.

A second group replicated Hosokawa's study, performing two-photon imaging on neurons labeleld with GPF in brain slices, before and after the perfusion of the same chemical LTP cocktail (Dunaevsky et al., 1999). No significant effect on spine numbers, densities, or even spine motility were detected, although, given the relatively low spatial resolution of two-photon microscopy, it cannot be ruled out that small changes in spine size or orientations could have occurred (figure 8.4; Tashiro and Yuste, unpublished experiments).

These results were challenged by two two-photon studies. In the first, Maletic-Savatic et al. (1999) used organotypic slices and local stimulation to investigate the effect of LTP on spinogenesis. Individual cells in these slices were visualized by infection of the slices with virus-eGFP constructs. These authors observed that a strong tetanus that would normally induce LTP led to local outgrowth of dendritic processes. The newly formed protrusions, however, were more akin to filopodia in that they were often more than 4 µm long and lacked a head. In some instances, however, these filopodia later turned into spinelike structures. The emergence of new protrusions could be blocked by agents such as APV, which interfere with LTP, although it was not clear whether the imaged neurons actually underwent LTP. Shortly afterwards, another study also reported that new spines can be formed in hippocampal tissue (Engert and Bonhoeffer, 1999). This study used a different strategy to pinpoint the locations where potential morphological changes could occur: In relatively thin organotypic slice cultures (Gähwihler, 1981), synaptic transmission was blocked by applying a medium with a relatively high concentration in $Cd^{2+}$ ions and low $Ca^{2+}$. This transmission blockade was then relieved only very locally (in an area of ~30 µm diameter) with a local superfusion system applying regular recording medium. In every instance of successful synaptic enhancement, new spines were generated, whereas practically no new spines appeared when the enhancement was not

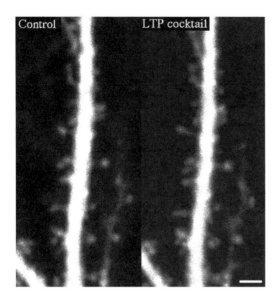

**Figure 8.4**
Imaging LTP. Frames from two-photon movie of a hippocampal pyramidal neuron, previously transfected with EGFP. (Left) Control. (Right) Same dendritic field, after the application of a cocktail of chemicals that induces LTP (see also Hosokawa et al., 1995). Note how chemical LTP has no notable effect on spine number or shape. Scale bar: 2 μm. Original data from Dunaevsky et al., 1999.

successful (or blocked). This study therefore reported that, in this specialized preparation, the functional enhancement of synapses was correlated with the generation of new spines.

Later in the same year, an EM study once more addressed the question of spinogenesis after LTP, but from a different angle. This study (Toni et al., 1999) was an extension of earlier work from the same lab (Buchs and Muller, 1996) using a different technique to select for the stimulated synapses and therefore the location in which morphological changes were expected to occur. Their assumption was that synapses that have just been subjected to a strong stimulus show an accumulation of electron-dense calcium precipitates in the postsynaptic spine. This precipitate is visible postsynaptically, and it was argued that this marks spines activated by the electrical stimulation. Toni et al. (1999) then reconstructed those spines, reporting that in many cases after stimulation there were pairs or triplets of marked spines making contact with the same presynaptic terminal (figure 8.5). Such multiple synapse boutons (MSBs) form separate synapses with two or more postsynaptic elements, instead of only one synapse with a single postsynaptic element, as is the case for most presynaptic boutons. As MSBs are rare normally, but are found after motor learning (Federmeier et al., 1994) and visual stimulation (Jones et al., 1997), it has been

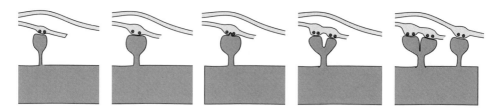

**Figure 8.5**
LTP induces multiple synapse boutons. In this model, LTP induces the appearance of pairs or triplets of spines making contact with the same presynaptic terminal. Such multiple synapse boutons would form separate synapses with two or more postsynaptic elements.

argued that they could be preferentially involved in the formation of new synapses (Knott and Holtmaat, 2008). Therefore, the data from Toni et al. were interpreted as evidence that new spines were generated under conditions of LTP-inducing stimulation.

Although these three studies reported a correlation between new spines and successful enhancement of synapses, they did not prove a causal link between LTP and new spines. In contrast with the Hosokawa and Dunaevsky studies, in which every spine was exposed to the chemical LTP cocktail, none of the three 1999 studies discussed demonstrated that the newly observed spines with their presumptive synapses contributed to the strength of the measured connection. In fact, the experiments of Maletic-Savatic et al. (1999) and Engert and Bonhoeffer (1999) actually prove that the changes in spine number cannot cause LTP because the synaptic enhancement occurs within minutes of the stimulation, whereas new spines appear only after roughly 30 minutes. Thus, using the temporal dissociation between both phenomena, one could use these same data to conclude that LTP is independent from of spinogenesis. At the same time, one could argue that the Hosowaka and Dunaevsky studies relied on a chemical manipulation that was not physiological.

A crucial experimental tool in solving this conundrum could be the ability to stimulate a single spine at will, while monitoring its morphology. This type of experiment has now become possible. As we discussed in chapter 7, calcium imaging of spines enables one to detect whether a spine is or is not activated by synaptic release, performing an optical quantal analysis (see figures 7.3 and 7.4). Moreover, the development of caged compounds that can be photoreleased with two-photon lasers (Ellis-Davies, 2003; Canepari et al., 2001; Matsuzaki et al., 2001; Fino et al., 2009), allows activation of any particular spine in the field of view.

## Imaging Increases in Spine Size during LTP

Matsuzaki et al. reexamined the relation between LTP and spine plasticity using two-photon uncaging of glutamate while simultaneously monitoring spine morphology with two-photon imaging (Matsuzaki et al., 2004). The experimental precision of the method allowed them to activate spines in a pinpoint fashion and examine carefully its morphological effects. After repetitive glutamate uncaging, the authors reported increases in the evoked synaptic currents that resembed LTP. Although they did not report the apperance of new spines, this enhancement was correlated with large increases (150–300%) in spine volume, specific to the stimulated spine. This correlation was likely causal because the potentiation occurred only in spines that enlarged, and because the amount of potentiation correlated with the magnitude of the enlargement. Also, the time course of the enlargement matched the time course of the potentiation.

The authors investigated the mechanisms of this enlargement and found that, like LTP, it depended on the activation of NMDAR, calmoduline, and CAMkinase-2 and was blocked by whole-cell dialysis and cytochalasin and thus involved active cytoskeletal rearragements. The authors then used glutamate uncaging to map the distribution and concentration of AMPA receptors and detected that AMPA receptors increased in the potentiated spines. Indeed, in previous work they had demonstrated a linear relation between spine size and number of AMPA receptors (Matsuzaki et al., 2001), in agreement with ultrastructural studies (Nusser et al., 1998). Finally, they described a different response among large, mushroom-type spines, in which the enlargement was only transient and potentiation does not occur.

Thus, this work lined up with the view that LTP is associated with morphological changes in spines, rather than with increases in spine number. Nevertheless, Masusaki et al. based their conclusions mostly on activation of spines with glutamate uncaging, in extracellular solutions without $Mg^{2+}$, thus making the NMDAR more active. These conditions could crucially differ from physiological synaptic release. Although they also reported increases in spine volumes after synaptic stimulation, a result also reported by Okamoto et al. (2004), they did not ascertained which spines were actually activated by their stimulation paradigm. This appears to be crucial, since neurons have thousands of spines whose morphologies could be changing spontaneously and extracellular synaptic stimulation engages spines that are not necessarily in the field of view. Therefore, it is difficult to correlate changes in spine morphology and electrophysiological responses of the neuron, unless one can demonstrate that the imaged spine was actually activated.

Indeed, a study published at the same time as the Masusaki et al. study arrived at a different conclusion (Lang et al., 2004). Using two-photon imaging of CA1 neurons in slices, and solutions with $Mg^{2+}$, the authors found that, after synaptic stimulation that elicited LTP, a subpopulation of spines increased their head volume. These spines, however, quickly returned to their original shape, even though the LTP was longer lasting. This study also did not report the appearance of new spines. Although Lang et al. did not establish that the spines that increased in size were the stimulated ones, the temporal dissociation between the synaptic enhancement and

the increases in spine size indicates that these two phenomena were not causally related. Thus, a more physiological stimulation than that used by Masusaki et al. only
generated transient enhancements.

Finally, a recent study has partly replicated the Masusaki et al. results, although
with the new twist that activation of nearby spines is necessary for local potentiation,
as if there were a dendritic activation threshold for LTP (Harvey and Svoboda,
2007).

## LTP and Spine Plasticity: A Model

In summary, the literature appears to be contradictory when the relation between
LTP and spines is analyzed. While some studies report increased numbers of spines,
others detect increases in the average size of the spine head or shortenings and widen-
ings of the neck, and yet other studies reveal no significant changes in spine densities
or shape. Also, given the well-known bias against negative data in science (which are
generally difficult to interpret and publish), there are probably many unpublished
studies that have detected no clear morphological change after LTP (see figure 8.4,
for example). Arguably, the ideal experiment, monitoring the potentiation of individual synapses and their associated spines in vivo, has yet to be done. Nevertheless,
new experimental methods are enabling more precise explorations of this idea.

At the same time, an answer is starting to emerge from this literature: As first suggested by Fifkova, LTP is associated with changes in spine shape, but not with
increases in spine number or density. LTP could increase the spine head volume and
also shorten and widen their spine necks (figure 8.2). These morphological changes
could be relatively strong (or perhaps easier to detect) in small spines, which have
fewer (or no) AMPA receptors, and could thus be the morphological reflection of
the so-called "silent synapses" (Isaac et al., 1995; Liao et al., 1995). LTP would
then generate increases in spine size, given that spine size is correlated with the
strength of synapse (figure 3.14), because of the direct relationship between spine volume and synaptic strength, reflected in an increased number of postsynaptic AMPA
receptor and presynaptic docked vesicles (Schikorski and Stevens, 1999). In addition,
the shortening and widening of the spine neck could also lead to greater synaptic
efficacy (see chapter 9). The changes in spine morphology and synaptic function
would, after all, be the same phenomenon. This model actually agrees very well
with the initial ultrastructural evidence that showed spine heads from stimulated
spines become larger and their necks shorter and wider (Desmond and Levy, 1986;
Fifkova and Van Harrefeld, 1977), with a concomitant increase in synaptic area
(Desmond and Levy, 1988).

Interestingly, small spines are particularly labile in long-term time-lapse experiments in vivo (Trachtenberg et al., 2002), so they could be more plastic. On the other

hand, larger spines, which have many more AMPA receptors and thus inject significantly more current, could be more dominant functionally, but less plastic. In fact, large spines appear to be remarkably resilient, lasting sometimes the entire adult life of the animal (Grutzendler et al., 2002). These large spines could both implement receptive field stability and be the morphological traces of memory. The fact that LTP could be preferentially generated in a subpopulation of spines may also partly explain the confusion in the literature of synaptic plasticity (or spine morphological plasticity), since different synapses or spines could behave quite differently.

This model therefore discards a significant contribution of new spines to LTP. As mentioned, spinogenesis, when reported, occurs only after LTP is in place and therefore, at most, could only help explain the late phase of LTP. But even that scenario is unlikely since the new spines would have to connect with the stimulated axon, something difficult to imagine as the trajectories of excitatory axons and postsynaptic dendrites are usually not parallel. One could imagine that the the new spine is generated exactly next to the potentiated spine, invoking bifurcating spines as an intermediate synaptic structure between a potentiated, perforated synapse and an additional spine generated in an MSB. But ultrastructurally, bifurcating spines on the same presynaptic axon are separated by other axons, something that makes the split spine model physically impossible (Fiala et al., 2002). Finally, the reported changes in spine number after LTP are too small to biophysically account for the larger increase in potentiated current measured.

How does one interpret the published evidence that synaptic stimulation can lead to the formation of new spines? One suggestion is that the spinogenesis found after synaptic stimulation represents a homeostatic reaction to the stimulation, unrelated to LTP. As argued in chapter 3, there is good evidence for a homeostatic regulation of spine density and size, since they are anticorrelated in all neurons and even within segments of a dendrite (Konur et al., 2003). This spine homeostasis could reflect synaptic homeostasis (Turrigiano et al., 1998; Turrigiano and Nelson, 2000). These phenomena are likely to be more important during early developmental stages, which are normally used in synaptic plasticity experiments. Finally, these new spines and presumably new synapses should eventually connect with axons and provide the circuit with novel pathways. This relatively unspecific form of plasticity, very different from the Hebbian learning rules, could endow the circuit with flexibility to encode novel computations.

**Morphological Plasticity of Spines: A Functional View**

After this focused review of the morphological consequences of LTP, it is time to step back and consider the larger issue of spines and plasticity. First, one should note that, besides LTP, other forms of synaptic plasticity have consequences for

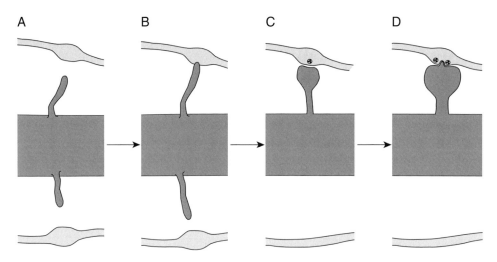

**Figure 8.6**
Spine development and LTP. This model incorporates ideas from spinogenesis, spine motility, and spine plasticity. In early development (A), dendritic filopodia seek neighboring axons, and, while, some eventually succeed in forming contacts with them (B, top), others are retracted (B, bottom). Eventually, those initial contacts are transformed in mature synapses on spines (C). After LTP, the spine head grows and the spine neck widens and shortens (D).

the morphology of spines. Long-term depression, for example, can generate morphological changes in spines, such as changes of the spine neck (Chen et al., 2004; Zhou et al., 2004), or even reduction in the number of spines (Nagerl et al., 2004), although, in other studies, LTD can occur without any significant changes of spine shape or number (see Sdrulla and Linden, 2007). One should also keep in mind that LTP and LTD, or more generally STDP, are just some of the probably many synaptic plasticity paradigms present in the CNS. It therefore seems that we are still in the early days of examining the question of the relation between synaptic plasticity and spine changes.

Nevertheless, it is interesting to speculate and bring into this discussion the conclusions reached when reviewing the development and the motility of spines (see chapters 5 and 6), together with their role as calcium compartments (see chapter 7), into a unified picture (figure 8.6). One could argue that most spines could arise from filopodial precursors, and actually represent those filopodia that have been successful at establishing a synaptic connection (figure 8.6A, B). But once spines emerge in development, and after the motility and pruning phase is finished, more spines are not generated, even under conditions that stimulate synaptic plasticity. Instead, synaptic plasticity (either STDP or other forms) would occur mosly as bidirectional alterations in synaptic strength, perhaps mediated by morphological regulation of the spine (and synaptic) structure (figure 8.6C, D).

After this developmental plasticity, the connectivity diagram of the nervous system becomes crystallized and the brain would essentially become hardwired. As Cajal put it, the "neural cement hardens," although his predictions that growth of neural protrusions would accompany learning appear less accurate that Tanzi's proposal, highlighting the strengthening or weakening of existing ones. Thus, the functional plasticity appearing during the adult life of the animals would essentially be based on changes in the strength of the connections, rather than on addition of new connections or elimination of existing ones. Instead of building new synaptic "dwellings," the brain enlarges (or reduces) existing ones. This implies that a structural limit to learning exists, such that the neural circuits can be altered only within the possibilities determined by their crystallized architecture.

Finally, one should mention that this scenario, where plasticity is achieved mostly through changes in the strength of existing synapses, corresponds very well with many models of associative neural network (Seung and Yuste, 2008). When viewed from this theoretical framework the function of spines becomes very clear: to implement local learning rules. In an artificial neural network, the connectivity, which is normally very distributed, is fixed and all learning occurs as a result of changes in the strength of the connections. But for this to occur, each connection needs to be altered independently of all the other ones. This change in input strength is controlled by a learning rule (Hebb, 1949), which is therefore input-specific. Spines could serve precisely that role: After helping to establish a distributed connectivity, they maintain a calcium compartment that confines synaptic plasticity to a single excitatory input. As we will see in the next two chapters, this idea fits well with the role of spines in independently integrating synaptic inputs.

# 9 Physiology

*The biochemical compartmentalization at individual spines is well demonstrated. At the same time, many theoretical studies have highlighted the role that spines could play in the electrical transformation of synaptic inputs. Recent data have demonstrated that spines indeed possess voltage-dependent conductances. Moreover, new experiments indicate that the spine neck can substantially filter membrane potential. Finally, spine sodium channels substantially amplify synaptic potentials and could enhance dendritic backpropagation. The purpose of the local amplification of the EPSP, followed by its subsequent filtering by the spine neck is still unclear, but may be related to enhancing the activation of NMDARs, while at the same time maximizing the number of inputs that a neuron can receive and preventing their interaction. In any case, spines appear to have a significant electrical role, one that could greatly influence synaptic transmission and plasticity, dendritic integration, and the function of many neural circuits.*

As explained in chapter 7, the introduction of imaging techniques has demonstrated that spines can serve as biochemical compartments. This compartmentalization, particularly in reference to calcium, can mediate the synapse-specific biochemistry associated with long-term plasticity (Lynch et al., 1983; Malenka et al., 1988; Yuste and Denk, 1995; Matsuzaki et al., 2004), thus giving a biochemical identity to the synapse, and could be a main *raison d'être* for spines. At the same time, since calcium compartmentalization can also occur without spines (Goldberg et al., 2003a), it is possible that spines could serve a separate function in the neuron, in addition to chemical compartmentalization. Among many possibilities, a long tradition of theoretical work has stressed the potential electrical function of spines (Coss and Perkel, 1985; Shepherd, 1996; reviewed in Tsay and Yuste, 2004). The basic idea is that spines, by virtue of their passive or active electrical properties, are endowed with electrical characteristics separate from those of the parent dendrite. Thus, in addition to being biochemical compartments, spines could also be electrical compartments.

If spines have an electrical role, they would have a major impact in the function of the neuron, given that spines are recipients of most excitatory inputs. Nevertheless, the electrical aspect of the function of spines has been virtually ignored in the last decade, due to low estimates of spine neck resistances, derived from passive models of spines (Harris and Kater, 1994; Harris and Stevens, 1989; Koch and Zador, 1993; Svoboda et al., 1996). Only recently has the tide started to turn, as a result of several lines of work. First, it has become clear that, as any dendritic membrane (Johnston et al., 1996; Yuste and Tank, 1996), spines have voltage-sensitive conductances, including calcium, potassium, and sodium channels (see chapters 4, 7, and below). Also, glutamate uncaging data have revealed that spines with longer necks have, on average, smaller synaptic potentials, as if the spine neck were filtering voltages (Araya et al., 2006b; Araya, Vogels, and Yuste, submitted). Finally, optical measurements of membrane potentials in spines have become possible (Nuriya et al., 2006), and are starting to demonstrate different electrical behavior of spines, compared with their parent dendrites (Araya et al., 2006b).

## Passive Models of Spines

The first proposal that spines may have an electrical function was by Cajal himself, who suggested that spines store electric energy (Ramón y Cajal, 1904). The thread was picked up 50 years later by Chang, who proposed that the spine neck had a high electrical resistance ($R_{neck}$) and therefore would attenuate synaptic inputs (Chang, 1952). This attenuation could diminish the functional impact of any given input, thus making neurons responsive only to combinations of synchronous inputs. A decade later, Llinás and Hillman highlighted the asymmetry in the electrical properties of a spine connected to a large dendrite: The small spine must have a high input resistance ($R_h$) and create an impedance mismatch between spine and dendrite. Because of this, spines would filter EPSPs and serve, as a DC source, to inject constant current (Llinás and Hillman, 1969).

Models of the electrical properties of spines can be divided into two categories, passive and active, according to whether they assume the presence of voltage-dependent conductances in spines (figures 9.1 and 9.2, plate 13). In particular, the pioneering work of Wilfrid Rall and his disciples has dominated theoretical studies of spines (Rall, 1970, 1974a, 1974b, 1978). Rall introduced cable theory and compartmental modeling to the analysis of dendrites and, with his coworkers, is responsible for creating a rich and lively literature that has influenced modern thinking on dendritic integration (Stuart et al., 1999). In a series of increasingly sophisticated models and analytical treatments, Rall and coworkers argued that the high spine resistance, relative to the dendritic one, would create a very large impedance mismatch

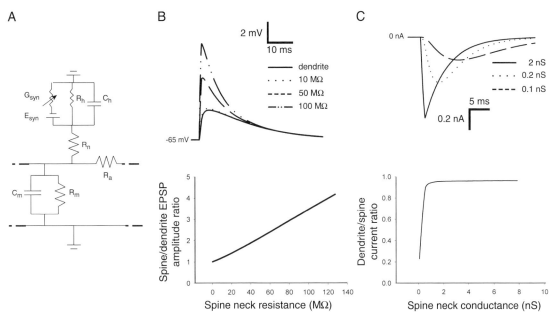

**Figure 9.1**
Passive model of a dendritic spine. (A) Circuit diagram of a passive spine with a synapse of conductance, $G_{syn}$, and reversal potential $E_{syn}$. The passive parameters of the spine are illustrated by its input resistance ($R_h$), spine head capacitance ($C_h$), and neck resistance ($R_n$); the adjacent dendrite is diagrammed by its axial resistance ($R_a$), membrane capacitance ($C_m$), and membrane resistance ($R_m$). (B) Results from numerical simulations demonstrate the amplification of the EPSP at the spine head and filtering of EPSPs by spines. Note how increasing spine neck resistance results in larger peak EPSP voltage differences between the spine and dendritic shaft (top); the peak EPSP spine/dendrite voltage ratio was found to be roughly linear to neck resistance (bottom). (C) Spine neck conductance affects the EPSC response seen at the dendrite (top). In order for significant attenuation of peak current in the dendrite to occur, spine neck conductances needed to approach values comparative to those of the synapse (<1 nS). Reprinted with permission from Tsay and Yuste, 2004.

(figure 9.1). While EPSPs would be attenuated by dendritic load on the spine, voltage signals propagating from dendrite into the spine should not be attenuated (Rall and Rinzel, 1971). Moreover, the spine neck length could modulate the extent of this attenuation, and this effect could be key for synaptic plasticity.

In complementary studies, Koch and Poggio modeled spines as small cylinders, with a small spine capacitance ($C_h$), a high spine head input resistance ($R_h$), a variable neck resistance ($R_n$), and a negligible neck capacitance ($C_n$), due to the small surface of the spine neck membrane (see figure 9.1; Koch and Poggio, 1983a, 1983b). They also concluded that spines could attenuate synaptic potentials and pointed out that the small spine volume could even saturate the EPSP as a result of the collapse of the $Na^+$ gradients across the spine membrane. As in the Rall studies, these electrical effects of the spine depended strongly on the spine neck geometry. Koch and Poggio also pointed out that the spines that received dual excitatory/inhibitory inputs could implement AND/NOT logical gating.

Therefore, if spines are passive electrical devices, their small size would create a sealed cable end with high input resistance ($R_h$) and very small capacitance ($C_h$) (Johnston and Wu, 1995). Because of this, there would not be a significant attenuation of the dendritic voltage pulses, although the spine could provide an attenuation of synaptic potentials. At the same time, the EPSP should be locally boosted by the spine head input resistance, with respect to the same EPSP injected in the dendritic shaft. Finally, there could be a significant decrease in the driving force of the EPSP, due to the large effect even small conductances can have on the ionic composition of the spine.

A key question for all these models is what is the exact value of the spine neck resistance ($R_n$), or its inverse term, the neck conductance ($G_n$), since its ratio with respect to the value of the synaptic conductance determines the amount of filtering the spine neck produces (Koch and Poggio, 1983a, 1983b). Estimates from models based on ultrastructural reconstructions suggest that the neck conductance ($G_n$) for rat hippocampal spines ranges from 18 to 138 nS (Harris and Stevens, 1989). A different estimate, based on actual measurements of diffusional coupling of dextrans between spine heads and dendrites in rat hippocampal and cerebellar spines, provides a lower bound of approximately 7 nS (Svoboda et al., 1996). These values seem much higher than those reported for synaptic conductances (0.05–0.1 nS; see Bekkers et al., 1990). Nevertheless, synaptic conductances are measured at the soma, and it is possible that voltage clamp underestimates synaptic conductances in spines (Johnston and Wu, 1995). Indeed, a recent experimental study has pointed out the difficulty in voltage clamping dendritic or spine conductances (Williams and Mitchell, 2008). In any case, the large difference in spine and synaptic conductances would, in principle, predict a relatively modest filtering of EPSP by spines, indicating that spines do not serve as electrical compartments, but primarily in chemical (calcium-based) compartmentalization (Harris and Kater, 1994; Koch and Zador, 1993). This theoretical calculations have been embraced by most researchers and, for the last decade, spine physiologists have concentrated on understanding the calcium dynamics of spines (Nimchinsky et al., 2002; Yuste et al., 2000).

We should also mention an important, yet often overlooked, conclusion from passive models of spines. Even if spines might not serve as fully independent electrical compartments, the overall geometry of spines could greatly affect the electrophysiology of the parent dendrites. Even assuming that their individual influence on a single EPSP is small, by their sheer number, spines can account for a significant amount of the dendritic membrane (Wilson, 1986). It has been argued that this "population" effect could be the main function of spines (Jaslove, 1992), lowering the input impedance and increasing the total capacitance of the neuron (Jaslove, 1992). This should result in a decreased average size of EPSPs and therefore also impact EPSP summation, effectively increasing the number of inputs a neuron can integrate. The proportionally larger increase in dendritic capacitance could also "slow down" the cell and make it a low-pass filter for trains of inputs, although one could also argue that the concomitant decrease in membrane resistance, as a consequence of a larger area, could cancel the effect of the capacitance. Nevertheless, as we discuss below, some comparative studies, together with the strong link between spines and slow NMDA receptors, support the possibility that spines are involved in low-pass filtering of inputs.

## Active Models of Spines

In the 1970s, pioneering experiments in Purkinje cells (Llinás and Nicholson, 1971) revealed that dendrites were active structures. This idea was incorporated into a new generation of proposals of electrical models of spines and dendrites (figure 9.2, plate 13; Rall, 1995; Rall and Segev, 1988). This new generation of models argued that active properties allowed spines to electrically isolate synaptic inputs (Diamond et al., 1970) or even generate local action potentials (APs), as a result of the spine head's high input resistance (Jack et al., 1975). Spines could act as synaptic amplifiers: An EPSP could generate spine APs if spines were endowed with sodium ($Na^+$) and potassium ($K^+$) channels at densities of four times those of the squid axon (Perkel, 1982; Perkel and Perkel, 1985). Rall and coworkers also generated active models of active spines and concluded that active spines could lead to a sixfold amplification of the amplitude of the EPSP and that generated APs could spread to neighboring spines, triggering a chain of AP events. This spread would be very sensitive to small changes in spine neck shape (Miller et al., 1985). The idea that small clusters of spines could become a focus of dendritic electrogenesis was further explored in a series of detailed models (Rall and Segev, 1987; 1988; Segev and Rall, 1988). Using channel models with kinetics derived from the squid $Na^+$ and delayed rectifier $K^+$ conductances, EPSPs in spines could approach 90 mV. This amplification in active spines could lead to an increased reliability in dendritic integration, while also economizing the number of receptors used. Spine APs, propagating through the dendrite in a saltatory fashion, were also modeled by Baer and Rinzel (1991) and Shepherd et al. (1985). Finally, Shepherd and Brayton raised the possibility that active spines could implement logical operations, for example, AND gates when two EPSPs occurs simultaneously on two active spines, OR gates when an EPSP fires a single active spine, and AND-NOT gates when an EPSP and an IPSP coincide at different dendritic position (Shepherd and Brayton, 1987).

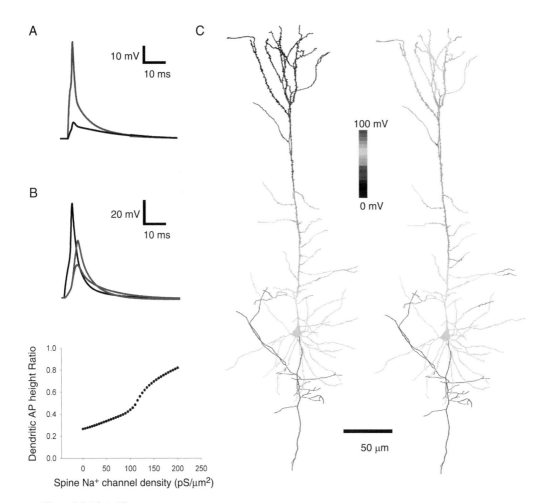

**Figure 9.2 (plate 13)**
Active models of spines. (A) Amplification of EPSP by spines. Single-spine model with high sodium channel densities ($\sim$7000 mS/cm$^2$) can elicit localized AP responses in the spine (red) but not in the dendrite (black). Note that in order for this to occur, spine neck resistances need to be high (>100 M$\Omega$) to provide sufficient electrical decoupling. (B) Moderately higher sodium channel densities ($\sim$200 mS/cm$^2$) globally in many spines can increase the efficacy of backpropagation. (Black) AP at soma; (blue) AP seen in apical dendrite 200 $\mu$m away, with weakly active spines ($G_{Na}$ = 40 mS/cm$^2$); (red) AP seen in apical dendrite with active spines ($G_{Na}$ = 200 mS/cm$^2$). Modulation of backpropagation does not require extensive electrical decoupling of spines. (C) The peak voltage response to a backpropagating action potential, represented by a color code. Backpropagation when Na channel densities in spines are relatively low (110 mS cm22) exhibits decremental invasion of the apical tree (left); with only moderately higher densities in spines (200 mS cm22), a backpropagating action potential is now able to invade the dendritic tree fully (right). Reprinted with permission from Tsay and Yuste, 2004.

## Active Conductances in Spines

These active models made it essential to investigate the nature and densities of dendritic and spine voltage-dependent conductances. More recently, the densities and gradients of $Na^+$ and $K^+$ channels present on dendritic trees of some cells types have been directly measured through whole-cell or cell-attached recordings from mammalian dendrites (Korngreen and Sakmann, 2000; Stuart et al., 1993; Stuart and Sakmann, 1994). Unfortunately, this technique appears to be limited to dendritic shafts, and electrical recordings of spine heads have not yet been achieved. However, compartmental models of dendrites have been built with channel densities and kinetics taken from recordings of dendritic patches. One consequence of these studies has been the characterization of backpropagation, where an action potential generated at the axon propagates in a retrograde manner along the dendritic tree (Stuart and Sakmann, 1994). Using multicompartmental models, Vetter et al. (2001) found that dendritic morphology greatly affects backpropagation. Since spines could constitute more than 50% of dendritic membrane, spine density could play an important role in regulating AP propagation in dendrites. In another recent model, pyramidal neurons could not sustain backpropagation when their dendrites expressed the measured densities and kinetics of $Na^+$ and $K^+$ channels (Tsay and Yuste, 2002). Only when the voltage-gated sodium channels on spines differed in either density or inactivation kinetics from those in the same dendrite was backpropagation possible. Interestingly, backpropagation in CA1 pyramidal cells appears to fall dichotomously into either non-backpropagating or backpropagating categories, and dendritic AP amplitude can be controlled by manipulation of dendritic channels (Golding and Spruston, 1998). Therefore, through modulation of spine sodium channels, backpropagation may be dynamically regulated.

A similar case could be made for the presence of $K^+$ channels in spines. Although multicompartmental models of spines with $K^+$ channels are only now starting to be generated, it is clear that the activation of spine $K^+$ channels could significantly shunt synaptic potentials (Vogels and Yuste, in prep.). Moreover, if $K^+$ channels were located in the spine neck, they could play a crucial role as gatekeepers of the synapse.

Therefore, the potential existence of $Na^+$ and $K^+$ channels in spines could endow spines with amplification or even electrogenic properties, which would have an enormous influence on synaptic integration or dendritic processing. But are there actually active conductances in spines? Although studies of this question are still preliminary, current evidence suggests that spines indeed have active conductances, and conclusions based solely on passive models, such as the lack of a significant electrical role of the spine, need to be reexamined.

A direct way to demonstrate the presence of active conductances is with structural techniques. Because of the small dimensions of the spines, and their close appositions to the synaptic terminals, light microscopy studies are of limited use and ultrastructural analyses are necessary. Immuno-ultrastructural techniques, although highly variable, have been applied to the localization of glutamatergic and GABA-ergic receptors on postsynaptic membranes, to the point where estimates of numbers or receptors for individual spines can be made (Nusser et al., 1998). A similar characterization of spine sodium, potassium, or calcium channels is only now beginning to be carried out, with some ultrastructural evidence of sodium and calcium channel subunits in the spine cytoplasm (Caldwell et al., 2000; Mills et al., 1994). Potassium channels have also been localized to spines, including SK2 (Adelman and Lujan, unpublished observations), GIRK (Jan et al., unpublished results), Kv4.2 (Kim et al., 2007), and also the nonselective cation channel HCN (Siegelbaum et al., personal communication).

An alternative method of localizing channels on spines is the biochemical purification of the PSD. As mentioned in chapter 4, proteomics analysis of PSD fractions is revealing a large diversity of conductances (Cheng et al., 2006; Grant et al., 2004; Husi et al., 2000; Li et al., 2004; Walikonis et al., 2000; Yoshimura et al., 2004), although these results need to be confirmed with proper ultrastructural methods.

Besides structural techniques, optical imaging techniques have been used to provide functional evidence for the existence of receptors and active conductances in spines, and also demonstrate that these receptors and channels are functional. Not surprisingly, calcium imaging experiments of spines under synaptic stimulation have confirmed that spines have functional NMDA and AMPA receptors (Kovalchuk et al., 2000; Yuste and Denk, 1995; Yuste et al., 1999). Also, estimates of the numbers of AMPA receptors for individual spines have been made using fluctuation analysis of the noise in the optical signals of calcium accumulations (Matsuzaki et al., 2001). In addition, based on the lack of delay of dendritic calcium accumulations after action potentials, and their larger amplitudes with respect to the accumulations on dendritic shaft, it has been concluded that the entire dendritic tree of pyramidal neurons (Yuste et al., 1994), including the spines (Segal, 1995; Yuste and Denk, 1995), is covered with VSCCs. Similar results have been obtained in Purkinje cells (Denk et al., 1995), and it could be a general phenomenon in the CNS. The number (<10, on average) of active VSCCs in individual spines has been estimated using fluctuation analysis of synaptic calcium responses (Sabatini and Svoboda, 2000). Surprisingly, these channels are estimated to have a density of VSCCs several times higher than the parent dendrite and to consist of specific subtypes (R-type). Moreover, GABAergic inputs seem to reduce the open probability of these channels, specifically in the spine but not in the dendrite. Indeed, it is clear that the spatial distribution and modulation of ion channels in spines can be regulated at the submicron level.

Sodium imaging of spines under synaptic stimulation or backpropagation APs has also been performed (Rose and Konnerth, 2001; Rose et al., 1999). Rose and Konnerth reported increases of up to 4 mM in sodium concentration after a train of backpropagating action potentials and concluded that spines were likely to have sodium channels because the kinetics of sodium accumulations in spines and dendrites are similar. Interestingly, during trains of EPSPs, sodium flows into spines and dendrites through activated NMDA receptors, with intraspine sodium concentrations reaching 30 to 100 mM. These accumulations were larger in a subtype of spines, providing further evidence for the heterogeneity of spines (Majewska et al., 2000a; Yuste et al., 1999). These sodium imaging data also demonstrated that trains of EPSPs, particularly when they elicit a suprathreshold response on the neuron, could collapse sodium gradients at a synapse. A saturation of the spine $Na^+$ gradient, predicted theoretically (Koch and Poggio, 1983a; 1983b; Qian and Sejnowski, 1989), could provide a mechanism for attenuation of EPSPs that would filter high-input frequencies.

Overall, these recent imaging experiments have confirmed some of the predictions of the active models of spines (Shepherd, 1996) and provide a functional counterpart to the ultrastructural studies.

Finally, a different approach to reveal the presence of conductances on spines is monitoring their effect on the activation of the synaptic input. The development of caged glutamate, particularly when photoreleased with two-photon excitation, has enabled turning on spines, while simultaneously monitoring the postsynaptic membrane potential via a patch electrode (Matsuzaki et al., 2001). Using this approach, Araya et al., recently investigated the effect of the TTX on spine potentials, finding that this sodium channel blocker significantly diminished them, yet had no effect on the potentials generated at dendritic shafts (figure 9.3, plate 14; Araya et al., 2007). The simplest interpretation is therefore that functional sodium channels exist in spines, and they can amplify local potentials, as predicted by some theoretical models mentioned earlier. These results from glutamate uncaging are likely to apply also to physiological synaptic potentials, since the intracellular perfusion of a sodium channel blocker produces a similar reduction on the amplitude of spontaneously occurring EPSPs (Araya, Vogels, and Yuste, submitted).

**Filtering of Membrane Potential by the Spine Neck**

Regardless of the exact complement of channels, one still could argue that the key question is whether spines behave as separate electrical compartments from the parent dendrite. In fact, a surprising result from these two-photon uncaging experiments indicates the spine neck can modulate the amplitude of spine potentials. After

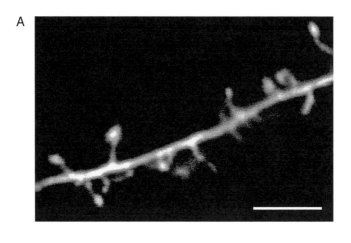

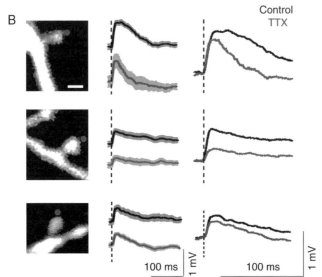

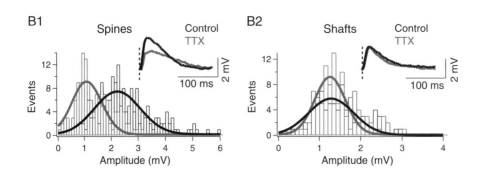

activating spines with caged glutamate, the somatic amplitude of the elicited potentials is inversely proportional to the length of the spine neck (Araya et al., 2006b). Thus, spines with longer necks generate very small, or even undetectable, somatic potentials, whereas spines with shorter neck generate much larger ones (figure 9.4). This effect was independent of the distance of the spine to the soma, indicating that the most significant filtering of the synaptic potentials was due to the spine neck and not to dendritic filtering.

These results were found with glutamate uncaging potentials, which are not entirely physiological, but they likely apply to EPSPs as well, since optical quantal analysis of synaptic potentials evoked by axonal stimulation reveal that spines with longer necks have smaller postsynaptic potentials than spines with shorter necks (Araya, Vogels and Yuste, submitted). Although the mechanisms responsible for this filtering are still unknown, the presence of potassium channels in the spine head and neck make them likely candidates, since even a few potassium channels can have a major impact in the spine/dendrite coupling (Vogels and Yuste, unpublished results).

On quick reflection, the strong modulation of spine potentials by the neck length could appears contrary to the well-demonstrated relation between the spine head volume and synaptic strength, as illustrated in figure 3.13. But because the spine neck length and head volume are actually uncorrelated (see figure 3.13D), their effects on synaptic strength should be independent. Indeed, in uncaging potentials, one can also find a correlation between spine head volume and uncaging potential amplitude, but only after filtering out the correlation between spine neck length and uncaging potentials (Araya and Yuste, unpublished observations). This suggests that it might be possible to calculate the synaptic strength of a synapse from the morphology of a spine. Specifically using the correlations between spine head volume and PSD size and between spine neck length and spine potential, one should be able to calculate the amplitude of the synaptic potential, knowing the spine head volume and neck length (and ideally also the neck diameter). Thus, it could become possible to analyze the morphology of a dendritic tree and reveal its functional input map.

**Figure 9.3 (plate 14)**
Spine sodium channels amplify spine potentials. The sodium channel blocker TTX reduces spine uncaging potentials. (A) Dendrite from a layer 5 pyramidal neuron, filled with a fluorescent indicator, whose spines where stimulated with two-photon glutamate uncaging. Scale bar: 5 μm. (B) Spine uncaging experiments. (Left) Red dots indicate site of laser uncaging. (Center) Uncaging potentials under control conditions (black traces) and in TTX (red traces). Dashed line is time of uncaging onset. Thicker traces are average of 10–15 depolarizations, and shaded areas illustrate SEM. (Right) Superimposition of average uncaging potentials. Note how TTX attenuates spine uncaging potentials. Scale bar: 1 μm. (B) Histogram of all individual uncaging potentials on spines (B1) and shafts (B2) in control and TTX. Note a shift toward smaller potentials caused by TTX in distribution of spine, but not shaft potentials, indicating that the TTX effect is specific to spines. Reprinted from Araya et al., 2007.

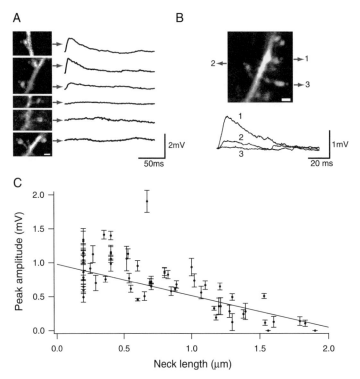

**Figure 9.4**
The spine neck filters spine potentials. (A) Examples of uncaging potentials in spines with short and long necks. Gray dots indicate the site of uncaging and traces corresponded to averages of 10 uncaging potentials for each spine. (B) Three neighboring spines (1, 2, and 3) with different neck lengths. Note the large difference in their uncaging potentials at the soma. (C) Plot of the uncaging potentials (peak amplitude) vs. neck length. Line is linear regression of the data. Reprinted from Araya et al., 2006a.

## Imaging Membrane Potential in a Spine

These results, showing a filtering of spine potentials by the spine neck, demonstrate that spines can be electrical compartments. Therefore it is key to directly measure membrane potential in spines. Indeed, the direct investigation of the electrical properties of spines and synapses is becoming possible through the use of voltage imaging techniques. There are two potential approaches to imaging voltage in neurons: One is the use of fluorescence voltage-sensitive dyes (Cohen, 1989), but a newer approach relies on second-harmonic generation (SHG), a nonlinear scattering that can report membrane potentials from membrane-bound chromophores (Lewis et al., 1999). Using SHG, Nuriya et al. recently reported the first measurements of membrane potential in spines (Nuriya et al., 2005). In this work, using intracellular injections of the styryl dye FM 4–64, the authors were able to image the invasion of backpropagated APs from dendrites into spine heads, reporting that amplitude at the spine was similar to that of their parent dendritic shafts (figure 9.5). Similar results, demonstrating the invasion of backpropagating action potentials into spines, have been recently obtained with fluorescence voltage-sensitive dyes (Palmer and Stuart, 2009; Konnerth et al., unpublished observations). Overall, these results agree with theoretical predictions based on the large impedance mismatch between spines and dendritic shafts, and give hope that voltage imaging may enable direct measurement of the spine potential achieved during synaptic activation of individual spines.

**The Electrical Function of Spines: A Functional Interpretation**

In summary, it is clear that spines are more than simple passive compartments; an abundance of recent structural and functional data demonstrates a rich diversity of ion channels on the spine head. Nevertheless, the spine repertoire of active conductances, particularly of sodium and potassium channels, needs to be better elucidated; the density values, subtypes, kinetics, and their subsequent influence on electrical behavior are of particular importance. Many experimental approaches appear possible. From immuno-EM localization studies of channels, to direct imaging of spine voltage, with either traditional voltage-sensitive indicators (Cohen, 1989) or second harmonic generation (figure 9.5; Millard et al., 2003; Nuriya et al., 2005), to genetic manipulation of spine density (Luo et al., 1996) or length (Tashiro et al., 2000), neurobiologists now have a host of techniques at their command to tackle this important problem. Even direct electrical recordings of spines may be possible, considering how *Caenorhabditis elegans* researchers can record from neuronal somata, not too different in size from large mammalian spines (Goodman and Lockery, 2000). Indeed, the electrical role of spines remains open and appears to be a rich field, one for which important key experiments are yet to be done. In particular, there are still two major unknown variables that could soon be directly measured: the spine neck resistance, and the membrane voltage at the head of the spine during physiological synaptic activation. These quantities are central to the role spines play in dendritic integration, yet they still can be only indirectly estimated.

Nevertheless, following the pioneering work of many theorists, the recent experimental evidence discussed above, although still in its infancy, is tantalizing and indicates that spines have a significant electrical influence of dendritic function. For example, the presence of sodium channels in spines appears to enable spines to carry out a significant amplification of the synaptic potentials (Araya et al., 2007), and also probably helps sustain dendritic backpropagation (Tsay and Yuste, 2002). Spine potassium channels, on the other hand, could be responsible for the filtering of

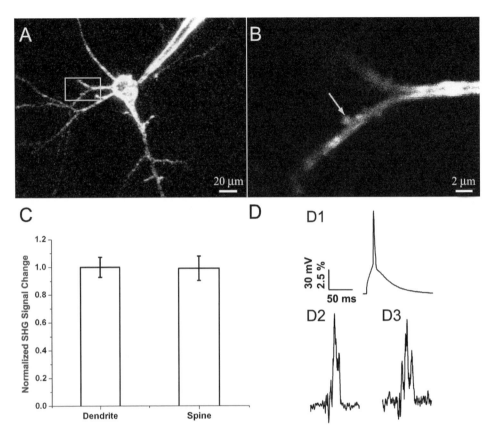

**Figure 9.5**
Imaging voltage in spines using second-harmonic generation (SHG). (A) SHG images of pyramidal neuron filled with the voltage-dependent SHG chromophore FM 4–64. (B) High-resolution image of a dendritic spine on the basal dendrite marked in (A). (C) Calibration of spine SHG signals under voltage-clamp condition. Normalized SHG signal changes upon voltage steps at spines and their parent dendrites are shown. There are no significant differences between the sensitivity of SHG at spines and dendrites. (D) SHG measurements of voltage in spines during backpropagating APs. A single AP was initiated by current injection at soma (shown in D1), and the resulting SHG signal changes were measured at soma (D2) and dendritic spines (D3). Reprinted with permission from Nuriya et al., 2006.

membrane potentials by the spine neck (Araya et al., 2006b). Moreover, the effect of spines on the cable properties of dendrites or the saturation of sodium gradients at the spine head by a train of synaptic activation could slow dendritic integration and make dendrites low-pass filters.

Reflecting on these recent results, there seems to be a fundamental paradox: After amplification, the spine neck appears to filter the EPSPs, as they traverse toward the dendritic shaft. What is the logic of this transformation? Why would spines systematically alter synaptic inputs, by first amplifying and then subsequently filtering EPSPs? What is the purpose of the electrical compartmentalization by spines? One speculation is that the electrical isolation of the synapse (its high neck resistance), or the local amplification of synaptic current by sodium channels, could enhance the EPSP, by generating a high-input impedance environment. Therefore, a similar dose of neurotransmitter could generate a larger postsynaptic depolarization.

But then, how would one explain the subsequent filtering by the spine neck? Perhaps this additional depolarization generated by the high neck resistance is locally necessary to release the magnesium block of NMDARs and enable the flux of calcium through NMDARs during subthreshold stimuli. As we discussed earlier, spines from pyramidal neurons are intimately associated with NMDARs (see chapter 4), and, since one needs substantial depolarization to release the $Mg^{2+}$ block (Nowack et al., 1984), it may be necessary for synaptic inputs to depolarize the postsynaptic membrane by more than a few millivolts, something that appears unlikely unless the region receiving the synaptic input is isolated from the rest of the neuron. At the same time, the local amplification should not be too strong, or the spines would not be able to distinguish between sub- and suprathreshold stimuli, which is something they can do (figure 7.5). If synapses were strong enough to unblock NMDARs, a given postsynaptic neuron might be able to functionally accommodate only a small number of them, before its response became saturated. By using spines, neurons could be solving both problems simultaneously: greatly increase the number of synapse they accommodate, while using the biophysical properties of NMDARs to their full advantage. The enhancement of NMDAR responses, however, cannot explain the electrical compartmentalization of spines that do not possess NMDARs, or that rely instead on $Ca^{2+}$-permeable AMPA receptors, such as mature Purkinje cells. At the same time, this idea will nicely fit with the overall structural logic of spines, which, as we argued in chapter 3, appear to be designed to maximize the number of inputs and thus enable a very distributed matrix of synaptic weights. Moreover, the local amplification of the synaptic depolarization by the spines can help explain the paradoxical influx of calcium through NMDARs that is measured under subthreshold synaptic stimulation, with somatic depolarizations in which the NMDARs should be clocked (Koester and Sakmann, 1998; Yuste et al., 1999).

Another possibility, which will be developed in chapter 10, that well complements the NMDA enhancement hypothesis is that the electrical compartmentalization generated by the spine neck serves to electrically isolate synapses from one another. The summation of EPSPs and, more generally, the integration of synaptic inputs, is the principal function of dendrites, so it may not be surprising that spines could play a fundamental role in this process. Indeed, as we will see, there is strong evidence supporting the view that spines enable a reliable, and linear, mode of dendritic integration.

In any case, from this discussion, one can conclude that the electrical role of spines has important repercussions for the function of the neuron, and it is likely that better knowledge of the electrical role of spines could change our understanding of how neurons work. Moreover, humans have spines that are much larger and have longer necks than those of rodents (Benavides-Piccione et al., 2002), so, given that the electrical compartmentalization of spines depends on the length of the spine neck (Araya et al., 2006b), it is likely that the electrical role spines play is even more important in humans.

# 10 Computation

*Spines appear to be designed to maximize connectivity and enable input-specific synaptic plasticity. Also, the spine neck electrically isolates synaptic inputs from each other, helping linearize their integration. These apparently disparate functions can be threaded together when viewed from the perspective of the circuits in which spiny neurons operate. Excitatory axons, which generally terminate on spines, have relatively straight trajectories, thus maximizing the innervating territories and dispersing information to a large number of recipient neurons. By enhancing connectivity, spines could help these circuits become more distributed. But to reap the full benefit of a distributed connectivity matrix, it appears necessary to integrate inputs faithfully and independently, to ensure that every input is tallied, and all possible information is extracted. Because of this, a linear summation regime would be quite desirable, since it would prevent input saturation. Finally, in distributed circuits it also seems necessary to maintain synaptic plasticity from one input independent from that of others, therefore keeping their functional individuality, which was the original goal of the circuit design. By enabling input-specific plasticity, spines would, in addition, provide distributed circuits with the ability to learn and be plastic. So, from this point of view, spines would not only make possible the wiring of a distributed circuit, but also help the accurate integration of its inputs and the individual tuning of their strengths. These are the properties that enable the basic computational capabilities of neural networks, which are also distributed circuit models with input-specific learning rules and, often, linear integration. Spines therefore could be viewed as anatomical signatures of a distributed neural network.*

In this final chapter I attempt to synthesize a coherent view of spine function, one that takes into account different aspects of the biology of spines. As mentioned in the introduction, my strategy to understand the function of spines is to consider them as elements within a circuit. In this respect, this chapter focuses mostly on the function of spines in neocortical circuits, my area of expertise, although I imagine that the function of the spines in other types of circuits is probably similar. Since there are scant data on many of these issues, this chapter is, by necessity, speculative, and many of the ideas presented here have not yet been confirmed experimentally.

**An Apparent Multitude of Spine Functions**

I start by reviewing the potential functions of spines, in a summary of the major conclusions drawn from the past chapters. I will not include references to the data discussed, but refer the reader to the appropriate chapters. The argument spans two levels of analysis: the biophysical level, revieweing some basic properties of neocortical neurons, and the anatomical level, analyzing their connectivity.

• *Spines must be key.*   As discussed in chapter 3, spines receive essentially all excitatory inputs, not just in neocortex, but also in many other regions of the brain. The number of spines is enormous: pyramidal neurons have about 20,000 spines and Purkinje cells can have up to 300,000. But because the dendritic shaft of mature pyramidal cells is essentially devoid of excitatory inputs, spines must have a particular function, rather than just serving as connecting devices. Otherwise, excitatory inputs could be made onto the shaft, thus saving the large expenditure of energy and structural components and developmental mechanisms necessary to build and maintain all the spines. Therefore, because of their prevalence, the particular function of the spines must be fundamental for the circuit.

• *Spines maximize the number of inputs.*   As argued in chapters 3 and 4, the dimensions of the spines are determined by the size of the synapse. Moreover, the number of glutamate receptors in a synapse can approach single-molecules. Thus, although spines can vary in size, overall they seem to be made as small as possible. This agrees well with the helical positioning of spines along the dendritic tree, since helixes are an efficient way to distribute linear structures in a volume. The purpose of this packing could be to help the neuron maximize the sampled neuropil and thus enhance its connectivity.

• *Spines define biochemical compartments.*   As reviewed in chapter 4, the molecular stucture of a spine is quite different from that of the parent dendritic shaft. The PSD is a veritable nanomachine with specific biochemical composition. Spines appear therefore designed to carry out particular biochemical reactions and, in pyramidal neurons, NMDAR-dependent biochemistry.

• *Spinogenesis can maximize synaptogenesis.*   Although it is not yet completely understood how spines develop, as discussed in chapters 5 and 6, the emergence and developmental motility of filopodia and spines could help in establishing synaptic connections. From the point of view of a circuit, this could help make every possible connection happen, thus filling the excitatory connectivity matrix. Moreover, by moving, spines may be able to change synaptic partners and choose between them, enabling the fine-tuning of the synaptic matrix.

• *Spine stability could mediate long-lasting memories.* As discussed in chapters 4 and 5, once spines emerge and make synaptic contacts, they can be remarkably stable, in some cases even lasting the entire adult life of the animal, like some memories. Therefore, spines could physically implement long-term memory storage. This does not mean that the only mechanism for long-term memory storage is long-term spine stability, but spines have ideal features to contribute to it, since they mediate synaptic contacts and can be stable for life.

• *Spines can mediate input-dependent synaptic plasticity.* As explained in chapter 7, by compartmentalizing calcium, spines may help to restrict synaptic plasticity to individual inputs. This plasticity probably has a morphological expression (chapter 8). This implies that the morphological diversity of spines could reflect their history as mediating input-specific learning rules. Nevertheless, calcium compartmentalization, and input-specific plasticity, also can occur in the absence of spines.

• *Spines could slow down neuronal integration.* As explained, spines may also have an electrical function, altering synaptic inputs and perhaps also the integrative properties of neurons (chapter 9). Interestingly, in pyramidal neurons spines are full of NMDA receptors, which are particularly slow compared to other excitatory receptors in the brain. Also, some spiny neurons have low-pass transfer properties, compared with nonspiny cells, which act more as high-pass filters.

• *Spines can be electrical compartments.* Moreover, as explained in chapter 9, spines can experience a different voltage regime from their parent dendrites. This electrical compartmentalization could isolate EPSPs from those occurring at neighboring synapses, effectively making spines a current injecting site, rather than a conductance-based input device.

**Spines Mediate Linear Integration**

Spines therefore can apparently serve for many things, and it is not obvious which one of these potential functions is more fundamental. One key to weaving together these functions is the fact that dendrites of pyramidal neurons summate their inputs linearly, whereby the joint activation of two inputs is exactly equal to the sum of their independent activity (figure 10.1A). In hippocampal pyramidal neurons from cultured or slice preparations, the arithmetic that dendrites use to sum excitatory inputs is remarkably linear and independent of the exact position of the input (Cash and Yuste, 1998, 1999). The linear summation has been confirmed in different types

A

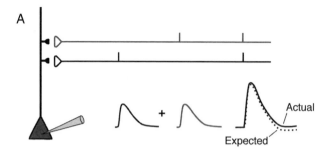

B

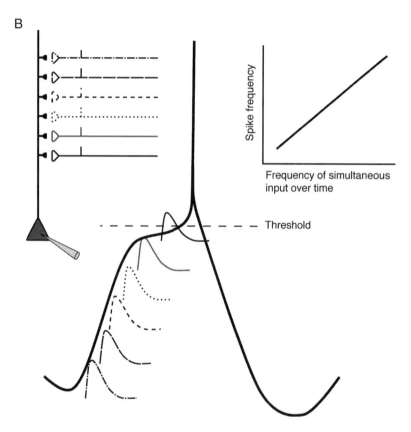

**Figure 10.1**
Linear integration of excitatory inputs. Diagram illustrating the linear summation of inputs by spines. (A) A pyramidal cell receives inputs from different excitatory neurons onto different spines. When both of them are activated together, the somatic response is linear (i.e., the actual response is equal to the expected sum of the individual responses). (B) When a sufficient number of inputs are added, action potential threshold is reached. In the spiking regime, the activation of additional inputs could still continue to produce a relatively linear increase in the action potential frequency. Reprinted from Yuste and Urban, 2004.

of neurons (Tamas and Szabadics, 2004; Tamas et al., 2003; H. Markram, pers. comm.). This linear integration could help neurons maintain a faithful transformation between input and output (figure 10.1B).

Moreover, recent experiments using two-photon glutamate uncaging have shown that activation of several spines simultaneously also generates a linear sum (Araya et al., 2006a; Gasparini and Magee, 2006), whereas activation of nonspiny regions in the dendritic shaft generates a significant interference, or electrical shunting, among inputs (figure 10.2; Araya et al., 2006a). The linear integration of activated spines is very robust and can occur even when they are literally next to each other (Araya et al., 2006a; Gasparini and Magee, 2006). Even though the exact mechanisms that mediate the linear summation of inputs are still not fully investigated, these results suggest that spines are involved in linearizing dendritic integration. As will be argued below, this linear integration could help us understand the global role of spines in circuits.

**Spines and Distributed Circuits**

Leaving the biophysics behind, the second part of my argument concerns the analysis of the microanatomy of the neocortex. Although the exact pattern of connections in the cortical microcircuit is still largely unknown, there is clear evidence that the excitatory circuit is very distributed, meaning that a given pyramidal neuron connects with, and receives inputs from, many other pyramidal cells. At the theoretical limit, as in some artificial neural network models (Seung and Yuste, 2010), every possible connection could be present. Below, I argue that spines can help make this connectivity matrix get closer to this theoretical limit, and that this strategy predicts that the integration of inputs in the circuit should be independent of each other.

• *Excitatory connections are weak.*    One interesting fact about cortical physiology is that connections between excitatory neurons are particularly weak (Abeles, 1991) and, for the most part, have depressing short-term dynamics (Abbott et al., 1997; Markram and Tsodyks, 1996). In the cases in which this has been examined carefully, with ultrastructural confirmation of synapses between connected neurons, the average number of synaptic contacts among corticocortical excitatory connections is generally fewer than 10. Moreover, each contact contributes at most a 1 mV depolarization to the soma, when it does not fail (Markram, 1997). These are very small depolarizations, given that the action potential threshold is approximately 20 mV higher than resting membrane potential. In addition, as with other central synapses, their probability of release is relatively low (Jack et al., 1994; Stratford et al., 1989).

• *Integration of many inputs is necessary to fire the neuron.*    On top of this, these weak and failing connections have generally depressing short-term synaptic plasticity (Abbott et al., 1997; Markram, 1997), so their influence might be even smaller at

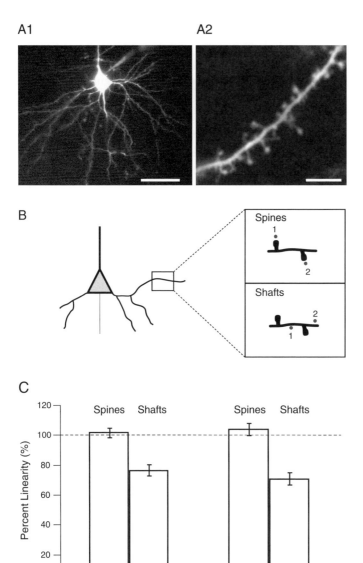

**Figure 10.2**
Linear summation of spine potentials. (A1) Layer 5 pyramidal cell filled with a fluorescence dye. Scale: 50 μm. (A2) Basal dendrite selected for uncaging. Scale bar: 5 μm. (B) Protocol for testing summation. Dots indicate the site of uncaging in spines or shaft locations. Uncaging was performed first at each spine or shaft location (1 or 2) and then in both spines or in both shaft locations. (C) Summary of results. Linearity is expressed as the ratio of the peak amplitude or area of the combined event to the expected values, calculated by adding the two separate events. Note how summation of spine potentials is linear but summation of two shaft potentials is already reduced by 30 to 40%. Data are presented as averages ± SEM. Reprinted from Araya et al., 2006b.

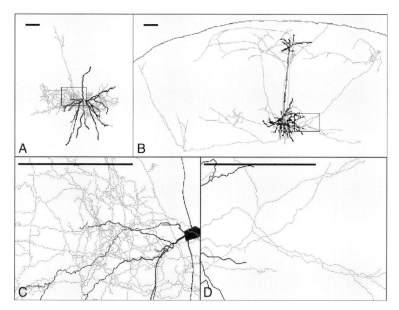

**Figure 10.3**
Differences in morphologies between excitatory and inhibitory axons. Comparison of axon morphologies
between pyramidal cells and GABAergic interneurons. Axons are drawn in light gray, dendrites in black.
Scale bars: 100 μm. Panels (A) and (C) show the same interneuron, (B) and (D) are the same pyramidal
cell. Both cells have 18,500 μm of axon. Boxes in (A) and (B) show areas from where magnified views were
taken. Note how pyramidal axons are relatively straight and cover large territories, when compared with
interneurons. Reprinted from Yuste and Urban, 2004.

steady state, when the circuit is continuously active. Because of these weak, depressing connections, summation of many cortical neurons is necessary to bring a postsynaptic cell to action potential threshold (Abeles, 1991). Moreover, if one also
considers the additional filtering caused by dendrites, and the potential role of inhibition at preventing spiking, one could argue that individual cortical inputs are
designed to have as little influence as possible in the firing of the postsynaptic neuron.
The corollary of this is that a neuron is designed to integrate as many inputs as possible.

• *Excitatory axons are relatively straight and innervate diffusely.*   In addition, axons
of excitatory neurons in the cortex traverse relatively extensive territories (compared
with their dendritic arbors) and innervate regions with low densities of contacts
(compared, for example, with axons of inhibitory cells; figure 10.3). Here I am refer-
ring strictly to local innervation, not the patchy axonal innervation observed over
longer (>1 mm) distances. Indeed, over small distances (<100 μm), axonal trajectories of pyramidal neurons (or parallel fibers in the cerebellum, for an even clearer example) are remarkably straight. This indicates that excitatory neurons distribute their

inputs across a large population of targets, but, in doing so, also minimize the total length of their axons by making them relatively straight. Besides economizing membrane and cytoplasm, shorter wire equals faster action potential transmission, so there could be a great evolutionary pressure in this design (Ramón y Cajal, 1899c).

• *Inhibitory axons are tortuous and innervate local regions.* Meanwhile, axons from inhibitory neurons appear to follow the opposite strategy, with clear differences in branching and arborization (figure 10.3A, C). Specifically, pyramidal neurons have straighter axons that fan out further, with fewer branch points, than interneurons (Yuste and Urban, 2004). Thus, pyramidal cells distribute their outputs broadly, innervating each target weakly, whereas interneurons concentrate their outputs onto a local territory of cells, yet innervate them strongly.

• *Spines could minimize the wiring while maximizing connectivity.* Spines not only protrude from the dendrite but also appear to be constantly moving, particularly during early developmental periods (see chapter 5). By allowing a dendrite to connect with a larger number of axons, spines would further serve to shorten the wire and sample a wider choice of axons. The role of spines in maximizing connectivity therefore is quite logical, but also makes sense if the circuit is distributed and weak. If connections were strong and focal, it would be a better strategy for any given axon to target the dendritic shaft, or the soma, of a neuron and then make as many contacts as possible, as indeed some inhibitory interneurons do. In the cerebellum, Purkinje cells illustrate the link between spiny cells and distributed connectivity matrixes: Because of the stunning orthogonal topology of the parallel fiber input, a given granule cell may contact hundreds of thousands of Purkinje cells, probably only once. Spines work as a sieve to catch these fibers, and the circuit achieves the maximum possible distributed connectivity. In networks of connected pyramidal neurons a similar principle could operate, although their axons are not orthogonal to the dendrites and the circuit is not so clearly laid out. Nevertheless, at least some pyramidal to pyramidal connections appear to be based on single contacts (CA3 to CA1, P. Somogy, pers. comm.), although others are mediated by a few contacts (Markram, 1997). Why a small number of contacts, rather than just one? Perhaps this could compensate for a low probability of release.

• *Spines could maximize input integration.* By using spines with NMDA receptors, which are quite slow, pyramidal neurons would slow down input integration and turn the millisecond spike signal of the presynaptic cell into a relatively long-lasting dendritic response. Slowing the signal is exactly what one would do if one wanted to integrate inputs over time. This integration is particularly slow when compared to the speed of the action potential generation and of its transmission through the axon of any neuron. Further, spines could also electrically isolate inputs and prevent their interaction and shunting, so that they could be integrated linearly. This would make the neuron resemble a low-pass processor that essentially keeps track of the integrated total current injected by the activated inputs.

• *Spiny neurons are individual integrating devices.* Therefore, the essential function of pyramidal cells, and of their elaborated dendritic trees full of spines, might be to keep a faithful tally of total injected current by all inputs per duty cycle. This cycle would last tens or even hundreds of milliseconds, the time necessary for NMDA receptors to close. During this time, the threshold could be reached by a fixed number of active inputs (figure 10.1B). The mathematical function that the pyramidal neurons implement could be to extract the integral of the input waveforms, and long time constants would be necessary for integration.

**Linear Integration and Distributed Connectivity**

After these considerations, we can now reconcile the role of spines at the biophysical and circuit levels, and realize that the apparently different functions that spines carry out could be, in reality, aspects of the same basic task. My proposal is that linear integration, distributed connectivity, and input-specific plasticity are intrinsically related functions. Moreover, these three features are essential functional properties of neural networks.

I will first address the relation between distributed connectivity and linear integration. A full connectivity goes hand in hand with linear summation of inputs. If neurons are associative elements and their circuits operate like a distributed circuit, one would probably want to sample the output of each element of the circuit independently. Linear integration thus would make sense to prevent interaction between inputs or saturation of the cell. Indeed, in the CNS, circuits in which neurons bear spines generally have a connectivity plan with a large input convergence (fan-in). This is evident in the Purkinje cells and some pyramidal neurons, where the typical number of connections between and incoming axon and the spiny cells is probably one, the theoretical maximum.

An advantage generally noted of distributed circuits is that they might make the nervous system more resilient. Whereas invertebrate species could survive and propagate by making many animals, vertebrates have a lot invested in each offspring, so it may be better to endow them with a particularly resilient nervous system by making many neurons (Stevens, 1998). This large connectivity, which by necessity has to be mediated by a large number of weak inputs, creates the constraint that all inputs need to be heard, and summing them linearly appears an ideal solution. Nonlinear summation would override, and seem contrary to, this "neuronal democracy," whereby all inputs are equally tallied. At the same time, this does not mean that all inputs should be exactly equal in weight, so the term "democracy" may not be an ideal one. Instead, these circuits could be a "plastic democracy," where the weight of the vote of each citizen could change over time, even though they would all be

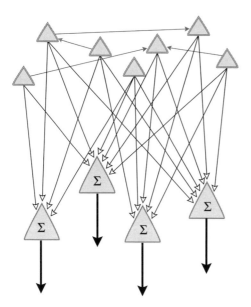

**Figure 10.4**
Model circuit of spiny excitatory neurons. The top layer of cells is connected to the bottom layer in a distributed connectivity. Neurons in the bottom layer integrate inputs linearly from the top layer.

taken into account. Nevertheless, the heterogeneity of spine sizes and synaptic strength, presumably a consequence of synaptic plasticity and the history of the synapse, would represent a set of scattered points around a mean baseline where inputs have generally a similar influence.

The use of such a simple algebraic summation is a necessary consequence of the distribution of information and inputs. A neuronal circuit where the information is maximally distributed, due to a large number of cells which are performing an equally important function, must ensure that all cells can influence the function of the circuit and therefore take maximum advantage of the distribution of information (figure 10.4). To ensure that all cells have an equal opportunity to influence the final computation, it seems natural that their inputs would be added linearly and that the postsynaptic cells are integrators. The neuronal democracy is therefore a direct consequence of having a large number of members.

## Distributed Connectivity and Input-Specific Plasticity

I will now reconcile the potential role of spines in synaptic plasticity with the proposal that the circuit is distributed. In a way, the argument stems directly from the previously discussed relation between distributed circuits and linear integration. Just as it appears important to register the functional effect of each input independently of the others, in order to take full advantage of a distributed connectivity matrix, it would make sense to keep the changes in the strength of each of these inputs from interfering with one another. If the synaptic plasticity elicited in one of the inputs to the neuron can alter the strength of the connections of other inputs, the neuron will lose the ability to tell these changes apart. This could impoverish the function of the cell over time. By using input-specific synaptic plasticity, the neuron has the ability to fine-tune each of its inputs, and extract the maximum possible information from their combinations. This strategy agrees well with linear integration, in which the neuron is trying also to maximize the information that it is extracting from the circuit, which again makes sense if the circuit is distributed.

Thus, distributed connectivity, linear integration, and input-specific synaptic plasticity appear to be following the same circuit logic. At this point I will briefly discuss theoretical studies of artificial neural networks. Rather than a digression from the main argument of the chapter, I will point out how the roles that I propose spines are playing are precisely the essential functional features that enable artificial neural networks to perform their computations.

### Distributed Connectivity and Neural Networks

Artificial neural networks are theoretical models of circuits of connected neurons that have been used to explore what classes of computational problems a neural circuit can solve (Churchland and Sejnowski, 1992; Dayan and Abbott, 2001; Rolls and Treves, 1998; Seung and Yuste, 2010). These neural network models are generally distributed circuits, in which a given neuron receives inputs from many other neurons in the network, and itself sends its output to many other neurons. There are as many types of artificial neural networks as there are practitioners in this field, but one can classify most neural networks into two major categories, depending on how their connectivity is laid out: either as a feedforward or a feedback circuit architecture. A feedforward neural network is one in which neurons are arranged in sequential layers, and the connections are unidirectional from one layer to the next. Therefore, the flow of information follows a single direction in the circuit, from its input to its output, and at each step there are no connections that return back to the previous layers of neurons. Because of this arrangement, feedforward networks are fast. Examples of these feedforward neural networks are the perceptrons (Rosenblatt, 1958), widely used for pattern recognition and categorization problems.

In feedback neural network models, on the other hand, connections are arranged in a recurrent fashion (Hopfield and Tank, 1986). That is, neurons can send their outputs back to the same neurons, or layers, from which they receive inputs, either directly or indirectly. Feedback neural networks therefore have circuit loops, and this generates reentrant patterns of activity that can be sustained by the network, even in the absence of external stimulation. In feedback networks, the input onto a network interacts with the intrinsic activity patterns to generate an output. An example of this class of neural networks is the model proposed by Hopfield (1982), also known as an attractor neural network, because its activity can persist in particular dynamic states called attractors. Attractor networks have multistability in their dynamics, and these stable or semistable states can be viewed as computational solutions. Feedback networks have been used as models for associative memory and for optimization problems (Hopfield and Tank, 1985; Rolls and Treves, 1998).

In neural networks, it is customary to represent the connectivity pattern of the circuit as a matrix, also known as the weight matrix. In it, each column represents connections from a particular presynaptic neuron and each row represents the inputs received by a particular postsynaptic cell. The diagonal of the matrix thus represents the connections that each neuron makes onto itself. In these matrices, the value of each element in the matrix corresponds to the synaptic weight of that particular connection. Thus, the entire connectivity diagram can be captured by a single weight matrix, and the role of each neuron becomes mathematically quite simple: to integrate all the values of its home row (i.e., its inputs) and feed the result to its target neurons. In some feedback network models this connectivity matrix is full, meaning that each neuron connects to, and receives connections from, all other neurons. This is the theoretical limit of a distributed circuit.

**Input Integration in Neural Networks**

How do neurons in a neural network integrate their inputs? In 1943, McCulloch and Pitts proposed a model by which neurons in an artificial neural network would integrate their inputs by a simple linear addition of their values, leading to a threshold firing (McCulloch and Pitts, 1943). In their simplification, these inputs could only have a binary value, a 1 (active) or a 0 (inactive). This linear integration was followed by an action potential; if the input sum was larger than a given threshold, the value of the activity of the postsynaptic neuron becomes 1. Therefore, integration in the McCulloch-Pitts (MP) model, also known as the linear-threshold model, is governed by the following equation:

$$x_i(t+1) = H\left(\sum_{j=1}^{N} W_{ij}x_j(t) - \theta_i\right), \tag{1}$$

where $x(t)$ represents the activity of neuron and $x(t+1)$ the activity at a next increment of time. $H$ is the Heaviside function defined by $H(u) = 1$ for $u \geqslant 0$ or $H(u) = 0$. Following the standard neural network nomenclature, $W_{ij}$ is the *strength* or *weight* of the synapse onto postsynaptic neuron $i$ from presynaptic neuron $j$, and $\theta_i$ is the fixed threshold of neuron $i$.

Using their model, McCulloch and Pitts proposed that the activity of each neuron coded the truth of some logical proposition. In other words, neurons (and by extension the brain) could perform formal logic. This is potentially of great importance, since formal logic is the base of any computation. Thus, a neural network built with simple linear integrating units could be very powerful. The simplicity and power of this model made it a classic reference in the subsequent literature on neural networks (for a review see McClelland and Rumelhart, 1986; Seung and Yuste, 2010). Indeed, in most neural network models integration is performed through the sum of the input values. These simple linearly integrating circuits, therefore, could be used as the foundation of calculus, logic and computation.

### Input-Specific Plasticity in Neural Networks

Neural networks are dynamical systems, i.e., they can change with time. In many neural network models, the values of the weight matrix are updated with each functional cycle of the activity of the circuit. The changes in synaptic weights are controlled by a learning rule, i.e., a function that normally depends on the state of the neuron or the network, and that is applied to the existing value of the synaptic weight to generate a new, updated value. Learning rules are applied to all the elements in the weight matrix, and in many models, they normally are input-selective, meaning that the change in one particular input does not influence other inputs. These learning rules can be supervised, when they depend on some extrinsic factor such as the overall performance of the network or the activity of a "teacher" input, or unsupervised, meaning that they operate at a local level, updating each synaptic weight independently of all the others. The Hebbian rule is a popular example of a learning rule, by which the synaptic weigth of a particular input changes if there is a temporal coincidence of the activity of the neuron generating that input and the neuron receiving the input, regardless of what the rest of the circuit is doing.

The presence of a learning rule is essential for the function of a neural network, since this enables it to change its synaptic matrix and thus adapt its circuit architecture to the particular computational problem that it is trying to solve. In fact, many neural network models start with a random distribution of synaptic weights in their matrices, which, in a training phase, becomes fine-tuned by the operation of its learning rule until its performance matches the desired task. Neural networks with an unsupervised learning rule become self-organizing systems, capable of learning a task and redistributing its connection strengths. The ability to evolve over time through changes in the weight matrix also enables neural networks to capture the statistical dependency of variables and link them together in a functional state, thus performing associative memory tasks.

**Dendritic Spines and Neural Networks**

I now put forward the hypothesis that spiny circuits are neural networks. Indeed, most neural network models have been inspired by brain anatomy and physiology, and at least to some, artificial neural networks are valid models for brain circuits. Here, not only will I embrace this idea, but I will argue that spines are precisely what enable these circuits to behave like neural networks.

Indeed, it seems that spines are ideally suited to provide brain circuits with the exact properties that give them their computational power as a neural network. First, by maximizing connectivity, they could help to fill in the weight matrix and approximate it to the desired theoretical maximum, increasing the sampling (or mixing) of connections as much as possible. Second, by enabling linear input summation, they could exactly implement the type of linear integration assumed by McCulloch-Pitts and most other mathematical models of networks. Finally, their role in compartmentalizing biochemistry and facilitating input-specific plasticity could make them physical repositories of input-specific learning rules.

In fact, many circuits that are dominated by spiny neurons have been modeled as neural networks (Rolls and Treves, 1998). For example, the cerebellar cortex, the dentate gyrus and CA1 region of the hippocampus have been modeled as perceptrons (Marr, 1969; 1971; Rolls and Treves, 1998). Other spiny circuits, such as the CA3 area of the hippocampus or the cerebral cortex, have been proposed to be essentially feedback attractor networks (Cossart et al., 2003; Douglas et al., 2004; Rolls and Treves, 1998). I would argue that the fact that these circuits are spiny is not a coincidence; on the contrary, spines are essentially linked to their function as neural networks. The abilities that these circuits have to solve organization, categorization, classification, or optimization problems, or to generate multistable dynamical states and temporal patterning of the activity, or to enable the association of sets of inputs, or to implement Boolean logic, could be based on the fact that they use spines. In this view, spines would not be an accidental design feature, but the functional components of these circuits, and precisely the ones that endow them with the properties that support their computational powers. In their multifaceted influence on the circuit, spines fit the neural network bill to a tee.

**Objections to the Proposal**

So far, in this chapter I have discussed the reasons why I believe that spines play a central role in the linearization of neuronal integration and how this goes hand in hand with the fact that, anatomically, spines receive distributed inputs and that they can also serve to biochemically isolate synapses and implement local synaptic plasticity. I then argued that these functional properties are precisely the ones that enable circuits with dendritic spines function as neural networks. I now examine the potential pitfalls and objections to these ideas with a critical eye, discussing alternative viewpoints. After all, the function of spines, and more generally, neural circuits, remains a relatively unknown subject for which current research is still in its infancy, and my proposal is a speculation that aims to help move forward our understanding of these topics.

I will first review some of these objections, discussing biophysical problems with linear integration or with the biochemical/plasticity input isolation, reviewing the special case of aspiny cells such as neocortical interneurons, and ending with the discussion of some circuit and computational problems that arise from this proposal. As the reader will see, the discussion of these issues raises many open questions that in principle could be investigated and solved.

**Biophysical Objections**

I have argued that pyramidal neurons and other spiny neurons appear to integrate inputs linearly, and that the electrical isolation of spines could serve to turn synaptic inputs into current-based synapses, which integrate by summing, rather than conductance-based synapses, which would shunt each other when integrating. Nevertheless, one could argue that the role that spines play in input linearization could be accidental and not causal. For example, the linearization of the summation could be achieved by a balance of active conductances (Cash and Yuste, 1998), something that does not necessarily need the electrical isolation of spines generated by the spine neck. From this point of view, the electrical isolation of spines could have a different function, such as generating a local amplification of the voltage signal at the synapse (see chapter 9). Also, although the differences between linear integration of spines and sublinear integration of dendritic shaft inputs are clear (figure 10.2; see Araya et al., 2006a), one could also counter-argue that the summation of uncaging potentials on dendritic shafts might be due to an entirely different set of mechanisms from those that control EPSPs summation in spines, so comparing spine and shaft integration may not be appropriate. Although, as pointed out earlier (Jack et al., 1975), electrical isolation between inputs leads to their linear integration, one cannot dispel these objections until more is known about the mechanisms underlying input summation in spines or shafts.

Another biophysical objection is that dendrites from spiny neurons can sustain local dendritic spikes (see figure 7.6 and Schiller et al., 2000; Yuste et al., 1994). Therefore, at least in some circumstances, integration of EPSPs could be nonlinear, and these nonlinearities could be used to enhance the computational possibilities on individual neurons (Mel, 1994). At the same time, however, these local dendritic spikes are elicited by stimulating clusters of synaptic inputs (Holthoff et al., 2004; Schiller et al., 2000), and it is presently unclear how common these patterns of stimulation are in vivo. In fact, the widely distributed axonal projections onto spiny neurons would appear to make the synchronous clustered activation of inputs quite improbable, compared with the distributed activation of different regions of the dendritic tree that would result from a distributed innervation pattern. In other words, since it requires a big barrage of localized input to make a local dendritic spike, if activity is not localized precisely on the dendrite, the neuron will just fire anyway, because other inputs in other dendrites will bring it to threshold. Based on my proposal, one would predict that stimulation of a neuron by sensory inputs in vivo would result in the activation of spatially uncorrelated patterns of spines in its dendritic tree. For stimuli whose spine patterns have stronger synaptic weights, a linear sum of their EPSPs would lead to the firing of the cell and determine its receptive field.

Nevertheless, dendritic spikes do occur occasionally, at least in vitro, and, interestingly, they can generate a very potent form of LTD, as if the neuron were to specifically diminish the weight of these clustered inputs (Holthoff et al., 2004). This strategy, weakening strong, clustered inputs, in fact could be ideal if one precisely wanted to make input innervation sparse and generate a more linear integration regime. Therefore, I would turn the argument around and propose that, although dendrites are capable of nonlinear behavior, such as dendritic spikes, these may be fine-tuning second-order mechanisms to promote or preserve an ultimate linear logic of their integration (figure 10.5). This argument follows the tradition of engineering of adding second-order hardware components to compensate nonlinearities to make a system linear and controllable (Mead, 1989).

A related issue is the presence of sodium channels in dendrites, or even in spines (Araya et al., 2007). Since these channels have a nonlinear dependency on voltage, their activation in spines by synaptic inputs could make linear integration difficult. Although this may seem potentially as countering linear summation, as argued above, the role of these and other nonlinear conductances in spines or dendrites is poorly understood and their effect on summation could depend on many factors, including how electrically isolated spines are from one another and exactly what range of voltages they experience. In fact, as argued before, hippocampal neurons can operate in an "active linearity" regime, by a compensation of conductances (Cash and Yuste, 1999).

Finally, one could argue that dendritic integration could be linear anyway, regardless of the presence or absence of spines, if inputs are very small or are too far from each other to interact electrically. Given the size of the dendritic tree relative to the size of single spine, if afferent axons connect without specificity with dendrites, statistically one would expect that most of the combination would result in distant activation of inputs, making them electrically isolated. This would make the role of spines in linearizing the input integration unnecessary. While this is likely the case for the situation in which the neuron is activated with few inputs, one should keep in mind

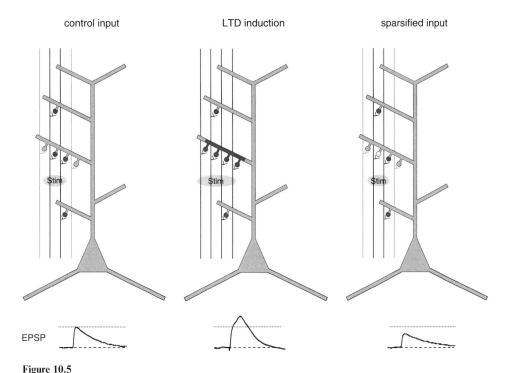

**Figure 10.5**
Local dendritic spikes can lead to sparsification of the connectivity. (Left) Weak stimulation triggers synaptic input to several individual spines at different locations of the dendritic tree. Some of the inputs can be clustered at the same part of the dendritic tree (middle left oblique branch). At the soma these inputs lead to a standard EPSP (bottom). (Middle) A single strong synaptic stimulus produces the activation of many coincident inputs to the same dendritic branch. The coincident activation of many spines at the same branch induces a local regenerative dendritic spike and a locally restricted dendritic calcium transient of large amplitude that generates LTD. (Right) The local dendritic spike induces synaptic depression of the synapses participating in the dendritic spike. This local LTD mechanism would depress neighboring inputs which are coincidentally active and eventually favor the distribution of coincident inputs over the dendritic tree.

that in vivo, neurons are likely bombarded constantly with hundreds of inputs within the integration time, sometimes up to a few hundreds of milliseconds, due to long, NMDAR-based conductances. In this physiological case, electrical interactions between inputs could become a real problem, since the dendrite could become saturated and electronically disconnected from the soma. In a theoretical study, Bernarder et al. (1994) highlighted this issue, proposing that calcium-activated conductances could help to prevent saturation and to linearize the input integration. The electrical isolation of inputs by the spine neck could be an alternative solution to the same problem, preventing the shunting of the dendritic tree by defending it from the changes in input conductance associated with massive barrages of synaptic inputs (Llinás and Nicholson, 1971).

**Biochemical and Plasticity Objections**

A different type of objection relates to the role of spines as biochemical compartments, and to this being the mechanism of input-specific synaptic plasticity. First,
spines are not completely isolated biochemically. Even for calcium, there is diffusion
of calcium from the spine head toward the dendrite, particularly significant for spines
with very short necks (figure 7.11; Majewska et al., 2000b). Other second messengers,
such as Ras, apparently can diffuse out of the spine in response to synaptic activity
(Yasuda et al., 2006). One could argue that the important biochemical compartmentalization is the one that matters functionally, so that the fact that a few calcium ions
or metabolites escape the spine may not have a strong functional significance. At the
same time, there is evidence for heterosynaptic plasticity in spiny neurons, whereby
synaptic plasticity in one spine can influence neighboring synapses (Bonhoeffer et al.,
1994; Schuman and Madison, 2001; Harvey and Svoboda, 2007). Therefore, synaptic
plasticity may not be completely input-specific, hinting at the possibility of learning rules that depend on the physical proximity of the synaptic weights or neurons,
something that theorists have postulated as a mechanism underlying self-assembly
of maps (Kohonen, 1990). At the same time, the manipulations that generate heterosynaptic plasticity are not based on physiological stimulations of the inputs, so it remains to be demonstrated whether these regimes are functional or the results depend
crucially on the stimulation protocols used. Also, if heterosynaptic plasticity were
physiological, one would need to weigh it versus homosynaptic plasticity (i.e., input-
specific) to discern its true importance in the normal functioning of the circuit.

**The Special Case of Cortical Interneurons**

Other objections to the theory arise from considerations about the morphological
structure of the neurons bearing—or not bearing—spines. In particular, in linking
the presence of spines to linear integration, or to distributed circuits, or input-specific
plasticity, one essentially leaves GABAergic interneurons out of the discussion of
how these circuits work. Given that nonspiny, or sparsely spiny, interneurons constitute approximately 20% of the cortical neurons, it is appropriate to consider, at least
briefly, how they integrate inputs, how their axons are organized, and what type of
plasticity they can sustain. The function of the spines, after all, might be clearly illustrated by comparing neurons with spines to those without them. Simply put, one
could argue that the three functional properties that I have proposed are linked to
the presence of dendritic spines, that is: distributed connectivity, linear input integration, and input-specific plasticity, should be absent in interneurons. As we'll see below, although this could be generally true, one should be cautious comparing or
extrapolating functional properties across cell types, since they could be endowed
with different mechanisms and follow a different circuit logic.

Indeed, interneurons are very different from pyramidal cells, and it may be inappropriate to compare them. Besides generally lacking spines and using a different neurotransmitter, they are also generated in the cerebral nuclei region of the early embryo and migrate into the cerebral cortex, so in a way they are a foreign population to the circuit (Anderson et al., 1997). Moreover, as opposed to pyramidal neurons, cortical interneurons are generally fast in their electrical properties (Makram et al., 2004) and they apparently lack slow currents, such as NMDARs or Ih, that could be key for input integration (see above).

The function of interneurons is still unclear. For example, interneurons could prevent overexcitation and saturation of excitatory cells, increase their dynamic range, and control their adaptation to different types of stimuli. Another idea could be that they essentially perform algebra on the spikes of pyramidal cells, carrying out subtraction or division operations, as a second computational layer imposed on the pyramidal cells (Marr, 1970). Indeed, the fact that the kinetics of EPSPs and IPSPs can be well matched to each other may not be a coincidence and suggests that the role of interneurons is related to modulating the function of pyramidal cells. In fact, I would go as far as proposing that pyramidal cells (or spiny neurons), form the "skeleton" of the circuit, which carries out the basic computation, whereas interneurons play a secondary, yet perhaps crucial, role in helping principal cells operate in their overall integrative regime. From this point of view, one should be able to understand the basic computational structure, or transfer function, of a circuit without discussing interneurons. One potential example of this is the remapping of grid cell receptive field onto hippocampal cells, where interneurons are apparently not needed for the computational transformation (Solstad et al., 2006).

In agreement with this, anatomically, interneurons appear to be following a completely different strategy than pyramidal neurons, which suggests that they are not contributing to the kernel of the computation. As pointed out above, axons from neocortical interneurons innervate local territories intensely, the opposite of the strategy of pyramidal neurons, which cover large territories. Also, interneuron axons generally do not target spines, although, as discussed in chapter 3, there are also some exceptions: Some inhibitory inputs occur on spines (as many as 10–20% of neocortical spines could have inhibitory inputs), and, conversely, some excitatory inputs occur on dendritic shafts. I do not have a good explanation for these exceptions. Further research is required on this special class of spines or inputs in order to better understand their functional differences.

But regardless of where their axons terminate or their circuit functions, why don't cortical interneurons have spines? Why not use the same strategy as pyramidal neurons, as GABAergic Purkinje cells do? Actually, to make it even more confusing, some interneurons do have spines, albeit always at significantly smaller densities than pyramidal neurons, while others do not (Fairen et al., 1984). It is quite mysterious why this is so. It is possible that spiny interneurons are carrying out a different circuit function, or that inputs contacting interneuron spines belong to a specific subtype. If one were to extrapolate from the argument made earlier in this book, linking spines with dense innervation, one could expect that interneurons should have an overall smaller innervation than spiny cells. This would be in line with Cajal's original hypothesis about spines enhancing connectivity (chapter 2) and with the potential role of spine development and motility in enhancing synaptogenesis (chapters 5 and 6). Linking this idea with the discussion above, if interneurons were to serve a monitoring role in the local circuit, they would not need an extensive connectivity, but only sample a representative proportion of local axons, so extensive innervation may not be necessary. Pyramidal neurons, on the other hand, would be interested in connecting with as many inputs as possible in order to fill the weight matrix. Nevertheless, it is possible, as we discussed in chapter 6, that the key advantage that spines provide would be not just to enhance connectivity, but to endow the dendrites with the ability to sample, and choose among, different axons, rather than to simply help establish synaptic connections. From this point of view, one would then expect that the overall innervation density of interneurons could be similar to that of pyramidal neurons, yet the interneuron inputs would be significantly less diverse.

In addition, following the argument made in this chapter, one could predict that, because they lack spines, interneurons might also integrate inputs differently from pyramidal cells, and also sustain different learning rules. Very little work has been done in characterizing input integration of GABAergic interneurons, but it is interesting that, in these measurements, integration of excitatory inputs in interneurons is sublinear if the inputs are close to each other, but linear if they are far away (further than 60 μm approximately; see figure 6d and e in Tamas et al., 2003). How about integration of inhibitory inputs by pyramidal neurons? The same work indicates that integration of these GABAergic inputs in pyramidal neurons, which for these type of interneurons apparently do not terminate on spines, is sublinear when these inputs are near each other but linear if they are far away (again, $>50$ μm approximately; Tamas et al., 2003). These results agree well with the comparison between dendritic integration of uncaging events on dendritic shafts and spines by pyramidal cells (Araya et al., 2006a) and with the general idea that the spine neck could help generate a linear sum of neighboring excitatory inputs (see figure 10.2).

Finally, one could use the comparison between pyramidal cells and interneurons to test or examine the link between spines and input-specific plasticity. By lacking spines, interneurons might also lack some of these same plasticity mechanisms. This simple reasoning is confounded by the fact that interneurons also are endowed with input-specific biochemical compartmentalization, as discussed in chapter 7 (figure 7.10). Moreover, in dendrites from interneurons calcium can accumulate with a spatial confinement similar to the dimensions of a dendritic spine (Goldberg et al., 2003a; Soler-Llavina and Sabatini, 2006). But then, one could argue that it is not just the spatial restriction of calcium that matters for input-specific synaptic plasticity, but the actual spatiotemporal concentration dynamics of the intracellular free calcium concentration and the subsequent biochemical reactions driven by it. In this respect, it appears that synaptically induced calcium accumulations in interneurons are significantly faster than those experienced by spines (Goldberg et al., 2003a). In fact, whereas most calcium accumulations in spines are due to influx through NMDARs (chapter 7), neocortical interneurons are suspiciously devoid of them, as well as lacking some key calcium-dependent enzymes, such as CAM-kinase II. Perhaps the ability to sustain an elevated concentration of calcium for a significant period of time is the key determinant in the role of spines in synaptic plasticity.

But do interneurons actually demonstrate input-specific synaptic plasticity? The answer from the literature seems controversial. The common view is that input-specific synaptic plasticity, such as LTP, is essentially absent in cortical interneurons (McBain et al., 1999). In fact, it has been argued that this is true precisely because they lack spines, in addition to certain postsynaptic molecular components. On the other hand, recent work argues for the existence of forms of long-term synaptic plasticity in interneurons, although with the caveat that this result might depends on the interneuron subtype (Kulmmann and Lamsa, 2007; Pelletier and Lacaille, 2008). Interestingly, some of the subtypes of interneurons that apparently have synaptic plasticity are precisely those that actually have some dendritic spines, such as the hippocampal O-LM cells (Pelletier and Lacaille, 2008). A study correlating the presence or absence of spines and of input-specific synaptic plasticity could help test this.

In summary, it is still unclear if neocortical interneurons can sample cortical connectivity as effectively as pyramidal cells, yet they appear to have significant differences with them in terms of linear integration and the expression of input-specific synaptic plasticity. At the same time, whether this could be solely explained by their lack of spines is far from being proven.

## Coda: A Single Function for Dendritic Spines

So arriving at the end, I recapitulate the main argument of the book: If one considers spines from a circuit perspective, rather than having many different functions, spines might actually serve one essential function, which is to implement a distributed form of computing. Spines would carry it out, quite remarkably, by using several complementary strategies. From this circuit viewpoint, apparently disconnected functions such as maximizing the distribution of information by receiving a large number of inputs (chapter 3), using motility during development to maximize the generation of a varied circuit (chapter 5), helping to physically isolate inputs to enable local biochemistry (chapter 3) and implementing calcium-mediated learning rules (chapters 6 and 7), and electrically isolating inputs to ensure their linear integration (chapters 9 and 10), would all be intrinsically linked, working toward the same goal.

Moreover, my proposal is that these functions are exactly the ones that make circuits with spines behave as neural networks. Spines could be viewed as the anatomical signatures of linearly integrating, distributed neural networks. Spines would endow neural circuits with the ability to perform Boolean logic, to implement associative memory, to have multistable dynamics, to become self-organized, and to become veritable learning machines. Spines would be the way the brain builds neural networks and generates emergent functional properties. When considering the complexity of these apparently different aspects of the spine function and their elegant interactions toward this joint aim, it is truly remarkable that nature has found this clever solution. Indeed, spines are used widely in many types of nervous systems (Brandon and Coss, 1982), so the "invention" of spines could be one of the key advances in the evolution of the nervous system.

In the second edition of his *Histology of the Nervous System*, when discussing the basic principles of the design of the brain, Cajal points out that the nervous system appears to have two basic patterns of axonal arborizations: a "crosswise or cruciate" axodendritic pattern, by which axons contact dendrites at orthogonal (i.e., 90 degrees) orientations, and a "parallel" axodendritic pattern, in which the axons make contacts with the dendrites, but follow a course parallel to them (Ramón y Cajal, 1904). Moreover, he argues that cruciate projections, like "telegraph wires," make very few contacts (or just one) with each neuron, and therefore appear designed to contact as many cells as possible. Parallel projections, on the other hand, selectively innervate few neurons, yet make many contacts on each of them, thus influencing them strongly. Examples of cruciate projections are cortical inputs onto striatal neurons and parallel fiber inputs to Purkinje cells, whereas parallel ones would be the climbing fiber projection to Purkinje cells, or the projection from some types of interneurons to excitatory neurons. With the hindsight of the ultrastructural studies published since Cajal, if one were to generalize within the enormous diversity of neurons and connectivity patterns in the nervous system, one could argue that cruciform projections normally terminate on spines, whereas parallel projections appear to avoid spines. This, of course, would be a natural consequence of the link between spines and distributed circuits. In a note of historical science fiction, it is fascinating to imagine what would have happened if Cajal had been alive only nine more years—long enough to read the seminal 1943 paper of McCulloch and Pitts, in which the theoretical foundation of distributed neural networks was laid out. I think Cajal would have immediately jumped at the link between dendritic spines, distributed circuits, and neural networks, and perhaps argued that those "impenetrable jungles" of the cerebral cortex could be, after all, functionally quite simple.

# References

Abbott, L. F., Varela, J. A., Sen, K., and Nelson, S. B. (1997). Synaptic depression and cortical gain control. *Science 275*, 220–224.

Abeles, M. (1991). *Corticonics*. Cambridge, UK: Cambridge University Press.

Abeles, M., Bergman, H., Margalit, E., and Vaadia, E. (1993). Spatiotemporal firing patterns in the frontal cortex of behaving monkeys. *J Neurophysiol 70*, 1629–1638.

Adams, R. D., and Victor, M. (1985). *Principle of Neurology*. New York: McGraw-Hill.

Ahmari, S., Buchanan, J., and Smith, S. (2000). Assembly of presynaptic active zones from cytoplasmic transport packets. *Nat Neurosci 3*, 445–451.

Airaksinen, M. S., Eiler, J., Garaschuk, O., Thoenen, H., and Konnerth, A. (1997). Ataxia and altered dendritic calcium signaling in mice carrying a targeted null mutation of the calbindin D28k gene. *Proc Natl Acad Sci USA 94*, 1488–1493.

Alcor, D., Gouzer, G., and Triller, A. (2009). Single-particle tracking methods for the study of membrane receptors dynamics. *Eur J Neurosci 30*, 987–997.

Alford, S., Frenguelli, B. G., Schofield, J. G., and Collingridge, G. L. (1993). Characterization of the CA2+ signals induced in hippocampal CA1 neurons by the synaptic activation of NMDA receptors. *J Physiol (Lond) 469*, 693–716.

Allbritton, N. L., Meyer, T., and Stryer, L. (1992). Range of messenger action of calcium ion and inositol 1,4,5-trisphosphate. *Science 258*, 1812–1815.

Allen, K. M., Gleeson, J. G., Bagrodia, S., Partington, M. W., MacMillan, J. C., Cerione, R. A., Mulley, J. C., and Walsh, C. A. (1998). PAK3 mutation in nonsyndromic X-linked mental retardation. *Nat Genet 20*, 25–30.

Allen, P. B., Ouimet, C. C., and Greengard, P. (1997). Spinophilin, a novel protein phosphatase 1 binding protein localized to dendritic spines. *Proc Natl Acad Sci USA 94*, 9956–9961.

Allison, D. W., Chervin, A. S., Gelfand, V. I., and Craig, A. M. (2000). Postsynaptic scaffolds of excitatory and inhibitory synapses in hippocampal neurons: Maintenance of core components independent of actin filaments and microtubules. *J Neurosci 20*, 4545–4554.

Allison, D. W., Gelfand, V. I., Spector, I., and Craig, A. M. (1998). Role of actin in anchoring postsynaptic receptors in cultured hippocampal neurons: Differential attachment of NMDA versus AMPA receptors. *J Neurosci 18*, 2423–2436.

Altman, J., and Anderson, W. J. (1972). Experimental reorganization of the cerebellar cortex. I. Morphological effects of elimination of all microneurons with prolonged X-irradiation started at birth. *J Comp Neurol 146*, 355–406.

Altman, J., and Bayer, S. A. (1997). *Development of the Cerebellar System*. Boca Raton, FL: CRC Press.

Alvarez, V., and Sabatini, B. (2007). Anatomical and physiological plasticity of dendritic spines. *Annu Rev Neurosci 30*, 79–97.

Amaral, D. G. (1979). Synaptic extensions from mossy fibers of the fascia dentata. *Anat Embryol 155*, 241–251.

Andersen, P., and Soleng, A. (1998). Long-term potentiation and spatial training are both associated with the generation of new excitatory synapses. *Brain Res Brain Res Rev 26*, 353–359.

Andersen, P., Silfvenius, H., Sundberg, S. H., and Sveen, O. (1980). A comparison of distal and proximal dendritic synapses on CA1 pyramids in guinea-pig hippocampal slices in vitro. *J Physiol (Lond) 307*, 273–299.

Anderson, S., Eisenstat, D., Shi, L., and Rubenstein, J. (1997). Interneuron migration from basal forebrain to neocortex: Dependence on Dlx genes. *Science 278*, 474–476.

Anderson, J. C., and Martin, K. A. (2001). Does bouton morphology optimize axon length? *Nat Neurosci 4*, 1166–1167.

Apperson, M. L., Moon, I. S., and Kennedy, M. B. (1996). Characterization of densin-180, a new brain-specific synaptic protein of the O-sialoglycoprotein family. *J Neurosci 16*, 6839–6852.

Aoki, C., Wu, K., Elste, A., Len, G., Lin, S., McAuliffe, G., and Black, I. B. (2000). Localization of brain-derived neurotrophic factor and TrkB receptors to postsynaptic densities of adult rat cerebral cortex. *J Neurosci Res 59*, 454–463.

Arai, Y., Ijuin, T., Takenawa, T., Becker, L. E., and Takashima, S. (2002). Excessive expression of synaptojanin in brains with Down syndrome. *Brain Devel 24*, 67–72.

Araya, R., Eisenthal, K. B., and Yuste, R. (2006a). Dendritic spines linearize the summation of excitatory potentials. *Proc Natl Acad Sci USA 103*, 18779–18804.

Araya, R., Jiang, J., Eisenthal, K. B., and Yuste, R. (2006b). The spine neck filters membrane potentials. *Proc Natl Acad Sci USA 103*, 17961–17966.

Araya, R., Nikolenko, V., Eisenthal, K. B., and Yuste, R. (2007). Sodium channels amplify spine potentials. *Proc Natl Acad Sci USA 104*, 12347–12352.

Arellano, J. I., Benavides-Piccione, R., De Felipe, J., and Yuste, R. (2007a). Ultrastructure of dendritic spines: Correlation between synaptic and spine morphologies. *Frontiers Neurosci 1*, 131–143.

Arellano, J. I., Espinosa, A., Fairen, A., Yuste, R., and De Felipe, J. (2007b). Non-synaptic dendritic spines in neocortex. *Neuroscience 145*, 464–469.

Ariens-Kapper, C. U., Huber, G. C., and Crosby, E. C. (1936). The comparative anatomy of the nervous system of vertebrates, including man. New York: Macmillan.

Asou, H., Hamada, K., Uyemura, K., Sakota, T., and Hayashi, K. (1994). How do oligodendrocytes ensheath and myelinate nerve fibers? *Brain Res Bull 35*, 359–365.

Baer, S. M., and Rinzel, J. (1991). Propagation of dendritic spikes mediated by excitable spines: A continuum theory. *J Neurophysiol 65*, 874–890.

Bahr, B. A., Staubli, U., Xiao, P., Chun, D., Ji, Z. X., Esteban, E. T., and Lynch, G. (1997). Arg-Gly-Asp-Ser-selective adhesion and the stabilization of long-term potentiation: Pharmacological studies and the characterization of a candidate matrix receptor. *J Neurosci 17*, 1320–1329.

Balice-Gordon, R. J., and Lichtman, J. W. (1984). Long-term synapse loss induced by focal blockade of postsynaptic receptors. *Nature 372*, 519–524.

Ballesteros-Yañez, I., Benavides-Piccione, R., Elston, G. N., Yuste, R., and Defelipe, J. (2006). Density and morphology of pyramidal cell dendritic spines in mouse neocortex. *Neuroscience 138*, 403–409.

Baptista, A. A., Hatten, M. E., Blazeski, R., and Mason, C. A. (1994). Cell-cell interactions influence survival and differentiation of Purkinje cells in vitro. *Neuron 12*, 243–260.

Barria, A., Muller, D., Derkach, V., Griffith, L. C., and Soderling, T. R. (1997). Regulatory phosphorylation of AMPA-type glutamate receptors by CaM-KII during long-term potentiation. *Science 276*, 2042–2045.

Batini, C., Pelstini, M., Thonasset, M., and Vigot, R. (1993). Cytoplasmic calcium buffer, calbindin-D28k, is regulated by excitatory amino acids. *Neuroreport 4*, 927–930.

Baude, A., Nusser, Z., Roberts, J. D., Mulvihill, E., McIlhinney, R. A., and Somogyi, P. (1993). The metabotropic glutamate receptor (mGluR1 alpha) is concentrated at perisynaptic membrane of neuronal subpopulations as detected by immunogold reaction. *Neuron 11*, 771–787.

Baudry, M., and Davis, J. L., eds. (1996). *Long-term Potentiation*. Cambridge, MA: MIT Press.

Bear, M. F., and Abraham, W. C. (1996). Long-term depression in hippocampus. *Annu Rev Neurosci 19*, 437–462.

Beesley, P. W., Mummery, R., and Tibaldi, J. (1995). N-cadherin is a major glycoprotein component of isolated rat forebrain postsynaptic densities. *J Neurochem 64*, 2288–2294.

Bekkers, J., Richerson, G. B., and Stevens, C. F. (1990). Origin of variability in quantal size in cultured hippocampal neurons and hippocampal slices. *Proc Natl Acad Sci USA 87*, 5359–5362.

Belichenko, P. V., Machanov, M. A., Fedorov, A. A., Krasnov, I. B., and Leontovich, T. A. (1990). Effects of space flight on dendrites of the neurons of the rat's brain. *Physiologist 33*, S12–15.

Benavides-Piccione, R., Ballesteros-Yáñez, I., De Felipe, J., and Yuste, R. (2002). Cortical area and species differences in dendritic spine morphology. *J Neurocytol 31*, 337–346.

Benavides-Piccione, R., Hamzei-Sichani, F., Ballesteros-Yánez, I., De Felipe, J., and Yuste, R. (2006). Dendritic size of pyramidal neurons differs among mouse cortical regions. *Cereb Cortex 16*, 990–1001.

Benson, D. L., Mandell, J. W., Shaw, G., and Banker, G. (1996). Compartmentation of alpha-internexin and neurofilament triplet proteins in cultured hippocampal neurons. *J Neurocytol 25*, 181–196.

Benson, D. L., and Tanaka, H. (1998). N-cadherin redistribution during synaptogenesis in hippocampal neurons. *J Neurosci 18*, 6892–6904.

Berkley, H. J. (1896). The psychical nerve cell in health and disease. *Bull Johns Hopkins Hosp 7*, 162–164.

Bernhardt, R., and Matus, A. (1984). Light and electron microscopic studies of the distribution of microtubule-associated protein 2 in rat brain: A difference between dendritic and axonal cytoskeletons. *J Comp Neurol 226*, 203–221.

Bernarder, O., Koch, C., and Douglas, R. J. (1994). Amplification and linearization of distal synaptic input to cortical pyramidal cells. *J Neurophysiol 72*, 2743–2753.

Berridge, M. J. (1998). Neuronal calcium signaling. *Neuron 21*, 13–26.

Berry, M., and Bradley, P. (1976). The growth of the dendritic trees of Purkinje cells in the cerebellum of the rat. *Brain Res 112*, 1–35.

Biederer, T., and Sudhof, T. C. (2001). CASK and protein 4.1 support F-actin nucleation on neurexins. *J Biol Chem 276*, 47869–47876.

Billuart, P., Bienvenu, T., Ronce, N., des Portes, V., Vinet, M. C., Zemni, R., et al. (1998). Oligophrenin-1 encodes a rhoGAP protein involved in X-linked mental retardation. *Nature 392*, 923–926.

Bliss, T. V. P., and Lømo, T. (1973). Long-lasting potentiation of synaptic transmission in the dentate area of the anaesthetized rabbit following stimulation of the perforant path. *J Physiol (Lond) 232*, 331–356.

Blomberg, F., Cohen, R., and Siekevitz, P. (1977). The structure of postsynaptic densities isolated from dog cerebral cortex. II. Characterization and arrangement of some of the major proteins within the structure. *J Cell Biol 86*, 831–845.

Bonhoeffer, T., Staiger, V., and Aertsen, A. (1989). Synaptic plasticity in rat hippocampal slice cultures: Local "Hebbian" conjunction of pre- and postsynaptic stimulation leads to distributed synaptic enhancement. *Proc Natl Acad Sci USA 86*, 8113–8117.

Bloodgood, B. L., and Sabatini, B. L. (2007a). Ca(2+) signaling in dendritic spines. *Curr Opin Neurobiol 17*, 345–351.

Bloodgood, B. L., and Sabatini, B. L. (2007b). Nonlinear regulation of unitary synaptic signals by CaV(2.3) voltage-sensitive calcium channels located in dendritic spines. *Neuron 53*, 249–260.

Bockers, T. M., Mameza, M. G., Kreutz, M. R., Bockmann, J., Weise, C., Buck, F., Richter, D., et al. (2001). Synaptic scaffolding proteins in rat brain. Ankyrin repeats of the multidomain Shank protein family interact with the cytoskeletal protein alpha-fodrin. *J Biol Chem 276*, 40104–40112.

Bourne, J. N., and Harris, K. M. (2008). Balancing structure and function at hippocampal dendritic spines. *Annu Rev Neurosci 31*, 37–67.

Bourne, J. N., Kirov, S. A., Sorra, K. E., and Harris, K. M. (2007a). Warmer preparation of hippocampal slices prevents synapse proliferation that might obscure LTP-related structural plasticity. *Neuropharmacology 52*, 55–59.

Bourne, J. N., Sorra, K. E., Hurlburt, J., and Harris, K. M. (2007b). Polyribosomes are increased in spines of CA1 dendrites 2 h after the induction of LTP in mature rat hippocampal slices. *Hippocampus 17*, 1–4.

Boyer, C., Schikorski, T., and Stevens, C. F. (1998). Comparison of hippocampal dendritic spines in culture and in brain. *J Neurosci 18*, 5294–5300.

Boynton, G. M., Engel, S. A., Glover, G. H., and Heeger, D. J. (1996). Linear systems analysis of functional magnetic resonance imaging in human V1. *J Neurosci 16*, 4207–4221.

Bradley, P. M., and Berry, M. (1976). The effects of reduced climbing and parallel fibre input on Purkinje cell dendritic growth. *Brain Res 109*, 133–151.

Bradley, P., and Horn, G. (1979). Neuronal plasticity in the chick brain: Morphological effects of visual experience on neurones in hyperstriatum accessorium. *Brain Res 162*, 148–153.

Braitenberg, V., and Schüz, A. (1998). Anatomy of the cortex, 2nd ed. Berlin: Springer.

Brakeman, P. R., Lanahan, A. A., O'Brien, R., Roche, K., Barnes, C. A., Huganir, R. L., and Worley, P. F. (1997). Homer: A protein that selectively binds metabotropic glutamate receptors. *Nature 386*, 284–288.

Brandon, J., and Coss, R. (1982). Rapid dendritic spine stem shortening during one-trial learning: The honeybee's first orientation flight. *Brain Res 252*, 51–61.

Bravin, M., Morando, L., Vercelli, A., Rossi, F., and Strata, P. (1999). Control of spine formation by electrical activity in the adult rat cerebellum. *Proc Natl Acad Sci USA 96*, 1704–1709.

Brecht, M., Schneider, M., Sakmann, B., and Margrie, T. W. (2004). Whisker movements evoked by stimulation of single pyramidal cells in rat motor cortex. *Nature 427*, 704–710.

Brizzee, K., Ordy, J., Kaack, M., and Beavers, T. (1980). Effect of prenatal ionizing radiation on the visual cortex and hippocampus of newborn squirrel monkeys. *J Neuropathol Exp Neurol 39*, 523–540.

Buchs, P., and Muller, D. (1996). Induction of long-term potentiation is associated with major ultrastructural changes of activated synapses. *Proc Natl Acad Sci USA 93*, 8040–8045.

Buchert, M., Schneider, S., Meskenaite, V., Adams, M. T., Canaani, E., Baechi, T., et al. (1999). The junction-associated protein AF-6 interacts and clusters with specific Eph receptor tyrosine kinases at specialized sites of cell-cell contact in the brain. *J Cell Biol 144*, 361–371.

Caceres, A., Payne, M. R., Binder, L. I., and Steward, O. (1983). Immunocytochemical localization of actin and microtubule-associated protein MAP2 in dendritic spines. *Proc Natl Acad Sci USA 80*, 1738–1742.

Calabrese, B., Wilson, M. S., and Halpain, S. (2006). Development and regulation of dendritic spine synapses. *Physiology 21*, 38–47.

Caldwell, J., Schallwe, K., Lasher, R., Peles, E., and Levisnon, S. (2000). Sodium channel Na(v)1.6 is localized at nodes of ranvier, dendrites, and synapses. *Proc Natl Acad Sci USA 97*, 5616–5620.

Canepari, M., Nelson, L., Papageorgiou, G., Corrie, J. E., and Ogden, D. (2001). Photochemical and pharmacological evaluation of 7-nitroindolinyl-and 4-methoxy-7-nitroindolinyl-amino acids as novel, fast caged neurotransmitters. *J Neurosci Methods 112*, 29–42.

Carandini, M., Heeger, D. J., and Movshon, J. A. (1997). Linearity and normalization in simple cells of the macaque primary visual cortex. *J Neurosci 17*, 8621–8644.

Cash, S., and Yuste, R. (1998). Input summation by cultured pyramidal neurons is linear and position-independent. *J Neurosci 18*, 10–15.

Cash, S., and Yuste, R. (1999). Linear summation of excitatory inputs by CA1 pyramidal neurons. *Neuron 22*, 383–394.

Caviness, V. S., and Sidman, R. L. (1972). Olfactory structures of the forbrain in the "reeler" mutant mouse. *J Comp Neurol 145*, 85–104.

Caviness, V. S. J., and Sidman, R. L. (1973). Time of origin of corresponding cell classes in the cerebral cortex of normal and mutant reeler mice: An autoradiographic analysis. *J Comp Neurol 148*, 141–151.

Cesa, R., Morando, L., and Strata, P. (2003). Glutamate receptor delta2 subunit in activity-dependent heterologous synaptic competition. *J Neurosci 23*, 2363–2370.

Cesa, R., and Strata, P. (2005). Axonal and synaptic remodeling in the mature cerebellar cortex. *Prog Brain Res 148*, 45–56.

Chan, S. L., and Mattson, M. P. (1999). Caspase and calpain substrates: Roles in synaptic plasticity and cell death. *J Neurosci Res 58*, 167–190.

Chang, H. T. (1952). Cortical neurons with particular reference to the apical dendrite. *Cold Spring Harbor Symp Quant Biol 17*, 189–202.

Chang, F., and Greenough, W. (1984). Transient and enduring morphological correlates of synaptic activity and efficacy change in the rat hippocampal slice. *Brain Res 309*, 35–46.

Chen, H. J., Rojas-Soto, M., Oguni, A., and Kennedy, M. B. (1998). A synaptic Ras-GTPase activating protein (p135 SynGAP) inhibited by CaM kinase II. *Neuron 20*, 895–904.

Chen, Y., Bourne, J., Pieribone, V. A., and Fitzsimonds, R. M. (2004). The role of actin in the regulation of dendritic spine morphology and bidirectional synaptic plasticity. *Neuroreport 15*, 829–832.

Cheng, D., Hoogenraad, C. C., Rush, J., Ramm, E., Schlager, M. A., Duong, D. M., et al. (2006). Relative and absolute quantification of postsynaptic density proteome isolated from rat forebrain and cerebellum. *Mol Cell Proteomics 5*, 1158–1170.

Cheng, X. T., Hayashi, K., and Shirao, T. (2000). Non-muscle myosin IIB-like immunoreactivity is present at the drebrin-binding cytoskeleton in neurons. *Neurosci Res 36*, 167–173.

Chittajallu, R., Braithwaite, S. P., Clarke, V. R., and Henley, J. M. (1999). Kainate receptors: Subunits, synaptic localization and function. *Trends Pharmacol Sci 20*, 26–35.

Chklovskii, D. B., Schikorski, T., and Stevens, C. F. (2002). Wiring optimization in cortical circuits. *Neuron 34*, 341–347.

Chung, H. J., Xia, J., Scannevin, R. H., Zhang, X., and Huganir, R. L. (2000). Phosphorylation of the AMPA receptor subunit GluR2 differentially regulates its interaction with PDZ domain-containing proteins. *J Neurosci 20*, 7258–7267.

Chung, H. J., Qian, X., Ehlers, M., Jan, Y. N., and Jan, L. Y. (2009). Neuronal activity regulates phosphorylation-dependent surface delivery of G protein-activated inwardly rectifying potassium channels. *Proc Natl Acad Sci USA 106*, 629–634.

Churchland, P. S., and Sejnowski, T. (1992). *The Computational Brain*. Cambridge, MA: MIT Press.

Cline, H. (2005). Synaptogenesis: A balancing act between excitation and inhibition. *Curr Biol 15*, R203–205.

Coghlan, V. M., Hausken, Z. E., and Scott, J. D. (1995). Subcellular targeting of kinases and phosphatases by association with bifunctional anchoring proteins. *Biochem Soc Trans 23*, 592–596.

Cohen, L. (1989). Optical approaches to neuronal function. In *Annual Review of Physiology*, ed. J. F. Hoffman and P. De Weer. Palo Alto, CA: Annual Review Inc., pp. 487–582.

Cohen, R. S., and Siekevitz, P. (1978). Form of the postsynaptic density. A serial section study. *J Cell Biol 78*, 36–46.

Colledge, M., Dean, R. A., Scott, G. K., Langeberg, L. K., Huganir, R. L., and Scott, J. D. (2000). Targeting of PKA to glutamate receptors through a MAGUK-AKAP complex. *Neuron 27*, 107–119.

Colonnier, M. (1968). Synaptic patterns on different cell types in the different laminae of the cat visual cortex. An electron microscope study. *Brain Res 9*, 268–287.

Communi, D., Vanweyenberg, V., and Erneux, C. (1997). D-myo-inositol 1,4,5-trisphosphate 3-kinase A is activated by receptor activation through a calcium:calmodulin-dependent protein kinase II phosphorylation mechanism. *Embo J 16*, 1943–1952.

Connor, J. A. (1986). Digital imaging of free calcium changes and of spatial gradients in growing processes in single, mammalian central nervous system cells. *Proc Natl Acad Sci USA 83*, 6179–6183.

Connor, J., and Diamond, M. (1982). A comparison of dendritic spine number and type on pyramidal neurons of the visual cortex of old adult rats from social or isolated environments. *J Comp Neurol 210*, 99–106.

Cooney, J. R., Hurlburt, J. L., Selig, D. K., Harris, K. M., and Fiala, J. C. (2002). Endosomal compartments serve multiple hippocampal dendritic spines from a widespread rather than a local store of recycling membrane. *J Neurosci 22*, 2215–2224.

Cornelisse, L. N., van Elburg, R. A. J., Meridith, R. M., Yuste, R., and Mansvelder, H. D. (2007). High speed two-photon imaging of calcium dynamics in dendritic spines: Consequences for spine calcium buffer capacity and influx kinetics. *J Comput Neurosci 8*, 65–85.

Cornell-Bell, A. H., Finkbeiner, S. M., Cooper, M. S., and Smith, S. J. (1990). Glutamate induces calcium waves in cultured astrocytes: Long-range glial signaling. *Science 247*, 470–473.

Cornell-Bell, A. H., Thomas, P. G., and Caffrey, J. M. (1992). $Ca^{2+}$ and filopodial responses to glutamate in cultured astrocytes and neurons. *Canad J Physiol Pharmacol 70*, S206–218.

Coss, R. G., and Perkel, D. H. (1985). The function of dendritic spines: A review of theoretical issues. *Behav Neural Biol 44*, 151–185.

Cossart, R., Aronov, D., and Yuste, R. (2003). Attractor dynamics of network UP states in neocortex. *Nature 423*, 283–289.

Cotman, C., Matthews, D., Taylor, D., and Lynch, G. (1973). Synaptic rearrangement in the dentate gyrus: Histochemical evidence of adjustments after lesions in immature and adult rats. *Proc Natl Acad Sci USA 70*, 3473–3477.

Cotman, C. W., and Nieto-Sampedro, M. (1984). Cell biology of synaptic plasticity. *Science 225*, 1287–1294.

Craig, A. M., and Boudin, H. (2001). Molecular heterogeneity of central synapses: Afferent and target regulation. *Nat Neurosci 4*, 569–578.

Craig, A. M., Graf, E. R., and Linhoff, M. W. (2006). How to build a central synapse: Clues from cell culture. *Trends Neurosci 29*, 8–20.

Crain, B., Cotman, C., Taylor, D., and Lynch, G. (1973). A quantitative electron microscopic study of synaptogenesis in the dentate gyrus of the rat. *Brain Res 63*, 195–204.

Crepel, F., and Mariani, J. (1976). Multiple innervation of Purkinje cells by climbing fibers in the cerebellum of the weaver mutant mouse. *J Neurobiol 7*, 579–582.

Crepel, F., Mariani, J., and Delhaye-Bouchaud, N. (1976). Evidence for multiple innervation of Purkinje cells by climbing fibers in the immature rat cerebellum. *J Neurobiol 7*, 567–578.

Crepel, L. (1971). Maturation of climbing fiber responses in the rat. *Brain Res 35*, 272–276.

Crick, F. (1982). Do spines twitch? *Trends Neurosci 5*, 44–46.

Dailey, M. E., and Smith, S. J. (1996). The dynamics of dendritic structure in developing hippocampal slices. *J Neurosci 16*, 2983–2994.

Dalva, M. B., Takasu, M. A., Lin, M. Z., Shamah, S. M., Hu, L., Gale, N. W., and Greenberg, M. E. (2000). EphB receptors interact with NMDA receptors and regulate excitatory synapse formation. *Cell 103*, 945–956.

Dayan, P., and Abbott, L. F. (2001). *Theoretical Neuroscience*. Cambridge, MA: MIT Press.

De Felipe, J., Marco, P., Fairen, A., and Jones, E. G. (1997). Inhibitory synaptogenesis in mouse somatosensory cortex. *Cereb Cortex 7*, 619–634.

Deller, T., Korte, M., Chabanis, S., Drakew, A., Schwegler, H., Stefani, G. G., et al. (2003). Synaptopodin-deficient mice lack a spine apparatus and show deficits in synaptic plasticity. *Proc Natl Acad Sci USA 100*, 10494–10499.

Deller, T., Merten, T., Roth, S. U., Mundel, P., and Frotscher, M. (2000). Actin-associated protein synaptopodin in the rat hippocampal formation: Localization in the spine neck and close association with the spine apparatus of principal neurons. *J Comp Neurol 418*, 164–181.

DeMarco, S. J., and Strehler, E. E. (2001). Plasma membrane Ca2+-atpase isoforms 2b and 4b interact promiscuously and selectively with members of the membrane-associated guanylate kinase family of PDZ (PSD95/Dlg/ZO-1) domain-containing proteins. *J Biol Chem 276*, 21594–21600.

Deng, J., and Dunaevsky, A. (2005). Dynamics of dendritic spines and their afferent terminals: Spines are more motile than presynaptic boutons. *Develop Biol 277*, 366–377.

Denk, W., Delaney, K. R., Gelperin, A., Kleinfeld, D., Strowbridge, B. W., Tank, D. W., and Yuste, R. (1994). Anatomical and functional imaging of neurons using 2-photon laser scanning microscopy. *J Neurosci Meth 54*, 151–162.

Denk, W., Strickler, J. H., and Webb, W. W. (1990). Two-photon laser scanning fluorescence microscopy. *Science 248*, 73–76.

Denk, W., Sugimori, M., and Llinás, R. (1995). Two types of calcium response limited to single spines in cerebellar Purkinje cells. *Proc Natl Acad Sci USA 92*, 8279–8282.

Derkach, V., Barria, A., and Soderling, T. R. (1999). Ca2+/calmodulin-kinase II enhances channel conductance of alpha-amino-3-hydroxy-5-methyl-4-isoxazolepropionate type glutamate receptors. *Proc Natl Acad Sci USA 96*, 3269–3274.

DeRobertis, E. D. P., and Bennett, H. S. (1955). Some features of the submicroscopic morphology of synapses in frog and earthworm. *J Biophy BiochemCytol 1*, 47–58.

Desmond, N., and Levy, W. (1986a). Changes in the numerical density of synaptic contacts with long-term potentiation in the hippocampal dentate gyrus. *J Comp Neurol 253*, 466–475.

Desmond, N., and Levy, W. (1986b). Changes in the postsynaptic density with long-term potentiation in the dentate gyrus. *J Comp Neurol 253*, 476–482.

Desmond, N., and Levy, W. (1988). Synaptic interface surface area increases with long-term potentiation in the hippocampal dentate gyrus. *Brain Res 453*, 308–314.

Desmond, N., and Levy, W. (1990). Morphological correlates of long-term potentiation imly the modification of existing synapses, not synpatogenesis, in the hippocampal dentate gyrus. *Synapse 5*, 139–143.

Desmond, N. L., and Levy, W. B. (1983). Synaptic associative potentiation/depression; an ultrastructural study in the hippocampus. *Brain Res 265*, 21–30.

Deuchards, J., West, D. C., and Thomson, A. (1994). Relationships between morphology and physiology of pyramid-pyramid single axon connections in rat neocortex in vitro. *J Neurophysiol 478*, 423–435.

Diamond, J., Gray, E. G., and Yasargil, G. M. (1970). The function of the dendritic spine: A hypothesis. In *Excitatory Synaptic Mechanisms*, ed. P. Andersen and J. K. S. Jansen. Oslo: Universitetsforlaget, pp. 175–187.

Dong, H., O'Brien, R. J., Fung, E. T., Lanahan, A. A., Worley, P. F., and Huganir, R. L. (1997). GRIP: A synaptic PDZ domain-containing protein that interacts with AMPA receptors. *Nature 386*, 279–284.

Dosemeci, A., and Reese, T. S. (1995). Effect of calpain on the composition and structure of postsynaptic densities. *Synapse 20*, 91–97.

Dougherty, K. D., and Milner, T. A. (1999). p75NTR immunoreactivity in the rat dentate gyrus is mostly within presynaptic profiles but is also found in some astrocytic and postsynaptic profiles. *J Comp Neurol 407*, 77–91.

Douglas, R. J., and Martin, K. A. C. (1998). Neocortex. In *The Synaptic Organization of the Brain*, ed. G. M. Shepherd. Oxford: Oxford University Press, pp. 459–511.

Douglas, R. J., Martin, K. A. C., and Markram, H. (2004). Neocortex. In *The Synaptic Organization of the Brain*, ed. G. M. Shepherd. Oxford: Oxford University Press, pp. 499–558.

Drake, C. T., Milner, T. A., and Patterson, S. L. (1999). Ultrastructural localization of full-length trkB immunoreactivity in rat hippocampus suggests multiple roles in modulating activity-dependent synaptic plasticity. *J Neurosci 19*, 8009–8026.

Dunaevsky, A., Blazeski, R., Yuste, R., and Mason, C. (2001). Spine motility with synaptic contact. *Nat Neurosci 4*, 685–686.

Dunaevsky, A., Tashiro, A., Majewska, A., Mason, C. A., and Yuste, R. (1999). Developmental regulation of spine motility in mammalian CNS. *Proc Natl Acad Sci USA 96*, 13438–13443.

Eccles, J. C., and Mc, I. A. (1953). The effects of disuse and of activity on mammalian spinal reflexes. *J Physiol 121*, 492–516.

Edwards, F. A. (1998). Dancing dendrites. *Nature 394*, 129–130.

Eilers, J., Callewaert, G., Armstrong, C., and Konnerth, A. (1995). Calcium signaling in a narrow somatic submembrane shell during synaptic activity in cerebellar Purkinje neurons. *Proc Natl Acad Sci USA 92*, 10272–10276.

Einheber, S., Schnapp, L. M., Salzer, J. L., Cappiello, Z. B., and Milner, T. A. (1996). Regional and ultrastructural distribution of the alpha 8 integrin subunit in developing and adult rat brain suggests a role in synaptic function. *J Comp Neurol 370*, 105–134.

Ellis-Davies, G. C. R. (2003). Development and application of calcium cages. *Meth Enymol 360A*, 226–238.

Elston, G. N., Benavides-Piccione, R., and De Felipe, J. (2005). A study of pyramidal cell structure in the cingulate cortex of the macaque monkey with comparative notes on inferotemporal and primary visual cortex. *Cereb Cortex 15*, 64–73.

Elston, G. N., and De Felipe, J. (2002). Spine distribution in cortical pyramidal cells: A common organizational principle across species. *Prog Brain Res 136*, 109–133.

Emptage, N., Bliss, T. V., and Fine, A. (1999). Single synaptic events evoke NMDA receptor-mediated release of calcium from internal stores in hippocampal dendritic spines. *Neuron 22*, 115–124.

Engert, F., and Bonhoeffer, T. (1997). Synapse specificity of long-term potentiation breaks down at short distances. *Nature 388*, 279–284.

Engert, F., and Bonhoeffer, T. (1999). Dendritic spine changes associated with hippocampal long-term synaptic plasticity. *Nature 399*, 66–70.

Erondu, N. E., and Kennedy, M. B. (1985). Regional distribution of type II calcium/calmodulin protein kinases in rat brain. *J Neurosci 5*, 3270–3277.

Ethell, I. M., Irie, F., Kalo, M. S., Couchman, J. R., Pasquale, E. B., and Yamaguchi, Y. (2001). EphB/syndecan-2 signaling in dendritic spine morphogenesis. *Neuron 31*, 1001–1013.

Ethell, I. M., Hagihara, K., Miura, Y., Irie, F., and Yamaguchi, Y. (2000). Synbindin, A novel syndecan-2-binding protein in neuronal dendritic spines. *J Cell Biol 151*, 53–68.

Ethell, I. M., Irie, F., Kalo, M. S., Couchman, J. R., Pasquale, E. B., and Yamaguchi, Y. (2001). EphB/syndecan-2 signaling in dendritic spine morphogenesis. *Neuron 31*, 1001–1013.

Ethell, I. M., and Pasquale, E. B. (2005). Molecular mechanisms of dendritic spine development and remodeling. *Prog Neurobiol 75*, 161–205.

Ethell, I. M., and Yamaguchi, Y. (1999). Cell surface heparan sulfate proteoglycan syndecan-2 induces the maturation of dendritic spines in rat hippocampal neurons. *J Cell Biol 144*, 575–586.

Fairen, A., De Felipe, J., and Regidor, J. (1984). Nonpyramidal neurons. In *Cerebral Cortex*, ed. A. Peters and E. G. Jones. New York: Plenum, pp. 201–253.

Fannon, A. M., and Colman, D. R. (1996). A model for central synaptic junctional complex formation based on the differential adhesive specificities of the cadherins. *Neuron 17*, 423–434.

Federmeier, K. D., Kleim, J. A., and Greenough, W. T. (2002). Learning-induced multiple synapse formation in rat cerebellar cortex. *Neurosci Lett 332*, 180–184.

Feng, J., Yan, Z., Ferreira, A., Tomizawa, K., Liauw, J. A., Zhuo, M., et al. (2000). Spinophilin regulates the formation and function of dendritic spines. *Proc Natl Acad Sci USA 97*, 9287–9292.

Feng, W., and Zhang, M. (2009). Organization and dynamics of PDZ-domain-related supramodules in the postsynaptic density. *Nat Rev Neurosci 10*, 87–99.

Fiala, J., Allwardt, B., and Harris, K. (2002). Dendritic spines do not split during hippocampal LTP or maturation. *Nat Neurosci 5*, 297–298.

Fiala, J. C., Feinberg, M., Popov, V., and Harris, K. M. (1998). Synaptogenesis via dendritic filopodia in developing hippocampal area CA1. *J Neurosci 18*, 8900–8911.

Fiala, J. C., and Harris, K. M. (1999). Dendrite structure. In *Dendrites*, ed. G. Stuart, N. Spruston, and M. Hausser. Oxford: Oxford University Press, pp. 1–34.

Fierro, L., and Llano, I. (1996). High endogenous calcium buffering in Purkinje cells from rat cerebellar slices. *J Physiol 496*, 617–625.

Fifkova, E. (1985). A possible mechanisms of morphometric change in dendritic spines induced by stimulation. *Cell Mol Neurobiol 5*, 47–63.

Fifkova, E., and Anderson, C. L. (1981). Stimulation-induced changes in dimensions of stalks of dendritic spines in the dentate molecular layer. *Exp Neurol 74*, 621–627.

Fifkova, E., and Van Harrefeld, A. (1977). Long-lasting morphological chnages in dendritic spines of dentate granular cells followeing stimualtion of the netorhinal area. *J Neurocytol 6*, 211–230.

Fifkova, E., and Delay, R. J. (1982). Cytoplasmic actin in neuronal processes as a possible mediator of synaptic plasticity. *J Cell Biol 95*, 345–350.

Fifkova, E., and Morales, M. (1992). Actin matrix of dendritic spines, synaptic plasticity, and long-term potentiation. *Int Rev Cytol 139*, 267–307.

Finch, E. A., and Augustine, G. J. (1998). Local calcium signalling by inositol-1,4,5-trisphosphate in Purkinje cell dendrites. *Nature 396*, 753–756.

Fine, A., Amos, W. B., Durbin, R. M., and McNaughton, P. A. (1988). Confocal microscopy: Applications in neurobiology. *Trends Neurosci 11*, 345–351.

Fischer, M., Kaech, S., Knutti, D., and Matus, A. (1998). Rapid actin-based plasticity in dendritic spine. *Neuron 20*, 847–854.

Fischer, M., Kaech, S., Wagner, U., Brinkhaus, H., and Matus, A. (2000). Glutamate receptors regulate actin-based plasticity in dendritic spines. *Nat Neurosci 3*, 887–894.

Fong, D. K., Rao, A., Crump, F. T., and Craig, A. M. (2002). Rapid synaptic remodeling by protein kinase C: Reciprocal translocation of NMDA receptors and calcium/calmodulin-dependent kinase II. *J Neurosci 22*, 2153–2164.

Fukata, Y., Oshiro, N., Kinoshita, N., Kawano, Y., Matsuoka, Y., Bennett, V., Matsuura, Y., and Kaibuchi, K. (1999). Phosphorylation of adducin by Rho-kinase plays a crucial role in cell motility. *J Cell Biol 145*, 347–361.

Furuichi, T., Furutama, D., Hakamata, Y., Nakai, J., Takeshima, H., and Mikoshiba, K. (1994a). Multiple types of ryanodine receptor/Ca2+ release channels are differentially expressed in rabbit brain. *J Neurosci 14*, 4794–4805.

Furuichi, T., Kohda, K., Miyawaki, A., and Mikoshiba, K. (1994b). Intracellular channels. *Curr Opin Neurobiol 4*, 294–303.

Fyhn, M., Hafting, T., Treves, A., Moser, M. B., and Moser, E. I. (2007). Hippocampal remapping and grid realignment in entorhinal cortex. *Nature 446*, 190–194.

Gabso, M., Neher, E., and Spira, M. E. (1997). Low mobility of the Ca2+ buffers in axons of cultured Aplysia neurons. *Neuron 18*, 473–481.

Gan, W., Kwon, E., Feng, G., Sanes, J., and Lichtman, J. (2003). Synaptic dynamism measured over minutes to months: Age-dependent decline in an autonomic ganglion. *Nat Neurosci 6*, 956–960.

Gahwiler, B. (1981). Organotypic monolayer cultures of nervous tissue. *J Neurosci Meth 4*, 329–342.

Gasparini, S., and Magee, J. (2006). State-dependent dendritic computation in hippocampal CA1 pyramidal neurons. *J Neurosci 26*, 2088–2100.

Geiger, B., Bershadsky, A., Pankov, R., and Yamada, K. M. (2001). Transmembrane crosstalk between the extracellular matrix–cytoskeleton crosstalk. *Nat Rev Mol Cell Biol 2*, 793–805.

Georgopoulos, A. P., Lurito, J. T., Petrides, M., Schwartz, A. B., and Massey, J. T. (1989). Mental rotation of the neuronal population vector. *Science 243*, 234–236.

Globus, A., and Scheibel, A. (1967). The effect of visual deprivation on cortical neurons: A Golgi study. *Exp Neurol 19*, 331–345.

Gold, J. I., and Shadlen, M. N. (2003). Banburismus and the brain: Decoding the relationship between sensory stimuli, decisions, and reward. *Neuron 36*, 299–308.

Goldberg, J., Tamas, G., Aronov, D., and Yuste, R. (2003a). Calcium microdomains in aspiny dendrites. *Neuron 40*, 807–821.

Goldberg, J., Yuste, R., and Tamas, G. (2003b). Ca2+ imaging of mouse neocortical interneurone dendrites: Contribution of Ca2+-permeable AMPA and NMDA receptors to subthreshold Ca2+ dynamics. *J Physiol 551*, 67–78.

Golding, N. L., and Spruston, N. (1998). Dendritic sodium spikes are variable triggers of axonal action potentials in hippocampal CA1 pyramidal neurons. *Neuron 21*, 1189–1200.

Goldman-Rakic, P. S. (1995). Cellular basis of working memory. *Neuron 14*, 477–485.

Goodman, M., and Lockery, S. (2000). Pressure polishing: A method for re-shaping patch pipettes during fire-polishing. *J Neurosci Meth 100*, 13–15.

Goto, S., Matsukado, Y., Mihara, Y., Inoue, N., and Miyamoto, E. (1986). The distribution of calcineurin in rat brain by light and electron microscopic immunohistochemistry and enzyme-immunoassay. *Brain Res 397*, 161–172.

Grant, S. G. N., Husi, H., Choudhary, J., Cumiskey, M., Blackstock, W., and Armstrong, J. D. (2004). The organization and integrative function of the post-synaptic proteome. In *Excitatory-Inhibitory Balance, Synapses, Circuits, Systems*, ed. T. K. Hensch, and M. Fagiolini. New York: Kluwer Academic/Plenum Press, pp. 13–44.

Gray, E. G. (1959a). Axo-somatic and axo-dendritic synapses of the cerebral cortex: An electron microscopic study. *J Anat 83*, 420–433.

Gray, E. G. (1959b). Electron microscopy of synaptic contacts on dendritic spines of the cerebral cortex. *Nature 183*, 1592–1594.

Greenough, W. T., and Volkmar, F. R. (1973). Pattern of dendritic branching in occipital cortex of rats reared in complex environments. *Exp Neurol 40*, 491–504.

Grutzendler, J., Kasthuri, N., and Gan, W. B. (2002). Long-term dendritic spine stability in the adult cortex. *Nature 420*, 812–816.

Guerini, D., Garcia-Martin, E., Gerber, A., Volbracht, C., Leist, M., Merino, C., and Carafoli, E. (1999). The expression of plasma membrane Ca2+ pump isoforms in cerebellar granule neurons is modulated by Ca2+. *J Biol Chem 274*, 1667–1676.

Guthrie, P. B., Segal, M., and Kater, S. B. (1991). Independent regulation of calcium revealed by imaging dendritic spines. *Nature 354*, 76–80.

Györke, I., and Györke, S. (1998). Regulation of the cardiac ryanodine receptor channel by luminal Ca2+ involves luminal Ca2+ sensing sites. *Biophys J 75*, 2801–2810.

Hahnloser, R., Kozhevnikov, A., and Fee, M. (2002). An ultra-sparse code underlies the generation of neural sequences in a songbird. *Nature 419*, 65–70.

Hall, A. (1994). Small GTP-binding proteins and the regulation of the actin cytoskeleton. *Annu Rev Cell Biol 10*, 31–54.

Hall, A. (1998). Rho GTPases and the actin cytoskeleton. *Science 279*, 509–514.

Hamada, S., and Yagi, T. (2001). The cadherin-related neuronal receptor family: A novel diversified cadherin family at the synapse. *Neurosci Res 41*, 207–215.

Harris, K. M. (1999). Structure, development, and plasticity of dendritic spines. *Curr Opin Neurobiol 9*, 343–348.

Harris, K. M., Jensen, F. E., and Tsao, B. (1992). Three-dimensional structure of dendritic spines and synapses in rat hippocampus (CA1) at postnatal day 15 and adult ages: Implications for the maturation of synaptic physiology and long-term potentiation. *J Neurosci 12*, 2685–2705.

Harris, K. M., and Kater, S. B. (1994). Dendritic spines: Cellular specializations imparting both stability and flexibility to synaptic function. *Annu Rev Neurosci 17*, 341–371.

Harris, K. M., and Stevens, J. K. (1988). Dendritic spines of rat cerebellar Purkinje cells: Serial electron microscopy with reference to their biophysical characteristics. *J Neurosci 8*, 4455–4469.

Harris, K. M., and Stevens, J. K. (1989). Dendritic spines of CA1 pyramidal cells in the rat hippocampus: Serial electron microscopy with reference to their biophysical characteristics. *J Neurosci 9*, 2982–2997.

Harvey, C. D., and Svoboda, K. (2007). Locally dynamic synaptic learning rules in pyramidal neuron dendrites. *Nature 450*, 1195–1200.

Hayashi, K., Ishikawa, R., Ye, L. H., He, X. L., Takata, K., Kohama, K., and Shirao, T. (1996). Modulatory role of drebrin on the cytoskeleton within dendritic spines in the rat cerebral cortex. *J Neurosci 16*, 7161–7170.

Hayashi, K., and Shirao, T. (1999). Change in the shape of dendritic spines caused by overexpression of drebrin in cultured cortical neurons. *J Neurosci 19*, 3918–3925.

Hayashi, Y., and Majewska, A. K. (2005). Dendritic spine geometry: Functional implication and regulation. *Neuron 46*, 529–532.

Hayashi, Y., Shi, S. H., Esteban, J. A., Piccini, A., Poncer, J. C., and Malinow, R. (2000). Driving AMPA receptors into synapses by LTP and CaMKII: Requirement for GluR1 and PDZ domain interaction. *Science 287*, 2262–2267.

Hebb, D. O. (1949). The Organization of Behavior. New York: Wiley.

Heeger, D., and Ress, D. (2002). What does fMRI tell us about neuronal activity? *Nat Rev Neurosci 3*, 142–151.

Heeger, D. J., Simoncelli, E. P., and Movshon, J. A. (1996). Computational models of cortical visual processing. *Proc Natl Acad Sci USA 93*, 623–627.

Helmchen, F., Imoto, K., and Sakmann, B. (1996). Ca2+ buffering and action potential-evoked Ca2+ signalling in dendrites of pyramidal neurons. *Biophys J 70*, 1069–1081.

Hering, H., and Sheng, M. (2001). Dendritic spines: Structure, dynamics and regulation. *Nat Rev Neurosci 2*, 880–888.

Hillman, D. E., Chen, S., Bing, R., Penniston, J. T., and Llinás, R. (1996). Ultrastructural localization of the plasmalemmal calcium pump in cerebellar neurons. *Neuroscience 72*, 315–324.

Hirai, H. (2000). Clustering of delta glutamate receptors is regulated by the actin cytoskeleton in the dendritic spines of cultured rat Purkinje cells. *Eur J Neurosci 12*, 563–570.

Hirano, A., and Dembitzer, H. M. (1973). Cerebellar alterations in the weaver mouse. *J Cell Biol 56*, 476–486.

Hirao, K., Hata, Y., Deguchi, M., Yao, I., Ogura, M., Rokukawa, C., et al. (2000). Association of synapse-associated protein 90/postsynaptic density-95-associated protein (SAPAP) with neurofilaments. *Genes Cells 5*, 203–210.

Hirao, K., Hata, Y., Ide, N., Takeuchi, M., Irie, M., Yao, I., et al. (1998). A novel multiple PDZ domain-containing molecule interacting with N-methyl-D-aspartate receptors and neuronal cell adhesion proteins. *J Biol Chem 273*, 21105–21110.

Holcman, D., and Triller, A. (2006). Modeling synaptic dynamics driven by receptor lateral diffusion. *Biophys J 91*, 2405–2415.

Hollmann, M., Hartley, M., and Heinemann, S. (1991). Ca2+ permeability of KA-AMPA—gated glutamate receptor channels depends on subunit composition. *Science 252*, 851–853.

Holmes, W. (1990). Is the function of dendritic spines to concentrate calcium? *Brain Res 519*, 338–342.

Holthoff, K., Kovalchuk, Y., Yuste, R., and Konnerth, A. (2004). Single-shock LTD by local dendritic spikes. *J Physiol (Lond) 560*, 27–36.

Holthoff, K., Tsay, D., Majewska, A., and Yuste, R. (2002a). Response: Raising the speed limit. *Trends Neurosci 25*, 441.

Holthoff, K., Tsay, D., and Yuste, R. (2002b). Calcium dynamics of spines depend on their dendritic location. *Neuron 33*, 425–437.

Holtmaat, A., De Paola, V., Wilbrecht, L., and Knott, G. W. (2008). Imaging of experience-dependent structural plasticity in the mouse neocortex in vivo. *Behav Brain Res 192*, 20–25.

Holtmaat, A., Wilbrecht, L., Knott, G. W., Welker, E., and Svoboda, K. (2006). Experience-dependent and cell-type-specific spine growth in the neocortex. *Nature 441*, 979–983.

Holtmaat, A. J., Trachtenberg, J. T., Wilbrecht, L., Shepherd, G. M., Zhang, X., Knott, G. W., and Svoboda, K. (2005). Transient and persistent dendritic spines in the neocortex in vivo. *Neuron 45*, 279–291.

Honkura, N., Matsuzaki, M., Noguchi, J., Ellis-Davies, G. C., and Kasai, H. (2008). The subspine organization of actin fibers regulates the structure and plasticity of dendritic spines. *Neuron 57*, 719–729.

Hoover, K. B., and Bryant, P. J. (2000). The genetics of the protein 4.1 family: Organizers of the membrane and cytoskeleton. *Curr Opin Cell Biol 12*, 229–234.

Hopfield, J. J. (1982). Neural networks and physical systems with emergent collective computational abilities. *Proc Natl Acad Sci USA 79*, 2554–2558.

Hopfield, J. J., and Tank, D. W. (1985). "Neural" computation of decisions in optimization problems. *Biol Cybern 52*, 141–152.

Hopfield, J. J., and Tank, D. W. (1986). Computing with neural circuits: A model. *Science 233*, 625–633.

Horch, H. W., Kruttgen, A., Portbury, S. D., and Katz, L. C. (1999). Destabilization of cortical dendrites and spines by BDNF. *Neuron 23*, 353–364.

Horner, A. J., and Andrews, T. J. (2009). Linearity of the fMRI response in catergory-selective regions of human visual cortex. *Human Brain Map 30*, 2628–2640.

Hosokawa, T., Bliss, T. V., and Fine, A. (1992). Persistence of individual dendritic spines in living brain slices. *Neuroreport 3*, 477–480.

Hosokawa, T., Rusakov, D. A., Bliss, T. V. P., and Fine, A. (1995). Repeated confocal imaging of individual dendritic spines in the living hippocampal slice: Evidence for changes in length and orientation associated with chemically induced LTP. *J Neurosci 15*, 5560–5573.

Houweling, A. R., and Brecht, M. (2008). Behavioural report of single neuron stimulation in somatosensory cortex. *Nature 451*, 65–68.

Hsueh, Y. P., Yang, F. C., Kharazia, V., Naisbitt, S., Cohen, A. R., Weinberg, R. J., and Sheng, M. (1998). Direct interaction of CASK/LIN-2 and syndecan heparan sulfate proteoglycan and their overlapping distribution in neuronal synapses. *J Cell Biol 142*, 139–151.

Huang, E. J., and Reichardt, L. F. (2001). Neurotrophins: Roles in neuronal development and function. *Annu Rev Neurosci 24*, 677–736.

Hume, R. I., Dingledine, R., and Heinemann, S. F. (1991). Identification of a site in glutamate receptor subunits that controls calcium permeability. *Science 253*, 1028–1031.

Hume, R. I., and Purves, D. (1981). Geometry of neonatal neurons and the regulation of synaptic elimination. *Nature 293*, 469–471.

Hunter, T. (1998). The Croonian Lecture 1997. The phosphorylation of proteins on tyrosine: Its role in cell growth and disease. *Phil Trans R Soc Lond B 353*, 583–605.

Huntley, G. W., Rogers, S. W., Moran, T., Janssen, W., Archin, N., Vickers, J. C., et al. (1993). Selective distribution of kainate receptor subunit immunoreactivity in monkey neocortex revealed by a monoclonal antibody that recognizes glutamate receptor subunits GluR5/6/7. *J Neurosci 13*, 2965–2981.

Husi, H., Ward, M. A., Choudhary, J. S., Blackstock, W. P., and Grant, S. G. (2000). Proteomic analysis of NMDA receptor-adhesion protein signaling complexes. *Nat Neurosci 3*, 661–669.

Ichtchenko, K., Hata, Y., Nguyen, T., Ullrich, B., Missler, M., Moomaw, C., and Sudhof, T. C. (1995). Neuroligin 1: A splice site-specific ligand for beta-neurexins. *Cell 81*, 435–443.

Ide, N., Hata, Y., Deguchi, M., Hirao, K., Yao, I., and Takai, Y. (1999). Interaction of S-SCAM with neural plakophilin-related Armadillo-repeat protein/delta-catenin. *Biochem Biophys Res Commun 256*, 456–461.

Ikegaya, Y., Aaron, G., Cossart, R., Aronov, D., Lampl, I., Ferster, D., and Yuste, R. (2004). Synfire chains and cortical songs: Temporal modules of cortical activity. *Science 304*, 559–564.

Irie, M., Hata, Y., Takeuchi, M., Ichtchenko, K., Toyoda, A., Hirao, K., et al. (1997). Binding of neuroligins to PSD-95. *Science 277*, 1511–1515.

Irvine, R. F., and Schell, M. J. (2001). Back in the water: The return of the inositol phosphates. *Nat Rev Mol Cell Biol 2*, 327–338.

Isaac, J., Nicoll, R., and Malenka, R. (1995). Evidence for silent synapses: Implications for the expression of LTP. *Neuron 15*, 427–434.

Izawa, I., Nishizawa, M., Ohtakara, K., and Inagaki, M. (2002). Densin-180 interacts with delta-catenin/neural plakophilin-related armadillo repeat protein at synapses. *J Biol Chem 277*, 5345–5350.

Jack, J. J. B., Noble, D., and Tsien, R. W. (1975). *Electric Current Flow in Excitable Cells*. London: Oxford University Press.

Jack, J. B., Larkman, A. U., Major, G., and Stratford, K. J. (1994). Quantal analysis of the synaptic excitation of CA1 hippocampal pyramidal cells. In *Molecular and Cellular Mechanisms of Neurotransmitter Release*, ed. L. Stjaerne, P. Greengard, S. Grillner, T. Hoekfelt, and D. Ottoson. New York: Raven Press, pp. 275–299.

Jack, J. J. B., Noble, D., and Tsien, R. W. (1975). *Electric Current Flow in Excitable Cells*. London: Oxford University Press.

Jacobson, M. (1991). *Developmental Neurobiology*, 3rd ed. New York: Plenum.

Jaffe, D., Fisher, S., and Brown, T. (1994). Confocal laser scanning microscopy reveals voltage-gated calcium signals within hippocampal dendritic spines. *J Neurobiol 25*, 220–233.

Jaslove, S. W. (1992). The integrative properties of spiny distal dendrites. *Neurosci 47*, 495–519.

Johnston, D., Magee, J. C., Colbert, C. M., and Christie, B. R. (1996). Active properties of neuronal dendrites. *Annu Rev Neurosci 19*, 165–186.

Johnston, D., and Wu, S. M.-S. (1995). *Foundations of Cellular Neurophysiology.* Cambridge, MA: MIT Press.

Jones, E. G., and Powell, T. P. S. (1969). Morphological variation in the dendritic spines of the neocortex. *J Cell Sci 5*, 509–529.

Jones, T. A., Klintsova, A. Y., Kilman, V. L., Sirevaag, A. M., and Greenough, W. T. (1997). Induction of multiple synapses by experience in the visual cortex of adult rats. *Neurobiol Learning Memory 68*, 13–20.

Jontes, J. D., Buchanan, J., and Smith, S. J. (2000). Growth cone and dendrite dynamics in zebrafish embryos: Early events in synaptogenesis imaged in vivo. *Nat Neurosci 3*, 231–237.

Jontes, J. D., and Smith, S. J. (2000). Filopodia, spines, and the generation of synaptic diversity. *Neuron 27*, 11–14.

Juraska, J., and Fifkova, E. (1979). An electron microscope study of the early postnatal development of the visual cortex of the hooded rat. *J Comp Neurol 183*, 257–267.

Kachar, B., Behar, T., and Dubois-Dalcq, M. (1986). Cell shape and motility of oligodendrocytes cultured without neurons. *Cell Tissue Res 244*, 27–38.

Kaech, S., Brinkhas, H., and Matus, A. (1999). Volatile anesthetics block actin-based motility in dendritic spines. *Proc Natl Acad Sci USA 96*, 10433–10437.

Kaech, S., Fischer, M., Doll, T., and Matus, A. (1997). Isoform specificity in the relationship of actin to dendritic spines. *J Neurosci 17*, 9565–9572.

Kalisman, N., Silberg, G., and Markram, H. (2005). The neocortical microcircuit as a tabula rasa. *Proc Natl Acad Sci USA 102*, 880–885.

Kater, S. B., Mattson, M. P., Cohan, C., and Connor, J. (1988). Calcium regulation of the neuronal growth cone. *Trends Neurosci 11*, 315–321.

Kato, A., Ozawa, F., Saitoh, Y., Fukazawa, Y., Sugiyama, H., and Inokuchi, K. (1998). Novel members of the Vesl/Homer family of PDZ proteins that bind metabotropic glutamate receptors. *J Biol Chem 273*, 23969–23975.

Katz, L. C., and Shatz, C. J. (1996). Synaptic activity and the construction of cortical circuits. *Science 274*, 1123.

Kay, K. N., Naselaris, T., Prenger, R. J., and Gallant, J. L. (2008). Identifying natural images from human brain activity. *Nature 452*, 352–355.

Kelly, P. T., and Cotman, C. W. (1978). Synaptic proteins. Characterization of tubulin and actin and identification of a distinct postsynaptic density polypeptide. *J Cell Biol 79*, 173–183.

Kelly, P. T., McGuinness, T. L., and Greengard, P. (1984). Evidence that the major postsynaptic density protein is a component of a Ca2+/calmodulin-dependent protein kinase. *Proc Natl Acad Sci USA 81*, 945–949.

Kennedy, M. B. (2000). Signal-processing machines at the postsynaptic density. *Science 290*, 750–754.

Kennedy, M. B., Beale, H. C., Carlisle, H. J., and Washburn, L. R. (2005). Integration of biochemical signalling in spines. *Nat Rev Neurosci 6*, 423–434.

Kennedy, M. B., Bennett, M. K., and Erondu, N. E. (1983). Biochemical and immunochemical evidence that the "major postsynaptic density protein" is a subunit of a calmodulin-dependent protein kinase. *Proc Natl Acad Sci USA 80*, 7357–7361.

Kim, E., Cho, K. O., Rothschild, A., and Sheng, M. (1996). Heteromultimerization and NMDA receptor-clustering activity of Chapsyn-110, a member of the PSD-95 family of proteins. *Neuron 17*, 103–113.

Kim, J., Jung, S., Clemens, A., Petralia, R., and Hoffman, D. (2007). Regulation of dendritic excitability by activity-dependent trafficking of the A-type K+ channel subunit Kv4.2 in hippocampal neurons. *Neuron 54*, 933–947.

Kim, J. H., Liao, D., Lau, L. F., and Huganir, R. L. (1998). SynGAP: A synaptic RasGAP that associates with the PSD-95/SAP90 protein family. *Neuron 20*, 683–691.

Kim, E., Naisbitt, S., Hsueh, Y. P., Rao, A., Rothschild, A., Craig, A. M., and Sheng, M. (1997). GKAP, a novel synaptic protein that interacts with the guanylate kinase-like domain of the PSD-95/SAP90 family of channel clustering molecules. *J Cell Biol 136*, 669–678.

Kirov, S., and Harris, K. (1999). Dendrites are more spiny on mature hippocampal neurons when synapses are inactivated. *Nat Neurosci 2*, 878–883.

Kirov, S., Sorra, K., and Harris, K. (1999). Slices have more synapses than perfusion-fixed hippocampus from both young and mature rats. *J Neurosci 19*, 2876–2886.

Kirov, S. A., Petrak, L. J., Fiala, J. C., and Harris, K. M. (2004). Dendritic spines disappear with chilling but proliferate excessively upon rewarming of mature hippocampus. *Neuroscience 127*, 69–80.

Klauck, T. M., Faux, M. C., Labudda, K., Langeberg, L. K., Jaken, S., and Scott, J. D. (1996). Coordination of three signaling enzymes by AKAP79, a mammalian scaffold protein. *Science 271*, 1589–1592.

Klee, C. B., Ren, H., and Wang, X. (1998). Regulation of the calmodulin-stimulated protein phosphatase, calcineurin. *J Biol Chem 273*, 13367–13370.

Knott, G., and Holtmaat, A. (2008). Dendritic spine plasticity—Current understanding from in vivo studies. *Brain Res Rev 58*, 282–289.

Knott, G. W., Holtmaat, A., Wilbrecht, L., Welker, E., and Svoboda, K. (2006). Spine growth precedes synapse formation in the adult neocortex in vivo. *Nat Neurosci 9*, 1117–1124.

Koch, C. (1999). Dendritic spines. In *Biophysics of Computation*, ed. C. Koch. New York: Oxford University Press, pp. 280–308.

Koch, C., and Poggio, T. (1983a). A theoretical analysis of electrical properties of spines. *Proc R Soc Lond B 213*, 455–477.

Koch, C., and Poggio, T. (1983b). Electrical properties of dendritic spines. *TINS 6*, 80–83.

Koch, C., and Zador, A. (1993). The function of dendritic spines—Devices subserving biochemical rather than electrical compartmentalization. *J Neuroscience 13*, 413–422.

Koester, H. J., and Sakmann, B. (1998). Calcium dynamics in single spines during coincident pre- and postsynaptic activity depend on relative timing of back-propagating action potentials and subthreshold excitatory postsynaptic potentials. *Proc Natl Acad Sci USA 95*, 9596–9601.

Kohmura, N., Senzaki, K., Hamada, S., Kai, N., Yasuda, R., Watanabe, M., Ishii, H., Yasuda, M., Mishina, M., and Yagi, T. (1998). Diversity revealed by a novel family of cadherins expressed in neurons at a synaptic complex. *Neuron 20*, 1137–1151.

Kohonen, T. (1990). Cortical maps. *Nature 346*, 24.

Konur, S., Rabinowitz, D., Fenstermaker, V. L., and Yuste, R. (2003). Systematic regulation of spine sizes and densities in pyramidal neurons. *J Neurobiol 56*, 95–112.

Konur, S., and Yuste, R. (2004a). Developmental regulation of spine and filopodial motility in primary visual cortex: Reduced effects of activity and sensory deprivation. *J Neurobiol 59*, 236–246.

Konur, S., and Yuste, R. (2004b). Imaging the motility of dendritic protrusions and axon terminals: Roles in axon sampling and synaptic competition. *Mol Cell Neurosci 27*, 427–440.

Korkotian, E., and Segal, M. (1998). Fast confocal imaging of calcium released from stores in dendritic spines. *Eur J Neurosci 10*, 2076–2084.

Korkotian, E., and Segal, M. (1999). Release of calcium from stores alters the morphology of dendritic spines in cultured hippocampal neurons. *Proc Natl Acad Sci USA 96*, 12068–12072.

Kornau, H. C., Schenker, L. T., Kennedy, M. B., and Seeburg, P. H. (1995). Domain interaction between NMDA receptor subunits and the postsynaptic density protein PSD-95. *Science 269*, 1737–1740.

Korngreen, A., and Sakmann, B. (2000). Voltage-gated K+ channels in layer 5 neocortical pyramidal neurones from young rats: Subtypes and gradients. *J Physiol 525 Pt 3*, 621–639.

Kose, A., Ito, A., Saito, N., and Tanaka, C. (1990). Electron microscopic localization of gamma- and beta II-subspecies of protein kinase C in rat hippocampus. *Brain Res 518*, 209–217.

Kovalchuk, Y., Eilers, J., Lisman, J., and Konnerth, A. (2000). NMDA receptor-mediated subthreshold Ca(2+) signals in spines of hippocampal neurons. *J Neurosci 20*, 1791–1799.

Kovalchuk, Y., Hanse, E., Kafitz, K. W., and Konnerth, A. (2002). Postsynaptic induction of BDNF-mediated long-term potentiation. *Science 295*, 1729–1734.

Kozloski, J., Hamzei-Sichani, F., and Yuste, R. (2001). Stereotyped position of local synaptic targets in neocortex. *Science 293*, 868–872.

Kullmann, D. M., and Lamsa, K. P. (2007). Long-term synaptic plasticity in hippocampal interneurons. *Nat Rev Neurosci 8*, 687–699.

Kuno, M., and Miyahara, J. T. (1969). Non-linear summation of unit synpatic potentials in spinal motor-neurons of the cat. *J Physiol 201*, 465–477.

Kutsche, K., Yntema, H., Brandt, A., Jantke, I., Nothwang, H. G., Orth, U., et al. (2000). Mutations in ARHGEF6, encoding a guanine nucleotide exchange factor for Rho GTPases, in patients with X-linked mental retardation. *Nat Genet 26*, 247–250.

Kwiatkowski, D. J. (1999). Functions of gelsolin: Motility, signaling, apoptosis, cancer. *Curr Opin Cell Biol 11*, 103–108.

Laatsch, R., and Cowan, W. (1066). Electron microscopic studies of the dentate gyrus of the rat. I. Normal structure with special reference to synaptic organization. *J Comp Neurol 128*, 359–395.

Lan, J. Y., Skeberdis, V. A., Jover, T., Grooms, S. Y., Lin, Y., Araneda, R. C., et al. (2001). Protein kinase C modulates NMDA receptor trafficking and gating. *Nat Neurosci 4*, 382–390.

Landis, D. M. D., and Reese, T. S. (1977). Structure of the Purkinje cell membrane in steggere and weaver mutant mice. *J Comp Neurol 171*, 247–260.

Lang, C., Barco, A., Zablow, L., Kandel, E. R., Siegelbaum, S. A., and Zakharenko, S. S. (2004). Transient expansion of synaptically connected dendritic spines upon induction of hippocampal long-term potentiation. *Proc Natl Acad Sci USA 101*, 16665–16670.

Larramendi, L. M. H. (1969). Analysis of synaptogenesis in the cerebellum of the mouse. In *Neurobiology of Cerebellar Evolution and Development*, ed. R. Llinás. Chicago: American Medical Association Education and Research Foundation, pp. 803–843.

Larramendi, L. M. H., and Victor, T. (1967). Synapses on the Purkinje cell spines in the mouse. An electron microscopic study. *Brain Res 5*, 247–260.

Laxson, L. C., and King, J. S. (1983). The development of the Purkinje cell in the cerebellar cortex of the opossum. *J Comp Neurol 214*, 290–308.

Lee, K., Oliver, M., Schottler, F., Creager, R., and Lynch, G. (1979a). Ultrastructural effetcs of repetitive synaptic stimulation in the hippocampal slice preparation: A preliminary report. *Exp Neurol 65*, 478–480.

Lee, K., Schottler, F., Oliver, M., and Lynch, G. (1979b). Synaptic change associated with the induction of long-term potentiation. *Anat Rec 193*, 601–602.

Lee, K. S., Schottler, F., Oliver, M., and Lynch, G. (1980). Brief bursts of high-frequency stimulation produce two types of structural change in rat hippocampus. *J Neurophysiol 44*, 247–258.

Lee, S. J., Escobedo-Lozoya, Y., Szatmari, E. M., and Yasuda, R. (2009). Activation of CaMKII in single dendritic spines during long-term potentiation. *Nature 458*, 299–304.

Lendvai, B., Stern, E., Chen, B., and Svoboda, K. (2000). Experience-dependent plasticity of dendritic spines in the developing rat barrel cortex in vivo. *Nature 404*, 876–881.

Leonard, A. S., Davare, M. A., Horne, M. C., Garner, C. C., and Hell, J. W. (1998). SAP97 is associated with the alpha-amino-3-hydroxy-5-methylisoxazole-4-propionic acid receptor GluR1 subunit. *J Biol Chem 273*, 19518–19524.

Leonard, A. S., Lim, I. A., Hemsworth, D. E., Horne, M. C., and Hell, J. W. (1999). Calcium/calmodulin-dependent protein kinase II is associated with the N-methyl-D-aspartate receptor. *Proc Natl Acad Sci USA 96*, 3239–3244.

Levy, W. B., and Steward, O. (1979). Synapses as associative memory elements in the hippocampal formation. *Brain Res 175*, 233–245.

Levy, W. B., and Desmond, N. L. (1985). Associative potentiation/depression in the hippocampal dentate gyrus. In *Electrical Activity of the Archicortex*, G. Buzsáki, and C. H. Vanderwolf, eds. Budapest: Akademiai Kiado, pp. 359–373.

Lewis, A., Khatchatouriants, A., Treinin, M., Chen, Z., Peleg, G., Friedman, N., et al. (1999). Second harmonic generation of biological interfaces: Probing membrane proteins and imaging membrane potential around GFP molecules at specific sites in neuronal cells of *C. elegans*. *Chem Phys 245*, 133–144.

Li, K. W., Hornshaw, M. P., Van der Schors, R. C., Watson, R., Tate, S., Casetta, B., et al. (2004). Proteomics analysis of rat brain postsynaptic density. *J Biol Chem 279*, 987–1002.

Li, Z., Van Aelst, L., and Cline, H. T. (2000). Rho GTPases regulate distinct aspects of dendritic arbor growth in Xenopus central neurons in vivo. *Nat Neurosci 3*, 217–225.

Liao, D., Hessler, N., and Malinow, R. (1995). Activation of postsynaptically silent synapses during pairing-induced LTP in CA1 region of hippocampal slice. *Nature 375*, 400–404.

Lin, M. T., Lujâan, R., Watanabe, M., Adelman, J. P., and Maylie, J. (2008). SK2 channel plasticity contributes to LTP at Schaffer collateral-CA1 synapses. *Nat Neurosci 11*, 170–177.

Lin, J. W., Wyszynski, M., Madhavan, R., Sealock, R., Kim, J. U., and Sheng, M. (1998). Yotiao, a novel protein of neuromuscular junction and brain that interacts with specific splice variants of NMDA receptor subunit NR1. *J Neurosci 18*, 2017–2027.

Linke, R., Soriano, E., and Frotscher, M. (1994). Transient dendritic appendages on differentiating septo-hippocampal neurons are not the sites of synaptogenesis. *Brain Res Dev Brain Res 83*, 67–78.

Lisman, J. (1989). A mechanism for the Hebb and anti-Hebb processes underlying learning and memory. *Proc Natl Acad Sci USA 86*, 9574–9578.

Liu, G., Choi, S., and Tsien, R. W. (1999). Variability of neurotransmitter concentration and nonsaturation of postsynaptic AMPA receptors at synapses in hippocampal cultures and slices. *Neuron 22*, 395–409.

Llinás, R., and Hillman, D. E. (1969). Physiological and morphological organization of the cerebellar circuits in various vertebrates. In *Neurobiology of Cerebellar Evolution and Development*, ed. R. Llinás. Chicago: American Medical Association Education and Research Foundation, pp. 43–73.

Llinás, R., and Nicholson, C. (1971). Electroresponsive properties of dendrites and somata in alligator Purkinje cells. *J Neurophysiol 34*, 532–551.

Llinás, R., and Sotelo, C., eds. (1992). *The Cerebellum Revisited*, 1st ed. New York: Springer-Verlag.

Llinás, R., Sugimori, M., and Silver, R. B. (1992). Microdomains of high calcium concentration in a presynaptic terminal. *Science 256*, 677–679.

Locke, J. (1669; 1996). *An Essay Concerning Human Understanding*. Indianapolis, IN: Hackett.

Lømo, T. (2003). The discovery of long-term potentiation. *Phil Trans Roy Soc Lond B 358*, 617–620.

Losonczy, A., and Magee, J. (2006). Integrative properties of radial oblique dendrites in hippocampal CA1 pyramidal neurons. *Neuron 50*, 291–307.

Lu, X., Rong, Y., and Baudry, M. (2000). Calpain-mediated degradation of PSD-95 in developing and adult rat brain. *Neurosci Lett 286*, 149–153.

Lu, X., Wyszynski, M., Sheng, M., and Baudry, M. (2001). Proteolysis of glutamate receptor-interacting protein by calpain in rat brain: Implications for synaptic plasticity. *J Neurochem 77*, 1553–1560.

Lujan, R., Nusser, Z., Roberts, J. D., Shigemoto, R., and Somogyi, P. (1996). Perisynaptic location of metabotropic glutamate receptors mGluR1 and mGluR5 on dendrites and dendritic spines in the rat hippocampus. *Eur J Neurosci 8*, 1488–1500.

Lujan, R., Maylie, J., and Adelman, J. P. (2009). New sites of action for GIRK and SK channels. *Nat Rev Neurosci 10*, 475–480.

Luo, L. (2000). Rho GTPases in neuronal morphogenesis. *Nat Rev Neurosci 1*, 173–180.

Luo, L., Hensch, T., Ackerman, L., Barbel, S., Jan, L., and Jan, Y. N. (1996). Differential effects of the Rac GTPase on Purkinje cell axons and dendritic trunks and spines. *Nature 379*, 837–840.

Lynch, G., Larson, J., Kelso, S., Barrionuevo, G., and Schottler, F. (1983). Intracellular injections of EGTA block induction of hippocampal long-term potentiation. *Nature 305*, 719–721.

Ma, W. J., Beck, J. M., Latham, P. E., and Pouget, A. (2006). Bayesian inference with probabilistic population codes. *Nat Neurosci 9*, 1432–1438.

MacLean, J. N., Watson, B. O., Aaron, G. B., and Yuste, R. (2005). Internal dynamics determine the cortical response to thalamic stimulation. *Neuron 48*, 811–823.

Maeda, H., Ellis-Davis, G. C. R., It, O. K., Miyashita, Y., and Kasai, H. (1999). Supralinear Ca2+ signaling by cooperative and mobile Ca2+ buffering in Purkinje neurons. *Neuron 24*, 989–1002.

Maffei, L., and Galli-Resta, L. (1990). Correlation in the discharges of neighboring rat retinal ganglion cells during prenatal life. *Proc Natl Acad USA 87*, 2861–2864.

Maffei, A., Nataraj, K., Nelson, S. B., and Turrigiano, G. G. (2006). Potentiation of cortical inhibition by visual deprivation. *Nature 443*, 81–84.

Magee, J. C., and Cook, E. P. (2000). Somatic EPSP amplitude is independent of synapse location in hippocampal pyramidal neurons. *Nat Neurosci 3*, 895–903.

Magee, J. C., and Johnston, D. (1997). A synaptically controlled, associative signal for hebbian plasticity in hippocampal neurons. *Science 275*, 209–212.

Mainen, Z., Malinow, R., and Svoboda, K. (1999). Synaptic calcium transients in single spines indicate that NMDA receptors are not saturated. *Nature 399*, 151–155.

Majewska, A., Brown, E., Ross, J., and Yuste, R. (2000a). Mechanisms of calcium decay kinetics in hippocampal spines: Role of spine calcium pumps and calcium diffusion through the spine neck in biochemical compartmentalization. *J Neurosci 20*, 1722–1734.

Majewska, A., and Sur, M. (2003). Motility of dendritic spines in visual cortex in vivo: Changes during the critical period and effects of visual deprivation. *Proc Natl Acad Sci USA 100*, 16024–16029.

Majewska, A., Newton, J. R., and Sur, M. (2006). Remodeling of synaptic structure in sensory cortical areas in vivo. *J Neurosci 26*, 3021–3029.

Majewska, A., Tashiro, A., and Yuste, R. (2000b). Regulation of spine calcium compartmentalization by rapid spine motility. *J Neurosci 20*, 8262–8268.

Malenka, R. C., Kauer, J. A., Perkel, D. J., and Nicoll, R. A. (1989). The impact of postsynaptic calcium on synaptic transmission—Its role in long-term potentiation. *Trends Neurosci 12*, 444–450.

Malenka, R. C., Kauer, J. A., Zucker, R. S., and Nicoll, R. A. (1988). Postsynaptic calcium is sufficient for potentiation of hippocampal slice transmission. *Science 242*, 81–84.

Malenka, R. C., and Nicoll, R. A. (1999). Long-term potentiation—A decade of progress? *Science 285*, 1870–1874.

Maletic-Savatic, M., Malinow, R., and Svoboda, K. (1999). Rapid dendritic morphogenesis in CA1 hippocampal dendrites induced by synaptic activity. *Science 283*, 1923–1927.

Malinow, R., and Malenka, R. C. (2002). AMPA receptor trafficking and synaptic plasticity. *Annu Rev Neurosci 25*, 103–126.

Mariani, J., Crepel, F., Mikoshiba, K., Changeux, J. P., and Sotelo, C. (1975). Anatomical, physiological and biochemical studies of the cerebellum from "reeler" mutant mouse. *Phil Trans Roy Soc B 281*, 1–28.

Marín-Padilla, M. (1967). Number and distribution of the apical dendritic spines of the layer 5 pyramidal cells in man. *J Comp Neurol 131*, 475–490.

Marín-Padilla, M. (1972). Structural abnormalities of the cerebral cortex in human chromosomal aberrations. *Brain Res 44*, 625–629.

Markram, H. (1997). A network of tufted layer 5 pyramidal neurons. *Cereb Cortex 7*, 523–533.

Markram, H., Lübke, J., Frotscher, M., Roth, A., and Sakmann, B. (1997a). Physiology and anatomy of synaptic connections between thick tufted pyramidal neurones in the developing rat neocortex. *J Physiol (Lond) 500*, 409–440.

Markram, H., Lübke, J., Frotscher, M., and Sakmann, B. (1997b). Regulation of synaptic efficacy by coincidence of postsynaptic APs and EPSPs. *Science 275*, 213–215.

Markram, H., Roth, A., and Helmchen, F. (1998). Competitive calcium binding: Implications for dendritic calcium signaling. *J Comput Neurosci 5*, 331 348.

Markram, H., Toledo-Rodriguez, M., Wang, Y., Gupta, A., Silberberg, G., and Wu, C. (2004). Interneurons of the neocortical inhibitory system. *Nat Rev Neurosci 5*, 793–807.

Markram, H., and Tsodyks, M. (1996). Redistribution of synaptic efficacy between neocortical pyramidal neurons. *Nature 382*, 807–810.

Marks, A., Tempst, P., Hwang, K., Taubman, M., Inui, M., Chadwick, C., et al. (1989). Molecular cloning and characterization of the ryanodine receptor/junctional channel complex cDNA from skeletal muscle sarcoplasmic reticulum. *Proc Natl Acad Sci USA 86*, 8683–8687.

Marr, D. (1969). A theory of cerebellar cortex. *J Physiol 202*, 437–470.

Marr, D. (1971). Simple memory: A theory for archicortex. *Phil Trans Roy Soc Lond B 262*, 23–81.

Marrs, G. S., Green, S. H., and Dailey, M. E. (2001). Rapid formation and remodeling of postsynaptic densities in developing dendrites. *Nat Neurosci 4*, 1006–1013.

Martone, M. E., Alba, S. A., Edelman, V. M., Airey, J. A., and Ellisman, M. H. (1997). Distribution of inositol-1,4,5-trisphosphate and ryanodine receptors in rat neostriatum. *Brain Res 756*, 9–21.

Mason, C. (1983). Postnatal maturation of neurons in the cat's lateral geniculate nucleus. *J Comp Neurol 217*, 458–469.

Mates, S., and Lund, J. (1983). Spine formation and maturation of type 1 synapses on spiny stellate neurons in primate visual cortex. *J Comp Neurol 221*, 91–97.

Matsuda, S., Mikawa, S., and Hirai, H. (1999). Phosphorylation of serine-880 in GluR2 by protein kinase C prevents its C terminus from binding with glutamate receptor-interacting protein. *J Neurochem 73*, 1765–1768.

Matsudaira, P. (1991). Modular organization of actin crosslinking proteins. *Trends Biochem Sci 16*, 87–92.

Matsuoka, Y., Hughes, C. A., and Bennett, V. (1996). Adducin regulation. Definition of the calmodulin-binding domain and sites of phosphorylation by protein kinases A and C. *J Biol Chem 271*, 25157–25166.

Matsuoka, Y., Li, X., and Bennett, V. (1998). Adducin is an in vivo substrate for protein kinase C: Phosphorylation in the MARCKS-related domain inhibits activity in promoting spectrin-actin complexes and occurs in many cells, including dendritic spines of neurons. *J Cell Biol 142*, 485–497.

Matsuzaki, M., Ellis-Davies, G. C., Nemoto, T., Miyashita, Y., Iino, M., and Kasai, H. (2001). Dendritic spine geometry is critical for AMPA receptor expression in hippocampal CA1 pyramidal neurons. *Nat Neurosci 4*, 1086–1092.

Matsuzaki, M., Honkura, N., Ellis-Davies, G. C., and Kasai, H. (2004). Structural basis of long-term potentiation in single dendritic spines. *Nature 429*, 761–766.

Matus, A. (2000). Actin-based plasticity in dendritic spines. *Science 290*, 754–758.

Matus, A., Ackermann, M., Pehling, G., Byers, H. R., and Fujiwara, K. (1982). High actin concentrations in brain dendritic spines and postsynaptic densities. *Proc Natl Acad Sci USA 79*, 7590–7594.

Mayford, M., Wang, J., Kandel, E. R., and O'Dell, T. J. (1995). CaMKII regulates the frequency-response function of hippocampal synapses for the production of both LTD and LTP. *Cell 81*, 891–904.

McBain, C. J., Freund, T. F., and Mody, I. (1999). Glutamatergic synapses onto hippocampal interneurons: Precision timing without lasting plasticity. *Trends Neurosci 22*, 228–235.

McClay, D. R. (1999). The role of thin filopodia in motility and morphogenesis. *Exp Cell Res 253*, 296–301.

McClelland, J. L., and Rumelhart, D. E. (1986). *Parallel Distributed Processing*. Cambridge, MA: MIT Press.

McCormick, D. A., Connors, B. W., Lighthall, J. W., and Prince, D. A. (1985). Comparative electrophysiology of pyramidal and sparsely spiny stellate neurons of the neocortex. *J Neurophysiol 54*, 782–806.

McCulloch, W. S., and Pitts, W. (1943). A logical calculus of the ideas immanent in nervous activity. *Bull Math Biol 52*, 99–115; discussion 173–197.

McKinney, R., Capogna, M., Durr, R., Gahwiler, B., and Thompson, S. (1999). Miniature synaptic events maintain dendritic spines via AMPA receptor activation. *Nat Neurosci 2*, 44–49.

Mead, C. (1989). *Analog VLSI and Neural Systems*. Reading, MA: Addison-Wesley.

Megias, M., Emri, Z., Freund, T. F., and Gulyas, A. I. (2001). Total number and distribution of inhibitory and excitatory synapses on hippocampal CA1 pyramidal cells. *Neuroscience 102*, 527–540.

Mehraein, P., Yamada, M., and Tarnowska-Dziduszko, E. (1975). Quantitative study on dendrites and dendritic spines in Alzheimer's disease and senile dementia. *Adv Neurol 12*, 453–458.

Mel, B. W. (1994). Information processing in dendritic trees. *Neur Comput 6*, 1031–1085.

Mèuller, B. M., Kistner, U., Kindler, S., Chung, W. J., Kuhlendahl, S., Fenster, S. D., et al. (1996). SAP102, a novel postsynaptic protein that interacts with NMDA receptor complexes in vivo. *Neuron 17*, 255–265.

Merchan-Perez, A. J., Rodriguez, R., Alonso-Nanclares, L., Schertel, A., and De Felipe, J. (2009). Counting synapses using FIB/SEM microscopy: A true revolution for ultrastructural volume reconstruction. *Frontiers Neuroanat 3*, 18.

Migaud, M., Charlesworth, P., Dempster, M., Webster, L. C., Watabe, A. M., Makhinson, M., et al. (1998). Enhanced long-term potentiation and impaired learning in mice with mutant postsynaptic density-95 protein. *Nature 396*, 433–439.

Millard, A. C., Campagnola, P., Mohler, W. A., Lewis, A., and Loew, L. (2003). Second harmonic imaging microscopy. *Methods Enzymol 361*, 47–69.

Miller, D. M., Shen, M. M., Shamu, C. E., Burglin, T. R., Ruvkun, G., Dubois, M. L., Ghee, M., and Wilson, L. (1992). C. elegans unc-4 gene encodes a homeodomain protein that determines the pattern of synaptic input to specific motor neurons. *Nature 355*, 841–845.

Miller, J. P., Rall, W., and Rinzel, J. (1985). Synaptic amplification by active membrane in dendritic spines. *Brain Res 325*, 325–330.

Miller, K. K., Verma, A., Snyder, S. H., and Ross, C. A. (1991). Localization of an endoplasmic reticulum calcium ATPase in rat brain by in situ hybridization. *Neuroscience 43*, 1–9.

Miller, M., and Peters, A. (1981). Maturation of rat visual cortex. II. A combined Golgi-electron microscope study of pyramidal neurons. *J Comp Neurol 203*, 555–573.

Miller, M. W. (1988). Development of projection and local circuit neurons in neocortex. In *Development and Maturation of Cerebral Cortex*, ed. A. Peters and E. G. Jones. New York: Plenum, pp. 133–166.

Miller, S., and Kennedy, M. (1985). Distinct forebrain and cerebellar isozymes of type II Ca2+/calmodulin-dependent protein kinase associate differently with the postsynaptic density fraction. *J Biol Chem 260*, 9039–9046.

Miller, S. G., and Kennedy, M. B. (1986). Regulation of brain type II Ca2+/Calmodulin-dependent protein kinase by autophosphorylation: A Ca2+-triggered molecular switch. *Cell 44*, 861–870.

Milner, B. (1966). Amnesia following operation on the temporal lobes. In *Amnesia: Clinical, Psychological and Medicolegal Aspects*, ed. C. W. M. Whitty, and O. L. Zangwill. Burlington, MA: Butterworths.

Mills, L. R., Niesen, C. E., So, A. P., Carlen, P. L., Spigelman, I., and Jones, O. T. (1994). N-type Ca2+ channels are located on somata, dendrites, and a subpopulation of dendritic spines on live hippocampal pyramidal neurons. *J Neurosci 14*, 6815–6824.

Morest, D. K. (1969a). The differentiation of cerebral dendrites: A study of the post-migratory neuroblast in the medial nucleus of the trapezoid body. *Z Anat Entwicklungsgesch 128*, 271–289.

Morest, D. K. (1969b). The growth of dendrites in the mammalian brain. *Z Anat Entwick Gesch 128*, 265–305.

Mori, H., Manabe, T., Watanabe, M., Satoh, Y., Suzuki, N., Toki, S., et al. (1998). Role of the carboxy-terminal region of the GluR epsilon2 subunit in synaptic localization of the NMDA receptor channel. *Neuron 21*, 571–580.

Mountcastle, V. B. (1957). Modality and topographic properties of single neurons of cat's somatosensory cortex. *J Neurophysiol 20*, 408–443.

Moser, M., Trommald, M., and Andersen, P. (1994). An increase in dendritic spine density on hippocampal CA1 pyramidal cells following spatial learning in adult rats suggests the formation of new synapses. *Proc Natl Acad Sci USA 91*, 12673–12675.

Moser, M., Trommald, M., Egeland, T., and P., A. (1997). Spatial training in a complex environment and isolation alter the spine distribution differently in rat CA1 pyramidal cells. *J Comp Neurol 380*, 373–381.

Movshon, J. A., Thompson, I. D., and Tolhurst, D. J. (1978). Spatial summation in the receptive fields of simple cells in the cat's striate cortex. *J Physiol 283*, 53–77.

Muller, D., Wang, C., Skibo, G., Toni, N., Cremer, H., Calaora, V., et al. (1996). PSA-NCAM is required for activity-induced synaptic plasticity. *Neuron 17*, 413–422.

Müller, W., and Connor, J. A. (1991). Dendritic spines as individual neuronal compartments for synaptic Ca2+ responses. *Nature 354*, 73–76.

Multani, P., Myers, R., Blume, H., Schomer, D., and Sotrel, A. (1994). Neocortical dendritic pathology in human partial epilepsy: A quantitative Golgi study. *Epilepsia 35*, 728–736.

Mundel, P., Heid, H. W., Mundel, T. M., Kruger, M., Reiser, J., and Kriz, W. (1997). Synaptopodin: An actin-associated protein in telencephalic dendrites and renal podocytes. *J Cell Biol 139*, 193–204.

Murakoshi, H., Lee, S. J., and Yasuda, R. (2008). Highly sensitive and quantitative FRET-FLIM imaging in single dendritic spines using improved non-radiative YFP. *Brain Cell Biol 36*, 31–42.

Murase, S., Mosser, E., and Schuman, E. M. (2002). Depolarization drives beta-Catenin into neuronal spines promoting changes in synaptic structure and function. *Neuron 35*, 91–105.

Murphy, T., Baraban, J., and Wier, W. (1995). Mapping miniature synaptic currents to single synapses using calcium imaging reveals heterogeneity in postsynaptic output. *Neuron 15*, 159–168.

Murphy, T. H., Baraban, J. M., Gil Wier, W., and Blatter, L. A. (1994). Visualization of quantal synaptic transmission by dendritic calcium imaging. *Nature 263*, 529–532.

Murthy, V. N., Sejnowski, T., and Stevens, C. (2000). Dynamics of dendritic calcium transients evoked by quantal release at excitatory hippocampal synapses. *Proc Natl Acad Sci USA 97*, 901–906.

Mussa-Ivaldi, F. A., and Bizzi, E. (2000). Motor learning through the combination of primitives. *Phil Trans R Soc Lond B 355*, 1755–1769.

Nabauer, M., Callewaert, G., Cleemann, L., and Morad, M. (1989). Regulation of calcium release is gated by calcium current, not gating charge, in cardiac myocytes. *Science 244*, 800–803.

Nagerl, U. V., Eberhorn, N., Cambridge, S. B., and Bonhoeffer, T. (2004). Bidirectional activity-dependent morphological plasticity in hippocampal neurons. *Neuron 44*, 759–767.

Naisbitt, S., Kim, E., Weinberg, R. J., Rao, A., Yang, F. C., Craig, A. M., and Sheng, M. (1997). Characterization of guanylate kinase-associated protein, a postsynaptic density protein at excitatory synapses that interacts directly with postsynaptic density-95/synapse-associated protein 90. *J Neurosci 17*, 5687–5696.

Naisbitt, S., Kim, E., Tu, J. C., Xiao, B., Sala, C., Valtschanoff, J., et al. (1999). Shank, a novel family of postsynaptic density proteins that binds to the NMDA receptor/PSD-95/GKAP complex and cortactin. *Neuron 23*, 569–582.

Naisbitt, S., Valtschanoff, J., Allison, D. W., Sala, C., Kim, E., Craig, A. M., et al. (2000). Interaction of the postsynaptic density-95/guanylate kinase domain-associated protein complex with a light chain of myosin-V and dynein. *J Neurosci 20*, 4524–4534.

Nakayama, A. Y., Harms, M. B., and Luo, L. (2000). Small GTPases Rac and Rho in the maintenance of dendritic spines and branches in hippocampal pyramidal neurons. *J Neurosci 20*, 5329–5338.

Nakayama, A. Y., and Luo, L. (2000). Intracellular signaling pathways that regulate dendritic spine morphogenesis. *Hippocampus 10*, 582–586.

Naraghi, M., and Neher, E. (1997). Linearized buffered Ca2+ diffusion in microdomains and its implications for calculation of [Ca2+] at the mouth of a calcium channel. *J Neurosci 17*, 6961–6973.

Neher, E. (1998). Usefulness and limitations of linear approximations to the understanding of Ca++ signals. *Cell Calcium 24*, 345–375.

Neher, E., and Augustine, G. J. (1992). Calcium gradients and buffers in bovine chromaffin cells. *J Physiol (Lond) 450*, 273–301.

Nevian, T., and Sakmann, B. (2004). Single spine Ca2+ signals evoked by coincident EPSPs and backpropagating action potentials in spiny stellate cells of layer 4 in the juvenile rat somatosensory barrel cortex. *J Neurosci 24*, 1689–1699.

Nevian, T., and Sakmann, B. (2006). Spine Ca2+ signaling in spike-timing-dependent plasticity. *J Neurosci 26*, 11001–11013.

Newey, S. E., Velamoor, V., Govek, E. E., and Van Aelst, L. (2005). Rho GTPases, dendritic structure, and mental retardation. *J Neurobiol 6*, 58–74.

Niethammer, M., Kim, E., and Sheng, M. (1996). Interaction between the C terminus of NMDA receptor subunits and multiple members of the PSD-95 family of membrane-associated guanylate kinases. *J Neurosci 16*, 2157–2163.

Nimchinsky, E., Sabatini, B. L., and Svoboda, K. (2002). Structure and function of dendritic spines. *Annu Rev Physiol 64*, 313–353.

Nishimune, A., Isaac, J. T., Molnar, E., Noel, J., Nash, S. R., Tagaya, M., et al. (1998). NSF binding to GluR2 regulates synaptic transmission. *Neuron 21*, 87–97.

Nishimura, S. L., Boylen, K. P., Einheber, S., Milner, T. A., Ramos, D. M., and Pytela, R. (1998). Synaptic and glial localization of the integrin alphavbeta8 in mouse and rat brain. *Brain Res 791*, 271–282.

Nishimura, W., Yao, I., Iida, J., Tanaka, N., and Hata, Y. (2002). Interaction of synaptic scaffolding molecule and Beta-catenin. *J Neurosci 22*, 757–765.

Noel, J., Ralph, G. S., Pickard, L., Williams, J., Molnar, E., Uney, J. B., et al. (1999). Surface expression of AMPA receptors in hippocampal neurons is regulated by an NSF-dependent mechanism. *Neuron 23*, 365–376.

Noguchi, J., Matsuzaki, M., Ellis-Davies, G. C., and Kasai, H. (2005). Spine-neck geometry determines NMDA receptor-dependent Ca2+ signaling in dendrites. *Neuron 46*, 609–622.

Nowack, L., Bregestovski, P., Ascher, P., Herbet, A., and Prochiantz, A. (1984). Magnesium gates glutamate-activated channels in mouse central neurons. *Nature 307*, 462–465.

Nuriya, M., Jiang, J., Nemet, B., Eisenthal, K. B., and Yuste, R. (2005). Imaging membrane potential in neurons with second harmonic generation. *Cold Spring Harbor Synaptic Plasticity Meeting 1*, 16.

Nuriya, M., Jiang, J., Nemet, B., Eisenthal, K. B., and Yuste, R. (2006). Imaging membrane potential in dendritic spines. *Proc Natl Acad Sci USA 103*, 786–790.

Nusser, Z., Cull-Candy, S., and Farrant, M. (1997). Differences in synaptic GABA(A) receptor number underlie variation in GABA mini amplitude. *Neuron 19*, 697–709.

Nusser, Z., Lujan, R., Laube, G., Roberts, J., Molnar, E., and Somogyi, P. (1998). Cell type and pathway dependence of synaptic AMPA receptor number and variability in the hippocampus. *Neuron 21*, 545–559.

O'Brien, J., and Unwin, N. (2006). Organization of spines on the dendrites of Purkinje cells. *Proc Natl Acad Sci USA 103*, 1575–1580.

O'Brien, R. J., and Fischbach, G. D. (1986). Characterization of excitatory amino acid receptors expressed by embryonic chick motoneurons in vitro. *J Neurosci 6*, 3275–3283.

Okabe, S., Miwa, A., and Okado, H. (2001a). Spine formation and correlated assembly of presynaptic and postsynaptic molecules. *J Neurosci 21*, 6105–6114.

Okabe, S., Urushido, T., Konno, D., Okado, H., and Sobue, K. (2001b). Rapid redistribution of the postsynaptic density protein PSD-Zip45 (Homer 1c) and its differential regulation by NMDA receptors and calcium channels. *J Neurosci 21*, 9561–9571.

Okamoto, K., Nagai, T., Miyawaki, A., and Hayashi, Y. (2004). Rapid and persistent modulation of actin dynamics regulates postsynaptic reorganization underlying bidirectional plasticity. *Nat Neurosci 7*, 1104–1112.

Omkumar, R. V., Kiely, M. J., Rosenstein, A. J., Min, K. T., and Kennedy, M. B. (1996). Identification of a phosphorylation site for calcium/calmodulin-dependent protein kinase II in the NR2B subunit of the N-methyl-D-aspartate receptor. *J Biol Chem 271*, 31670–31678.

Osten, P., Khatri, L., Perez, J. L., Kohr, G., Giese, G., Daly, C., et al. (2000). Mutagenesis reveals a role for ABP/GRIP binding to GluR2 in synaptic surface accumulation of the AMPA receptor. *Neuron 27*, 313–325.

Ostroff, L. E., Fiala, J. C., Allwardt, B., and Harris, K. M. (2002). Polyribosomes redistribute from dendritic shafts into spines with enlarged synapses during LTP in developing rat hippocampal slices. *Neuron 35*, 535–545.

Ouimet, C. C., da Cruz e Silva, E. F., and Greengard, P. (1995). The alpha and gamma 1 isoforms of protein phosphatase 1 are highly and specifically concentrated in dendritic spines. *Proc Natl Acad Sci USA 92*, 3396–3400.

Ouimet, C. C., McGinness, T. L., and Greengard, P. (1984). Immunocytochemical localization of calcium/calmodulin-dependent potein kinase II in rat brain. *Proc Natl Acad Sci USA 81*, 5604–5608.

Pak, D. T., Yang, S., Rudolph-Correia, S., Kim, E., and Sheng, M. (2001). Regulation of dendritic spine morphology by SPAR, a PSD-95-associated RapGAP. *Neuron 31*, 289–303.

Palay, S. L. (1956). Synapses in the central nervous system. *J Biophysiol Biochem Cytol 2*, 193–201.

Palay, S. L., and Chan-Palay, V. (1974). *Cerebellar Cortex.* New York: Springer.

Palmer, L. M., and Stuart, G. J. (2009). Membrane potential changes in dendritic spines during action potentials and synaptic input. *J Neurosci 29*, 6897–6903.

Papa, M., Bundman, M. C., Greenberger, V., and Segal, M. (1995). Morphological analysis of dendritic spine development in primary cultures of hippocampal neurons. *J Neurosci 15*, 1–11.

Papa, M., and Segal, M. (1996). Morphological plasticity in dendritic spines of cultured hippocampal neurons. *Neuroscience 71*, 1005–1011.

Park, M., Salgado, J. M., Ostroff, L., Helton, T. D., Robinson, C. G., Harris, K. M., and Ehlers, M. D. (2006). Plasticity-induced growth of dendritic spines by exocytic trafficking from recycling endosomes. *Neuron 52*, 817–830.

Parnass, Z., Tashiro, A., and Yuste, R. (2000). Analysis of spine morphological plasticity in developing hippocampal pyramidal neurons. *Hippocampus 10*, 561–568.

Parnavelas, J., Globus, A., and Kaups, P. (1973). Continuous illumination from birth affects spine density of neurons in the visual cortex of the rat. *Exp Neurol 40*, 742–747.

Passafaro, M., Nakagawa, T., Sala, C., and Sheng, M. (2003). Induction of dendritic spines by an extracellular domain of AMPA receptor subunit GluR2. *Nature 424*, 677–681.

Passafaro, M., Sala, C., Niethammer, M., and Sheng, M. (1999). Microtubule binding by CRIPT and its potential role in the synaptic clustering of PSD-95. *Nat Neurosci 2*, 1063–1069.

Patel, S. N., and Stewart, M. G. (1988). Changes in the number and structure of dendritic spines 25 hours after passive avoidance training in the domestic chick, *Gallus domesticus. Brain Res 449*, 34–46.

Pelletier, J. G., and Lacaille, J. C. (2008). Long-term synaptic plasticity in hippocampal feedback inhibitory networks. *Prog Brain Res 169*, 241–250.

Penzes, P., Johnson, R. C., Sattler, R., Zhang, X., Huganir, R. L., Kambampati, V., et al. (2001). The neuronal Rho-GEF Kalirin-7 interacts with PDZ domain-containing proteins and regulates dendritic morphogenesis. *Neuron 29*, 229–242.

Perez, J. L., Khatri, L., Chang, C., Srivastava, S., Osten, P., and Ziff, E. B. (2001). PICK1 targets activated protein kinase C-alpha to AMPA receptor clusters in spines of hippocampal neurons and reduces surface levels of the AMPA-type glutamate receptor subunit 2. *J Neurosci 21*, 5417–5428.

Perkel, D. H. (1982). Functional role of dendritic spines. *J Physiol (Paris) 78*, 695–699.

Perkel, D. H., and Perkel, D. J. (1985). Dendritic spines: Role of active membrane in modulating synaptic efficacy. *Brain Res 325*, 331–335.

Perlmutter, L. S., Siman, R., Gall, C., Seubert, P., Baudry, M., and Lynch, G. (1988). The ultrastructural localization of calcium-activated protease "calpain" in rat brain. *Synapse 2*, 79–88.

Persohn, E., and Schachner, M. (1987). Immunoelectron microscopic localization of the neural cell adhesion molecules L1 and N-CAM during postnatal development of the mouse cerebellum. *J Cell Biol 105*, 569–576.

Persohn, E., and Schachner, M. (1990). Immunohistological localization of the neural adhesion molecules L1 and N-CAM in the developing hippocampus of the mouse. *J Neurocytol 19*, 807–819.

Peterlin, Z. A., Kozloski, J., Mao, B., Tsiola, A., and Yuste, R. (2000). Optical probing of neuronal circuits with calcium indicators. *Proc Natl Acad Sci USA 97*, 3619–3624.

Peters, A., and Kaiserman-Abramof, I. R. (1969). The small pyramidal neuron of the rat cerebral cortex. The synapses upon dendritic spines. *Z Zellforsch Mikrosk Anat 100*, 487–506.

Peters, A., and Kaiserman-Abramof, I. R. (1970). The small pyramidal neuron of the rat cerebral cortex. The perikaryon, dendrites and spines. *Am J Anat 127*, 321–356.

Peters, A., Palay, S. L., and Webster, H. D. (1991). *The Fine Structure of the Nervous System: Neurons and Their Supporting Cells*, 3rd ed. New York: Oxford University Press.

Peters, A., Paley, S. L., and Webster, H. D. F. (1976). *The Fine Structure of the Nervous System.* Philadelphia: Saunders.

Petersen, C., Malenka, R., Nicoll, R., and Hopfield, J. (1998). All-or-none potentiation at CA3-CA1 synapses. *Proc Natl Acad Sci USA 95*, 4732–4737.

Petrak, L. J., Harris, K. M., and Kirov, S. A. (2005). Synaptogenesis on mature hippocampal dendrites occurs via filopodia and immature spines during blocked synaptic transmission. *J Comp Neurol 484*, 183–190.

Petrozzino, J., Pozzo Miller, L., and Connor, J. (1995). Micromolar Ca2+ transients in dendritic spines of hippocampal pyramidal neurons in brain slice. *Neuron 14*, 1223–1231.

Poirazi, P., and Mel, B. W. (2001). Impact of active dendrites and structural plasticity on the memory capacity of neural tissue. *Neuron 29*, 779–796.

Pokorny, J., and Yamamoto, T. (1981). Postnatal ontogenesis of hippocampal CA1 area in rats. II. Development of ultrastructure in stratum lacunosum and moleculare. *Brain Res Bull 7*, 121–130.

Pollard, T. D., and Borisy, G. G. (2003). Cellular motility driven by assembly and disassembly of actin filaments. *Cell 112*, 453–465.

Popov, V., and Bocharova, L. (1992). Hibernation-induced structural changes in synaptic contacts between mossy fibres and hippocampal pyramidal neurons. *Neuroscience 48*, 53–62.

Popov, V., Bocharova, L., and Bragin, A. (1992). Repeated changes of dendritic morphology in the hippocampus of ground squirrels in the course of hibernation. *Neuroscience 48*, 45–51.

Portera-Cailliau, C., Pan, D. T., and Yuste, R. (2003). Activity-regulated dynamic behavior of early dendritic protrusions: Evidence for different types of dendritic filopodia. *J Neurosci 23*, 7129–7142.

Portera-Cailliau, C., and Yuste, R. (2001). On the function of dendritic filopodia. *Rev Neurol 33*, 1158–1166.

Portera-Cailliau, C., and Yuste, R. (2004). Espinas y filopodios. *Mente y cerebro. 9*, 10–21.

Pozzo-Miller, L., Inoue, T., and Murphy, D. (1999). Estradiol increases spine density and NMDA-dependent Ca2+ transients in spines of CA1 pyramidal neurons from hippocampal slices. *J Neurophysiol 81*, 1404–1411.

Purpura, D. (1974). Dendritic spine "dysgenesis" and mental retardation. *Science 186*, 1126–1128.

Purves, D., and Hadley, R. (1985). Changes in the dendritic branching of adult mammalian neurones revealed by repeated imaging in situ. *Nature 315*, 404–406.

Purves, D., Hadley, R., and Voyvodic, J. (1986). Dynamic changes in the dendritic geometry of individual neurons visualized over periods of up to three months in the superior cervical ganglion of living mice. *J Neurosci 6*, 1051–1060.

Purves, D., and Lichtman, J. W. (1985). *Principles of Neural Development* Sunderland, MA: Sinauer Associates.

Qian, N., and Sejnowski, T. J. (1989). An electro-diffusion model for computing membrane potentials and ionic concentrations in branching dendrites, spines and axons. *Biol Cybern 62*, 1–15.

Rakic, P., Bourgeois, J. P., Eckenhoff, M. F., Zecevic, N., and Goldman-Rakic, P. S. (1986). Concurrent overproduction of synapses in diverse regions of the primate cerebral cortex. *Science 232*, 232–235.

Rakic, P., and Sidman, R. L. (1973). Organization of cerebellar cortex secondary to deficits of granule cells in weaver mutant mice. *J Comp Neurol 152*, 133–162.

Rall, W. (1970). Cable properties of dendrites and effects of synaptic location. In *Excitatory Mechanisms, Proceeding of the 5th International Meeting of Neurobiologists*, ed. P. Andersen, and J. Jansen. Oslo: Universitets Forlaget, pp. 175–187.

Rall, W. (1974a). Dendritic spines and synaptic potency. In *Studies in Neurophysiology*, ed. R. Porter. Cambridge: Cambridge University Press, pp. 203–209.

Rall, W. (1974b). Dendritic spines, synaptic potency and neuronal plasticity. In *Cellular Mechanisms Subserving Changes in Neuronal Activity*, ed. C. D. Woody, K. A. Brown, T. J. Crow, and J. D. Knispel. Los Angeles: Brain Information Services, pp. 13–21.

Rall, W. (1978). Dendritic spines and synaptic potency. In *Studies in Neurophysiology*, ed. R. Porter. Cambridge: Cambridge University Press, pp. 203–209.

Rall, W. (1995). *The Theoretical Foundation of Dendritic Function*. Cambridge, MA: MIT Press.

Rall, W., and Rinzel, J. (1971). Dendritic spine function and synaptic attenuation calculations. *Soc Neurosci Abst 1*, 64.

Rall, W., and Segev, I. (1987). Functional possibilities for synapses on dendrites and on dendritic spines. In *Synaptic Function*, ed. G. E. Edelman, W. F. Gall, and W. M. Cowan. New York: Wiley, pp. 605–637.

Rall, W., and Segev, I. (1988). Excitable dendritic spine clusters: Nonlinear synaptic processing. In *Computer Simulation in Brain Science*, ed. R. M. J. Cotterill. Cambridge: Cambridge University Press, pp. 26–43.

Ramón y Cajal, S. (1888). Estructura de los centros nerviosos de las aves. *Rev Trim Histol Norm Pat 1*, 1–10.

Ramón y Cajal, S. (1891a). Significación fisiológica de las expansiones protoplásmicas y nerviosas de la sustancia gris. *Revista de ciencias médicas de Barcelona 22*, 23.

Ramón y Cajal, S. (1891b). Sur la structure de l'ecorce cerebrale de quelques mamiferes. *La Cellule 7*, 124–176.

Ramón y Cajal, S. (1893). Neue darstellung vom histologischen bau des centralnervensystem. *Arch Anat Entwick, AnatAbt Supplement 1893*, 319–428.

Ramón y Cajal, S. (1894). La fine structure des centres nerveux. The Croonian Lecture. *Proc Roy Soc Lond 55*, 443–468.

Ramón y Cajal, S. (1896a). Le bleu de methylene dans les centres nerveaux. *Rev Trim Microgr 1*, 21–82.

Ramón y Cajal, S. (1896b). Les epines collaterales des cellules du cerveau colorees au bleu de methylene. *Rev Trim Microgr 1*, 5–19.

Ramón y Cajal, S. (1897). *Reglas y consejos sobre la investigacion cientifica: Tonicos de la voluntad.* Madrid.

Ramón y Cajal, S. (1899a). Estudios sobre la cortexa cerebral humana. Corteza visual. *Rev Trim Microgr 4*, 1–63.

Ramón y Cajal, S. (1899b). Estudios sobre la cortexa cerebral humana. Estructura de la cortex motriz del hombre y mamiferos. *Rev Trim Microgr 4*, 117–200.

Ramón y Cajal, S. (1899c). *La Textura del Sistema Nerviosa del Hombre y los Vertebrados*, 1st ed. Madrid: Moya.

Ramón y Cajal, S. (1900a). Estudios sobre la cortexa cerebral humana. Esctructura de la corteza acustica. *Rev Trim Microgr 5*, 129–183.

Ramón y Cajal, S. (1900b). Estudios sobre la cortexa cerebral humana. Estructura de la corteza cerebral olfativa del hombre y mamiferos. *Rev Trim Microgr 6*, 1–150.

Ramón y Cajal, S. (1904). *La Textura del Sistema Nerviosa del Hombre y los Vertebrados*, 2nd ed. Madrid: Moya.

Ramón y Cajal, S. (1923). *Recuerdos de mi vida: Historia de mi labor científica*. Madrid: Alianza Editorial.

Ramón y Cajal, S. (1933). *Neuronismo o reticularismo? Las pruebas objetivas de la unidad anatomica de las celulas nerviosas.* Madrid: Instituto Cajal.

Rao, A., and Craig, A. M. (2000). Signaling between the actin cytoskeleton and the postsynaptic density of dendritic spines. *Hippocampus 10*, 527–541.

Ramón y Cajal, S. (1934). Les preuves objectives de l'unite anatomique des cellules nerveuses. In *Revista Trimestral Micrografica*. Madrid: Travaux du laboratoire de recherches biologiques de l'Universite de Madrid, pp. 1–137.

Rausch, G., and Scheich, H. (1982). Dendritic spine loss and enlargement during maturation of the speech control system in the mynah bird (*Gracula religiosa*). *Neurosci Lett 29*, 129–133.

Richards, D. A., De Paola, V., Caroni, P., Gahwiler, B. H., and McKinney, R. A. (2004). AMPA-receptor activation regulates the diffusion of a membrane marker in parallel with dendritic spine motility in the mouse hippocampus. *J Physiol 558*, 503–512.

Ritzenthaler, S., and Chiba, A. (2003). Myopodia (postsynaptic filopodia) participate in synaptic target recognition. *J Neurobiol 55*, 31–40.

Robinson, T. E., and Kolb, B. (1999). Alterations in the morphology of dendrites and dendritic spines in the nucleus accumbens and prefrontal cortex following repeated treatment with amphetamine or cocaine. *Eur J Neurosci 11*, 1598–1604.

Roche, K. W., and Huganir, R. L. (1995). Synaptic expression of the high-affinity kainate receptor subunit KA2 in hippocampal cultures. *Neuroscience 69*, 383–393.

Roelandse, M., Welman, A., Wagner, U., Hagmann, J., and Matus, A. (2003). Focal motility determines the geometry of dendritic spines. *Neuroscience 121*, 39–49.

Rolls, E. T., and Treves, A. (1998). *Neural Networks and Brain Function*, 1st ed. Oxford: Oxford University Press.

Rose, C., and Konnerth, A. (2001). NMDA receptor-medited Na+ signals in spines and dendrites. *J Neurosci 21*, 4207–4214.

Rose, C., Kovalchuk, Y., Eilers, J., and Konnerth, A. (1999). Two-photon Na+ imaging in spines and fine dendrites of central neurons. *Pflugers Arch 439*, 201–207.

Rosenblatt, F. (1958). The perceptron: A probabilistic model for information storage and organization in the brain. *Psychol Rev 65*, 386–408.

Rosenmund, C., and Stevens, C. F. (1996). Definition of the readily releasable pool of vesicles at hippocampal synapses. *Neuron 16*, 1197–1207.

Ruchhoeft, M. L., Ohnuma, S., McNeill, L., Holt, C. E., and Harris, W. A. (1999). The neuronal architecture of Xenopus retinal ganglion cells is sculpted by rho-family GTPases in vivo. *J Neurosci 19*, 8454–8463.

Ruiz-Marcos, A., and Valverde, F. (1969). The temporal evolution of the distribution of dendritic spines in the visual cortex of normal and dark raised mice. *Exp Brain Res 8*, 284–294.

Sabatini, B. L., Oertner, T. G., and Svoboda, K. (2002). The life cycle of Ca(2+) ions in dendritic spines. *Neuron 33*, 439–452.

Sabatini, B. L., and Svoboda, K. (2000). Analysis of calcium channels in single spines using optical fluctuation analysis. *Nature 408*, 589–593.

Saito, Y., Song, W. J., and Murakami, F. (1997). Preferential termination of corticorubral axons on spine-like dendritic protrusions in developing cat. *J Neurosci 17*, 8792–8803.

Sanes, J., and Lichtman, J. (1999). Development of the vertebrate neuromuscular junction. *Annu Rev Neurosci 22*, 389–442.

Santamaria, F., Wils, S., De Schutter, E., and Augustine, G. J. (2006). Anomalous diffusion in Purkinje cell dendrites caused by spines. *Neuron 52*, 635–648.

Satoh, A., Nakanishi, H., Obaishi, H., Wada, M., Takahashi, K., Satoh, K., Hirao, K., Nishioka, H., Hata, Y., Mizoguchi, A., et al. (1998). Neurabin-II/spinophilin. An actin filament-binding protein with one pdz domain localized at cadherin-based cell-cell adhesion sites. *J Biol Chem 273*, 3470–3475.

Satoh, K., Yanai, H., Senda, T., Kohu, K., Nakamura, T., Okumura, N., Matsumine, A., Kobayashi, S., Toyoshima, K., and Akiyama, T. (1997). DAP-1, a novel protein that interacts with the guanylate kinase-like domains of hDLG and PSD-95. *Genes Cells 2*, 415–424.

Scheiffele, P., Fan, J., Choih, J., Fetter, R., and Serafini, T. (2000). Neuroligin expressed in nonneuronal cells triggers presynaptic development in contacting axons. *Cell 101*, 657–669.

Schell, M. J., Erneux, C., and Irvine, R. F. (2001). Inositol 1,4,5-trisphosphate 3-kinase A associates with F-actin and dendritic spines via its N terminus. *J Biol Chem 276*, 37537–37546.

Scheuss, V., Yasuda, R., Sobczyk, A., and Svoboda, K. (2006). Nonlinear [Ca2+] signaling in dendrites and spines caused by activity-dependent depression of Ca2+ extrusion. *J Neurosci 26*, 8183–8194.

Schikorski, T., and Stevens, C. (1999). Quantitative fine-structural analysis of olfactory cortical synapses. *Proc Natl Acad Sci USA 96*, 4107–4112.

Schikorski, T., and Stevens, C. (2001). Morphological correlates of functionally defined synaptic vesicle populations. *Nat Neurosci 4*, 391–395.

Schiller, J., Major, G., Koester, H. J., and Schiller, Y. (2000). NMDA spikes in basal dendrites of cortical pyramidal neurons. *Nature 404*, 285–289.

Schiller, J., Schiller, Y., and Clapham, D. (1998). NMDA receptors amplify calcium influx into dendritic spines during associative pre- and postsynaptic activation. *Nat Neurosci 1*, 114–118.

Schuman, E. M., and Madison, D. V. (1991). A requirement for the intercellular messenger nitric oxide in long-term potentiation. *Science 254*, 1503–1506.

Schuman, E. M., and Madison, D. V. (1994). Communication of synaptic potentiation between synapses of the hippocampus. *Adv Second Messenger Phosphoprotein Res 29*, 507–520.

Schüz, A. (1981). Prenatal development and postnatal changes in the guinea pig cortex: Microscopic evaluation of a natural deprivation experiment. I. Prenatal development (in German). *J Hirnforsch 22*, 93–111.

Schuster, T., Krug, M., Stalder, M., Hackel, N., Gerardy-Schahn, R., and Schachner, M. (2001). Immunoelectron microscopic localization of the neural recognition molecules L1, NCAM, and its isoform NCAM180, the NCAM-associated polysialic acid, beta1 integrin and the extracellular matrix molecule tenascin-R in synapses of the adult rat hippocampus. *J Neurobiol 49*, 142–158.

Schwartzkroin, P. A., Kunkel, D. D., and Mathers, L. H. (1982). Development of rabbit hippocampus: Anatomy. *Dev Brain Res 2*, 453–486.

Sdrulla, A. D., and Linden, D. J. (2007). Double dissociation between long-term depression and dendritic spine morphology in cerebellar Purkinje cells. *Nat Neurosci 10*, 546–548.

Segal, M. (1995). Fast imaging of [Ca]i reveals presence of voltage-gated calcium channels in dendritic spines of cultured hippocampal neurons. *J Neurophys 74*, 484–488.

Segal, M., and Andersen, P. (2000). Dendritic spines shaped by synaptic activity. *Curr Opin Neurobiol 10*, 582–586.

Segev, I., and Rall, W. (1988). Computational study of an excitable dendritic spine. *J Neurophysiol 60*, 499–523.

Seung, H. S., and Yuste, R. (2010). Neural networks. In *Principles of Neural Science*, ed. E. R. Kandel and T. J. Jessel. New York: McGraw-Hill.

Sharp, A. H., McPherson, P. S., Dawson, T. M., Aoki, C., Campbell, K. P., and Snyder, S. H. (1993). Differential immunohistochemical localization of inositol 1,4,5-trisphosphate- and ryanodine-sensitive Ca2+ release channels in rat brain. *J Neurosci 13*, 3051–3063.

Shatz, C. J., and Stryker, M. P. (1988). Prenatal tetrodotoxin infusion blocks segregation of retinogeniculate afferents. *Science 242*, 87–89.

Shen, K., and Meyer, T. (1999). Dynamic control of CaMKII translocation and localization in hippocampal neurons by NMDA receptor stimulation. *Science 284*, 162–166.

Shen, K., Teruel, M. N., Subramanian, K., and Meyer, T. (1998). CaMKIIbeta functions as an F-actin targeting module that localizes CaMKIIalpha/beta heterooligomers to dendritic spines. *Neuron 21*, 593–606.

Shen, L., Liang, F., Walensky, L. D., and Huganir, R. L. (2000). Regulation of AMPA receptor GluR1 subunit surface expression by a 4.1N-linked actin cytoskeletal association. *J Neurosci 20*, 7932–7940.

Sheng, M., and Hoogenraad, C. C. (2007). The postsynaptic architecture of excitatory synapses: A more quantitative view. *Annu Rev Biochem 76*, 823–847.

Sheng, M., and Kim, E. (2000). The Shank family of scaffold proteins. *J Cell Sci 113*, 1851–1856.

Sheng, M., and Sala, C. (2001). PDZ domains and the organization of supramolecular complexes. *Annu Rev Neurosci 24*, 1–29.

Shepherd, G. M. (1990). *The Synaptic Organization of the Brain.* Oxford: Oxford University Press.

Shepherd, G. M. (1991). *Foundations of the Neuron Doctrine.* Oxford: Oxford University Press.

Shepherd, G. M. (1996). The dendritic spine: A multifunctional integrative unit. *J Neurophysiol 75*, 2197–2210.

Shepherd, G. M., and Brayton, R. K. (1987). Logic operations are properties of computer-simulated interactions between excitable dendritic spines. *Neuroscience 21*, 151–165.

Shepherd, G. M., Brayton, R. K., Miller, J. P., Segev, I., Rinzel, J., and Rall, W. (1985). Signal enhancement in distal cortical dendrites by means of interactions betrween active dendritic spines. *Proc Natl Acad Sci USA 82*, 2192–2195.

Shields, S. M., Ingebritsen, T. S., and Kelly, P. T. (1985). Identification of protein phosphatase 1 in synaptic junctions: Dephosphorylation of endogenous calmodulin-dependent kinase II and synapse-enriched phosphoproteins. *J Neurosci 5*, 3414–3422.

Shimada, A., Mason, C. A., and Morrison, M. E. (1998). TrkB signaling modulates spine density and morphology independent of dendrite structure in cultured neonatal Purkinje cells. *J Neurosci 18*, 8559–8570.

Sik, A., Gulacsi, A., Lai, Y., Doyle, W. K., Pacia, S., Mody, I., and Freund, T. F. (2000). Localization of the A kinase anchoring protein AKAP79 in the human hippocampus. *Eur J Neurosci 12*, 1155–1164.

Siman, R., Baudry, M., and Lynch, G. (1984). Brain fodrin: Substrate for calpain I, an endogenous calcium-activated protease. *Proc Natl Acad Sci USA 81*, 3572–3576.

Siman, R., and Noszek, J. C. (1988). Excitatory amino acids activate calpain I and induce structural protein breakdown in vivo. *Neuron 1*, 279–287.

Skeberdis, V. A., Chevaleyre, V., Lau, C. G., Goldberg, J. H., Pettit, D. L., Suadicani, S. O., et al. (2006). Protein kinase A regulates calcium permeability of NMDA receptors. *Nat Neurosci 9*, 501–510.

Skoff, R. P., and Hamburger, V. (1974). Fine structure of dendritic and axonal growth cones in embryonic chick spinal cord. *J Comp Neurol 153*, 107–148.

Skydsgaard, M., and Hounsgaard, J. (1994). Spatial integration of local transmitter responses in motoneurons of the turtle spinal cord in vitro. *J Physiol 479*, 233–246.

Snyder, S. H., Lai, M. M., and Burnett, P. E. (1998). Immunophilins in the nervous system. *Neuron 21*, 283–294.

Sobczyk, A., Scheuss, V., and Svoboda, K. (2005). NMDA receptor subunit-dependent [Ca2+] signaling in individual hippocampal dendritic spines. *J Neurosci 25*, 6037–6046.

Sobel, E. C., and Tank, D. W. (1994). In vivo Ca2+ dynamics in a cricket auditory neuron: An example of chemical computation. *Science 263*, 823–826.

Soderling, T. R. (2000). CaM-kinases: Modulators of synaptic plasticity. *Curr Opin Neurobiol 10*, 375–380.

Soler-Llavina, G. J., and Sabatini, B. L. (2006). Synapse-specific plasticity and compartmentalized signaling in cerebellar stellate cells. *Nat Neurosci 9*, 798–806.

Solstad, T., Moser, E. I., and Einevoll, G. T. (2006). From grid cells to place cells: A mathematical model. *Hippocampus 16*, 1026–1031.

Sommer, B., Kohler, M., Sprengel, R., and Seeburg, P. H. (1991). RNA editing in brain controls a determinant of ion flow in glutamate-gated channels. *Cell 67*, 11–19.

Somogyi, P., Tamas, G., Lujan, R., and Buhl, E. (1998). Salient features of synaptic organisation in the cerebral cortex. *Brain Res Rev 26*, 113–135.

Song, I., Kamboj, S., Xia, J., Dong, H., Liao, D., and Huganir, R. L. (1998). Interaction of the N-ethylmaleimide-sensitive factor with AMPA receptors. *Neuron 21*, 393–400.

Song, J. Y., Ichtchenko, K., Sudhof, T. C., and Brose, N. (1999). Neuroligin 1 is a postsynaptic cell-adhesion molecule of excitatory synapses. *Proc Natl Acad Sci USA 96*, 1100–1105.

Sorra, K., and Harris, K. (1998). Stability in synapse number and size at 2 hr after long-term potentiation in hippocampal area CA1. *J Neurosci 18*, 658–671.

Sotelo, C. (1975). Anatomical, physiological and biochemical studies of the cerebellum from mutant mice. II Morphological study of cerebellar cortical neurons and circuits in the weaver mouse. *Brain Res 84*, 19–44.

Sotelo, C. (1977). Formation of presynaptic dendrites in the rat cerebellum following neonatal X-irradiation. *Neuroscience 2*, 275–283.

Sotelo, C. (1978). Purkinje cell ontogeny: Formation and maintenance of spines. *Prog Brain Res 48*, 149–170.

Sotelo, C. (1990). Cerebellar synaptogenesis: What we can learn from mutant mice. *J Exp Biol 153*, 225–279.

Sotelo, C., Hillman, D. E., Zamora, A. J., and Llinás, R. (1975). Climbing fiber deafferentation: Its actions on Purkinje cell dendritic spines. *Brain Res 175*, 574–581.

Spacek, J. (1985a). Three-dimensional analysis of dendritic spines. II. Spine apparatus and other cytoplasmic components. *Anat Embryol 171*, 235–243.

Spacek, J. (1985b). Three-dimensional analysis of dendritic spines. III. Glial sheath. *Anat Embryol 171*, 245–252.

Spacek, J., and Harris, K. M. (1997). Three-dimensional organization of smooth endoplasmic reticulum in hippocampal CA1 dendrites and dendritic spines of the immature and mature rat. *J Neurosci 17*, 190–203.

Spacek, J., and Hartmann, M. (1983). Three-dimensional analysis of dendritic spines. I. Quantitative observations related to dendritic spine and synaptic morphology in cerebral and cerebellar cortices. *Anat Embryol 167*, 289–310.

Spencer, W. (1862). *First Principles*. London: Williams and Norgate.

Srivastava, S., Osten, P., Vilim, F. S., Khatri, L., Inman, G., States, B., et al. (1998). Novel anchorage of GluR2/3 to the postsynaptic density by the AMPA receptor-binding protein ABP. *Neuron 21*, 581–591.

Star, E. N., Kwiatkowski, D. J., and Murthy, V. N. (2002). Rapid turnover of actin in dendritic spines and its regulation by activity. *Nat Neurosci 5*, 239–246.

Stauffer, T. P., Guerini, D., and Carafoli, E. (1995). Tissue distribution of the four gene products of the plasma membrane Ca2+ pump. A study using specific antibodies. *J Biol Chem 270*, 12184–12190.

Stauffer, T. P., Guerini, D., Celio, M. R., and Carafoli, E. (1997). Immunolocalization of the plasma membrane Ca2+ pump isoforms in the rat brain. *Brain Res 748*, 21–29.

Steigerwald, F., Schulz, T. W., Schenker, L. T., Kennedy, M. B., Seeburg, P. H., and Kèohr, G. (2000). C-Terminal truncation of NR2A subunits impairs synaptic but not extrasynaptic localization of NMDA receptors. *J Neurosci 20*, 4573–4581.

Stepanyants, A., Hof, P. R., and Chklovskii, D. B. (2002). Geometry and structural plasticity of synaptic connectivity. *Neuron 34*, 275–288.

Stevens, C., and Zador, A. (1998). Input synchrony and the irregular firing of cortical neurons. *Nat Neurosci 1*, 210–217.

Stevens, C. F. (1998). Neuronal diversity: Too many cell types for comfort? *Curr Biol 8*, R708–710.

Steward, O., Davis, L., Dotti, C., Phillips, L., Rao, A., and Banker, G. (1988). Protein synthesis and processing in cytoplasmic microdomains beneath postsynaptic sites on CNS neurons. A mechanism for establishing and maintaining a mosaic postsynaptic receptive surface. *Mol Neurobiol 2*, 227–261.

Steward, O., and Levy, W. B. (1982). Preferential localization of polyribosomes under the base of dendritic spines in granule cells of the dentate gyrus. *J Neurosci 2*, 284–291.

Steward, O., and Schuman, E. M. (2001). Protein synthesis at synaptic sites on dendrites. *Annu Rev Neurosci 24*, 299–325.

Strack, S., Barban, M. A., Wadzinski, B. E., and Colbran, R. J. (1997). Differential inactivation of postsynaptic density-associated and soluble $Ca^{2+}$/calmodulin-dependent protein kinase II by protein phosphatases 1 and 2A. *J Neurochem 68*, 2119–2128.

Strack, S., and Colbran, R. J. (1998). Autophosphorylation-dependent targeting of calcium/calmodulin-dependent protein kinase II by the NR2B subunit of the N-methyl-D-aspartate receptor. *J Biol Chem 273*, 20689–20692.

Strack, S., McNeill, R. B., and Colbran, R. J. (2000). Mechanism and regulation of calcium/calmodulin-dependent protein kinase II targeting to the NR2B subunit of the N-methyl-D-aspartate receptor. *J Biol Chem 275*, 23798–23806.

Stratford, K., Mason, A., Larkman, A., Major, G., and Jack, J. J. (1989). The modelling of pyramidal neurons in the visual cortex. In *The Computing Neuron*, ed. R. Durbin, C. Miall, and G. Mitchinson. Workingham, England: Addison-Wesley, pp. 296–322.

Stuart, G., Spruston, N., and Hausser, M., eds. (1999). *Dendrites*. Oxford: Oxford University Press.

Stuart, G., Spruston, N., Sakmann, B., and Häusser, M. (1997). Action potential initiation and backpropagation in neurons of the mammalian CNS. *Trends Neurosci 20*, 125–131.

Stuart, G. J., Dodt, H.-U., and Sakmann, B. (1993). Patch clamp recording from the soma and dendrites of neurons in brain slices using infrared video microscopy. *Plfuegers Arch 423*, 511–518.

Stuart, G. J., and Sakmann, B. (1994). Active propagation of somatic action potentials into neocortical pyramidal cell dendrites. *Nature 367*, 69–72.

Suzuki, T., Mitake, S., Okumura-Noji, K., Shimizu, H., Tada, T., and Fujii, T. (1997). Excitable membranes and synaptic transmission: Postsynaptic mechanisms. Localization of alpha-internexin in the postsynaptic density of the rat brain. *Brain Res 765*, 74–80.

Svoboda, K., Tank, D. W., and Denk, W. (1996). Direct measurement of coupling between dendritic spines and shafts. *Science 272*, 716–719.

Swindale, N. V. (1981). Dendritic spines only connect. *Trends Neurosci 4*, 240–241.

Tada, T., and Sheng, M. (2006). Molecular mechanisms of dendritic spine morphogenesis. *Curr Opin Neurobiol 16*, 95–101.

Takechi, H., Eilers, J., and Konnerth, A. (1998). A new class of synaptic response involving calcium release in dendritic spines. *Nature 396*, 757–760.

Takeichi, M. (1990). Cadherins: A molecular family important in selective cell-cell adhesion. *Annu Rev Biochem 59*, 237–252.

Takeichi, M. (1995). Morphogenetic roles of classic cadherins. *Curr Opin Cell Biol 7*, 619–627.

Takeuchi, M., Hata, Y., Hirao, K., Toyoda, A., Irie, M., and Takai, Y. (1997). SAPAPs. A family of PSD-95/SAP90-associated proteins localized at postsynaptic density. *J Biol Chem 272*, 11943–11951.

Takumi, Y., Ramâirez-Leâon, V., Laake, P., Rinvik, E., and Ottersen, O. P. (1999). Different modes of expression of AMPA and NMDA receptors in hippocampal synapses. *Nat Neurosci 2*, 618–624.

Tamas, G., and Szabadics, J. (2004). Summation of unitary IPSPs elicited by identified axo-axonic interneurons. *Cereb Cortex 14*, 823–826.

Tamas, G., Szabadics, J., and Somogyi, P. (2003). Cell type- and subcellular position-dependent summation of unitary postsynaptic potentials in neocortical neurons. *J Neurosci 22*, 740–747.

Tang, L., Hung, C. P., and Schuman, E. M. (1998). A role for the cadherin family of cell adhesion molecules in hippocampal long-term potentiation. *Neuron 20*, 1165–1175.

Tank, D. W., Delaney, K. D., and Regehr, W. G. (1995). The quantitative analysis of presynaptic calcium dynamics that contribute to short-term synaptic enhancement. *J Neurosci 15*, 7940–7952.

Tanzi, G. (1893). I fatti i le indizioni nell'odierna istologi del sistema nervoso. *Riv Sper Freniatr 19*, 419–472.

Tashiro, A., Dunaevsky, A., Blazeski, R., Mason, C. A., and Yuste, R. (2003). Bidirectional regulation of hippocampal mossy fiber filopodial motility by kainate receptors: A two-step model of synaptogenesis. *Neuron 38*, 773–784.

Tashiro, A., Minden, A., and Yuste, R. (2000). Regulation of dendritic spine morphology by the Rho family of small GTPases: Antagonistic roles of Rac and Rho. *Cereb Cortex 10*, 927–938.

Tashiro, A., and Yuste, R. (2004). Regulation of dendritic spine motility and stability by Rac1 and Rho kinase: Evidence for two forms of spine motility. *Mol Cell Neurosci 26*, 429–440.

Tashiro, A., and Yuste, R. (2008). Role of Rho GTPases in the morphogenesis and motility of dendritic spines. *Methods Enzymol 439*, 285–302.

Tessier-Lavigne, M., and Goodman, C. S. (1996). The molecular biology of axon guidance. *Science 274*, 1123–1133.

Tello, J. F. (1907). Degeneration et regeneration des plaques motrices après la section des nerfs. *Travaux du Laboratoire de Recherches Biologiques de l'Université de Madrid 5*, 117–149.

Threadgill, R., Bobb, K., and Ghosh, A. (1997). Regulation of dendritic growth and remodeling by Rho, Rac, and Cdc42. *Neuron 19*, 625–634.

Togashi, H., Abe, K., Mizoguchi, A., Takaoka, K., Chisaka, O., and Takeichi, M. (2002). Cadherin regulates dendritic spine morphogenesis. *Neuron 35*, 77–89.

Tomita, S., Adesnik, H., Sekiguchi, M., Zhang, W., Wada, K., Howe, J. R., et al. (2005). Stargazin modulates AMPA receptor gating and trafficking by distinct domains. *Nature 435*, 1052–1058.

Toni, N., Buchs, P., Nikonenko, I., Bron, C., and D., M. (1999). LTP promotes formation of multiple spine synapses between a single axon terminal and a dendrite. *Nature 402*, 421–425.

Toni, N., Teng, E. M., Bushong, E. A., Aimone, J. B., Zhao, C., Consiglio, A., et al. (2007). Synapse formation on neurons born in the adult hippocampus. *Nat Neurosci 10*, 727–734.

Torres, R., Firestein, B. L., Dong, H., Staudinger, J., Olson, E. N., Huganir, R. L., et al. (1998). PDZ proteins bind, cluster, and synaptically colocalize with Eph receptors and their ephrin ligands. *Neuron 21*, 1453–1463.

Trachtenberg, J. T., Chen, B. E., Knott, G. W., Feng, G., Sanes, J. R., Welker, E., and Svoboda, K. (2002). Long-term in vivo imaging of experience-dependent synaptic plasticity in adult cortex. *Nature 420*, 788–794.

Trommald, M., Hulleberg, G., and Andersen, P. (1996). Long-term potentiation is associated with new excitatory spine synapses on rat dentate granule cells. *Learn Mem 3*, 218–228.

Trommald, M., and Hulleberg, G. (1997). Dimensions and density of dendritic spines from rat dentate granule cells based on reconstructions from serial electron micrographs. *J Comp Neurol 377*, 15–28.

Trommald, M., Vaaland, J. L., Blackstad, T. W., and Andersen, P. (1990). Dendritic spine changes in rat dentate granule cells associated with long-term potentiation. In *Neurotoxicity of Excitatory Amino Acids*, ed. A. Guidotti. New York: Raven Press, pp. 163–174.

Tsay, D., and Yuste, R. (2002). Role of dendritic spines in action potential backpropagation: A numerical simulation study. *J Neurophysiol 88*, 2834–2845.

Tsay, D., and Yuste, R. (2004). On the electrical function of spines. *Trends Neurosci 27*, 77–83.

Tsien, R. Y. (1989). Fluorescent probes of cell signaling. *Annu Rev Neurosci 12*, 227–253.

Tu, J. C., Xiao, B., Naisbitt, S., Yuan, J. P., Petralia, R. S., Brakeman, P., et al. (1999). Coupling of mGluR/Homer and PSD-95 complexes by the Shank family of postsynaptic density proteins. *Neuron 23*, 583–592.

Tu, J. C., Xiao, B., Yuan, J. P., Lanahan, A. A., Leoffert, K., Li, M., et al. (1998). Homer binds a novel proline-rich motif and links group 1 metabotropic glutamate receptors with IP3 receptors. *Neuron 21*, 717–726.

Turrigiano, G. G., Leslie, K. R., Desai, N. S., Rutherford, L. C., and Nelson, S. B. (1998). Activity-dependent scaling of quantal amplitude in neocortical neurons. *Nature 391*, 892–896.

Turrigiano, G. G., and Nelson, S. B. (2000). Hebb and homeostasis in neuronal plasticity. *Curr Opin Neurobiol 10*, 358–364.

Uchida, N., Honjo, Y., Johnson, K. R., Wheelock, M. J., and Takeichi, M. (1996). The catenin/cadherin adhesion system is localized in synaptic junctions bordering transmitter release zones. *J Cell Biol 135*, 767–779.

Ullian, E. M., Christopherson, K. S., and Barres, B. A. (2004). Role for glia in synaptogenesis. *Glia 47*, 209–216.

Ursitti, J. A., Martin, L., Resneck, W. G., Chaney, T., Zielke, C., Alger, B. E., and Bloch, R. J. (2001). Spectrins in developing rat hippocampal cells. *Brain Res Dev Brain Res 129*, 81–93.

Valverde, F. (1967). Apical dendritic spines of the visual cortex and light deprivation in the mouse. *Exp Brain Res 3*, 337–352.

Valverde, F. (1971). Rate and extent of recovery from dark rearing in the visual cortex of the mouse. *Brain Res 33*, 1–11.

Van Harrefeld, A., and Fifkova, E. (1975). Swelling of dendritic spines in the fascia dentata after simulation of the preforant fibers as a mechanism of post-tetatnin potentiation. *Exp Neurol 49*, 736–749.

Vardinon-Friedman, H., Bresler, T., Garner, C., and Ziv, N. (2000). Assembly of new individual excitatory synapses time course and temporal order of synaptic molecule recruitment. *Neuron 27*, 57–79.

Vaughn, J., Henrikson, C., and Grieshaber, J. (1974). A quantitative study of synapses on motor neuron dendritic growth cones in developing mouse spinal cord. *J Cell Biol 60*, 664–672.

Vaughn, J. E. (1989). Fine structure of synaptogenesis in the vertebrate central nervous system. *Synapse 3*, 255–285.

Verhage, M., Maia, A., Plomp, J., Brussaard, A., Heeroma, J., Vermeer, H., et al. (2000). Synaptic assembly of the brain in the absence of neurotransmitter secretion. *Science 287*, 864–869.

Vetter, P., Roth, A., and Hausser, M. (2001). Propagation of action potentials in dendrites depends on dendritic morphology. *J Neurophysiol 85*, 926–937.

Vinade, L., Petersen, J. D., Do, K., Dosemeci, A., and Reese, T. S. (2001). Activation of calpain may alter the postsynaptic density structure and modulate anchoring of NMDA receptors. *Synapse 40*, 302–309.

Volfovsky, N., Parnas, H., Sega, l. M., and Korkotian, E. (1999). Geometry of dendritic spines affects calcium dynamics in hippocampal neurons: Theory and experiments. *J Neurophysiol 82*, 450–462.

Waites, C. L., Craig, A. M., and Garner, C. C. (2005). Mechanisms of vertebrate synaptogenesis. *Annu Rev Neurosci 28*, 251–274.

Walensky, L. D., Blackshaw, S., Liao, D., Watkins, C. C., Weier, H. U., Parra, M., et al. (1999). A novel neuron-enriched homolog of the erythrocyte membrane cytoskeletal protein 4.1. *J Neurosci 19*, 6457–6467.

Walikonis, R. S., Jensen, O. N., Mann, M., Provance, D. W., Jr., Mercer, J. A., and Kennedy, M. B. (2000). Identification of proteins in the postsynaptic density fraction by mass spectrometry. *J Neurosci 20*, 4069–4080.

Walikonis, R. S., Oguni, A., Khorosheva, E. M., Jeng, C. J., Asuncion, F. J., and Kennedy, M. B. (2001). Densin-180 forms a ternary complex with the (alpha)-subunit of Ca2+/calmodulin-dependent protein kinase II and (alpha)-actinin. *J Neurosci 21*, 423–433.

Walsh, F. S., and Doherty, P. (1997). Neural cell adhesion molecules of the immunoglobulin superfamily: Role in axon growth and guidance. *Annu Rev Cell Dev Biol 13*, 425–456.

Walsh, M. J., and Kuruc, N. (1992). The postsynaptic density: Constituent and associated proteins characterized by electrophoresis, immunoblotting, and peptide sequencing. *J Neurochem 59*, 667–678.

Walsh, M. K., and Lichtman, J. W. (2003). In vivo time-lapse imaging of synaptic takeover associated with naturally occurring synapse elimination. *Neuron 37*, 67–73.

Walton, P. D., Airey, J. A., Sutko, J. L., Beck, C. F., Mignery, G. A., Sudhof, T. C., et al. (1991). Ryanodine and inositol trisphosphate receptors coexist in avian cerebellar Purkinje neurons. *J Cell Biol 113*, 1145–1157.

Wandell, B. A. (1995). *Foundations of Vision*. Sunderland, MA: Sinauer.

Wang, H., and Macagno, E. (1997). The establishment of peripheral sensory arbors in the leech: In vivo time-lapse studies reveal a highly dynamic process. *J Neurosci 17*, 2408–2419.

Wang, S. S., Denk, W., and Hausser, M. (2000). Coincidence detection in single dendritic spines mediated by calcium release. *Nat Neurosci 3*, 1266–1273.

Weed, S. A., and Parsons, J. T. (2001). Cortactin: Coupling membrane dynamics to cortical actin assembly. *Oncogene 20*, 6418–6434.

Weiss, G. M., and Pysh, J. J. (1978). Evidence for loss of Purkinje cell dendrites during late development: A morphometric Golgi analysis in the mouse. *Brain Res 154*, 219–230.

Wen, Q., and Chklovskii, D. B. (2008). A cost-benefit analysis of neuronal morphology. *J Neurophysiol 99*, 2320–2328.

Wenzel, J., Otani, S., Desmond, N., and Levy, W. Rapid development of somatic spines in stratum granulosum of the adult hippocampus in vitro. *Brain Res 656*, 127–134.

Wessberg, J., and Nicolelis, M. (2004). Optimizing a linear algorithm for real-time robotic control using chronic cortical ensemble recordings in monkeys. *J Cogn Neurosci 16*, 1022–1035.

Westphal, R. S., Tavalin, S. J., Lin, J. W., Alto, N. M., Fraser, I. D., Langeberg, L. K., et al. (1999). Regulation of NMDA receptors by an associated phosphatase-kinase signaling complex. *Science 285*, 93–96.

Westrum, L. E., Jones, D. H., Gray, E. G., and Barron, J. (1980). Microtubules, dendritic spines and spine appratuses. *Cell Tissue Res 208*, 171–181.

Wickens, J. (1988). Electrically coupled but chemically isolated synapses: Dendritic spines and calcium in a rule for synaptic modification. *Prog Neurobiol 31*, 507–528.

Wigstrom, H., Gustafsson, B., Huang, Y.-Y., and Abraham, W. C. (1986). Hippocampal long-term potentiation is induced by pairing single afferent volleys with intracellularly injected depolarizing current pulses. *Acta Physiol Scand 126*, 317–319.

Williams, S. R., and Mitchell, S. J. (2008). Direct measurement of somatic voltage clamp errors in central neurons. *Nat Neurosci 11*, 790–798.

Wilson, C. J. (1986). Three dimensional analysis of dendritic spines by means of HVEM. *J Electron Microsci 35 (Suppl.)*, 1151–1155.

Winder, D. G., and Sweatt, J. D. (2001). Roles of serine/threonine phosphatases in hippocampal synaptic plasticity. *Nat Rev Neurosci 2*, 461–474.

Wisniewski, K., Segan, S., Miezejeski, C., Sersen, E., and Rudelli, R. (1991). The Fra(X) syndrome: Neurological, electrophysiological, and neuropathological abnormalities. *Am J Med Genet 38*, 476–480.

Witcher, M. R., Kirov, S. A., and Harris, K. M. (2007). Plasticity of perisynaptic astroglia during synaptogenesis in the mature rat hippocampus. *Glia 55*, 13–23.

Wolf, M., Burgess, S., Misra, U. K., and Sahyoun, N. (1986). Postsynaptic densities contain a subtype of protein kinase C. *Biochem Biophys Res Commun 140*, 691–698.

Woolley, C. S., and McEwen, B. S. (1994). Estradiol regulates hippocampal dendritic spine density via an N-methyl-D-aspartate receptor-dependent mechanism. *J Neurosci 14*, 7680–7687.

Woolley, C. S., Gould, E., Frankfurt, M., and McEwen, B. S. (1990). Naturally occurring fluctuation in dendritic spine density on adult hippocampal pyramidal neurons. *J Neurosci 10*, 4035–4039.

Wong, R. O. L., Yamawaki, R. M., and Shatz, C. L. (1992). Synaptic contacts and the transient dendritic spines of developing retinal ganglion cells. *Eur J Neurosci 4*, 1387–1397.

Wong, W. T., Faulkner-Jones, B. E., Sanes, J. R., and Wong, R. O. (2000). Rapid dendritic remodeling in the developing retina: Dependence on neurotransmission and reciprocal regulation by Rac and Rho. *J Neurosci 20*, 5024–5036.

Woodring, P. J., and Garrison, J. C. (1997). Expression, purification, and regulation of two isoforms of the inositol 1,4,5-trisphosphate 3-kinase. *J Biol Chem 272*, 30447–30454.

Wu, K., Xu, J. L., Suen, P. C., Levine, E., Huang, Y. Y., Mount, H. T., et al. (1996). Functional trkB neurotrophin receptors are intrinsic components of the adult brain postsynaptic density. *Brain Res Mol Brain Res 43*, 286–290.

Wyszynski, M., Lin, J., Rao, A., Nigh, E., Beggs, A. H., Craig, A. M., and Sheng, M. (1997). Competitive binding of alpha-actinin and calmodulin to the NMDA receptor. *Nature 385*, 439–442.

Wyszynski, M., Valtschanoff, J. G., Naisbitt, S., Dunah, A. W., Kim, E., Standaert, D. G., Weinberg, R., and Sheng, M. (1999). Association of AMPA receptors with a subset of glutamate receptor-interacting protein in vivo. *J Neurosci 19*, 6528–6537.

Xia, J., Zhang, X., Staudinger, J., and Huganir, R. L. (1999). Clustering of AMPA receptors by the synaptic PDZ domain-containing protein PICK1. *Neuron 22*, 179–187.

Xiao, B., Tu, J. C., Petralia, R. S., Yuan, J. P., Doan, A., Breder, C. D., et al. (1998). Homer regulates the association of group 1 metabotropic glutamate receptors with multivalent complexes of homer-related, synaptic proteins. *Neuron 21*, 707–716.

Xiao, B., Tu, J. C., and Worley, P. F. (2000). Homer: a link between neural activity and glutamate receptor function. *Curr Opin Neurobiol 10*, 370–374.

Yamashita, T., Tucker, K. L., and Barde, Y. A. (1999). Neurotrophin binding to the p75 receptor modulates Rho activity and axonal outgrowth. *Neuron 24*, 585–593.

Yang, T., and Shadlen, M. N. (2007). Probabilistic reasoning by neurons. *Nature 447*, 1075–1080.

Yasuda, R., Harvey, C. D., Zhong, H., Sobczyk, A., van Aelst, L., and Svoboda, K. (2006). Supersensitive Ras activation in dendrites and spines revealed by two-photon fluorescence lifetime imaging. *Nat Neurosci 9*, 283–291.

Yoshimura, Y., Aoi, C., and Yamauchi, T. (2000). Investigation of protein substrates of Ca(2+)/calmodulin-dependent protein kinase II translocated to the postsynaptic density. *Brain Res Mol Brain Res 81*, 118–128.

Yoshimura, Y., Sogawa, Y., and Yamauchi, T. (1999). Protein phosphatase 1 is involved in the dissociation of Ca2+/calmodulin-dependent protein kinase II from postsynaptic densities. *FEBS Lett 446*, 239–242.

Yoshimura, Y., Yamauchi, Y., Shinkawa, T., Taoka, M., Donai, H., Takahashi, N., et al. (2004). Molecular constituents of the postsynaptic density fraction revealed by proteomic analysis using multidimensional liquid chromatography-tandem mass spectrometry. *J Neurochem 88*, 759–768.

Yuste, R. (2005). Origin and classification of neocortical interneurons. *Neuron 48*, 524–527.

Yuste, R., and Bonhoeffer, T. (2001). Morphological changes in dendritic spines associated with long-term synaptic plasticity. *Annu Rev Neurosci*, 1071–1089.

Yuste, R., and Denk, W. (1995). Dendritic spines as basic units of synaptic integration. *Nature 375*, 682–684.

Yuste, R., Gutnick, M. J., Saar, D., Delaney, K. D., and Tank, D. W. (1994). Calcium accumulations in dendrites from neocortical neurons: An apical band and evidence for functional compartments. *Neuron 13*, 23–43.

Yuste, R., and Majewska, A. (2001). On the function of dendritic spines. *Neuroscientist 7*, 387–395.

Yuste, R., Majewska, A., Cash, S., and Denk, W. (1999). Mechanisms of calcium influx into spines: Heterogeinity among spines, coincidence detection by NMDA receptors and optical quantal analysis. *J Neurosci 19*, 1976–1987.

Yuste, R., Majewska, A., and Holthoff, K. (2000). From form to function: Calcium compartmentalization in dendritic spines. *Nat Neurosci 3*, 653–659.

Yuste, R., and Tank, D. W. (1996). Dendritic integration in mammalian neurons, a century after Cajal. *Neuron 16*, 701–716.

Yuste, R., and Urban, R. (2004). Dendritic spines and linear networks. *J Physiol (Paris) 98*, 479–486.

Zamanillo, D., Sprengel, R., Hvalby, O., Jensen, V., Burnashev, N., Rozov, A., Kaiser, K. M., Kèoster, H. J., Borchardt, T., Worley, P., et al. (1999). Importance of AMPA receptors for hippocampal synaptic plasticity but not for spatial learning. *Science 284*, 1805–1811.

Zhang, L., Tao, H., Holt, C., Harris, W., and Poo, M. (1998). A critical window for cooperation and competition among developing retinotectal synapses. *Nature 395*, 37–44.

Zhang, W., and Benson, D. L. (2000). Development and molecular organization of dendritic spines and their synapses. *Hippocampus 10*, 512–526.

Zhang, W., Vazquez, L., Apperson, M., and Kennedy, M. B. (1999). Citron binds to PSD-95 at glutamatergic synapses on inhibitory neurons in the hippocampus. *J Neurosci 19*, 96–108.

Zheng, J. Q., Felder, M., Connor, J. A., and Poo, M. M. (1994). Turning of nerve growth cones induced by neurotransmitters. *Nature 368*, 140–144.

Zhou, Q., Homma, K. J., and Poo, M. M. (2004). Shrinkage of dendritic spines associated with long-term depression of hippocampal synapses. *Neuron 44*, 749–757.

Ziv, N., and Smith, S. (1996). Evidence for a role of dendritic filopodia in synaptogenesis and spine formation. *Neuron 17*, 91–102.

Ziv, N. E., and Garner, C. C. (2001). Principles of glutamatergic synapse formation: Seeing the forest for the trees. *Curr Opin Neurobiol 11*, 536–543.

Zohary, E., Shadlen, M. N., and Newsome, W. T. (1994). Correlated neuronal discharge rate and its implications for psychophysical performance. *Nature 370*, 140–143.

Zuo, Y., Yang, G., Kwon, E., and Gan, W. B. (2005). Long-term sensory deprivation prevents dendritic spine loss in primary somatosensory cortex. *Nature 436*, 261–265.

# Source Notes

Chapter 2 is revised from the text that originally appeared in Yuste, R. (2002). History of neuroscience: The discovery of dendritic spines, *IBRO History of Neuroscience* [http://www.ibro.info/Pub/Pub_Main _Display.asp?LC_Docs_ID=3532].

Chapter 3 is based on Tashiro, A., and Yuste, R. (2003). Structure and molecular organization of spines. *Histol Histopathol 18*, 617–634.

Chapter 4 is based on Tashiro, A., and Yuste, R. (2003). Structure and molecular organization of spines. *Histol Histopathol 18*, 617–634.

Chapter 5 is based on Yuste, R., and Bonhoeffer, T. (2004). Genesis of spines: insights from ultrastructural and imaging studies. *Nature Neurosci Rev 5*, 24–34 and Portera-Cailliau, C., and Yuste, R. (2001). On the function of dendritic filopodia. *Rev Neurol 33*, 1158–1166.

Chapter 6 is revised from Bonhoeffer, T., and Yuste, R. (2002). Spine motility: Phenomenology, mechanisms and function. *Neuron 35*, 1019–1027.

Chapter 7 is updated from Yuste, R., Majewska, A., and Holthoff, K. (2000). From form to function: Calcium compartmentalization in spines. *Nature Neurosci 3*, 653–659.

Chapter 8 is updated from Yuste, R., and Bonhoeffer, T. (2001). Morphological changes in spines associated with long-term synaptic plasticity. *Annu Rev Neurosci 24*, 1071–1089.

Chapter 9 is updated from a modified version of Tsay, D., and Yuste, R. (2004). On the electrical function of spines. *TINS 27*, 77–83.

Some sections of chapter 10 appeared in Yuste, R., and Urban, A. (2005). Spines and linear networks. *J Physiol (Paris) 98*, 479–486.

# Index